T0186851

# Human Saliva:
# Clinical Chemistry
# and
# Microbiology

## Volume I

Editor

**Jorma O. Tenovuo, D.Odont.**

Professor and Chairman
Department of Oral Biology
Institute of Dentistry
University of Turku
Turku, Finland

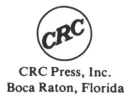

CRC Press, Inc.
Boca Raton, Florida

**Library of Congress Cataloging-in-Publication Data**

Human saliva.

    Bibliography: p.
    Includes index
    1. Saliva — Analysis.  2. Saliva — Microbiology
I. Tenovuo, Jorma O.
RB52.5.H86 1989    616.07'56   88-36218
ISBN 0-8493-6391-8 (v.1)
ISBN 0-8493-6392-6 (v.2)

Direct all inquires to CRC Press, Inc., 2000 Corporate Blvd., N.W., Boca Raton, Florida, 33431.

© 1989 by CRC Press, Inc.

International Standard Book Number 0-8493-6391-8 (v.1)
International Standard Book Number 0-8493-6392-6 (v.2)

Library of Congress Card Number 88-36218
Printed in the United States

# PREFACE

In daily talk the word "saliva" is used to describe the combined fluids present in the mouth. However, in its strict sense this word refers only to the hypotonic, watery fluid secreted by the major and minor salivary glands. Expressions like "whole saliva", "mixed saliva", and "oral fluid" are used in scientific purposes to represent the combined fluids of the mouth. Indeed, whole saliva is a mixture of pure glandular saliva, gingival crevicular fluid, oral epithelial cells, microorganisms, food remnants, etc.

Saliva is not only a pleasant lubricant which makes oral functions — such as speech, mastication, and swallowing — easier but also a fluid with many important functions in the maintenance of oral and general health. Although saliva is not considered an essential fluid for life in man, it protects the human body, and in particular oral tissues, against numerous noxious and harmful agents. Therefore, it is not surprising that decreased, or even completely ceased, saliva flow brings along discomfort and many health problems. The number of people suffering from hyposalivation or xerostomia is relatively high, due to the widespread use of drugs with flow -reducing side effects. Many oral, and possibly also systemic symptoms, are related to these untoward changes in the normal salivary function. On the other hand, some systemic diseases and hormonal changes can alter the flow and composition of saliva, even so that in many cases saliva analyses have diagnostic value.

In addition to the documented relationship between saliva and some local or systemic diseases, also the excretion of various compunds — hormones, drugs, pollutants, etc. — into saliva has gained increasing scientific interest. Compared to blood or urine, saliva is easy to collect which makes for frequent monitoring of excreted substances possible. Furthermore, the amount detectable in saliva has been interpreted to represent the biologically active fraction of a particular compound.

These examples show that salivary chemistry and microbiology have become in many laboratories as part of their daily practice. However, the information of the origin of various salivary compounds, their normal values, age dependency, relation to flow rate, diseases or hormonal status, assay problems, etc., is hard to find. This book is meant to cover the current knowledge of these factors and in this way serve both scientists and clinicians with the relevant information needed in planning, performing, and interpreting saliva analyses.

**Jorma Tenovuo**
Editor

## THE EDITOR

**Dr. Jorma Tenovuo** is Docent of Dental Biochemistry and Acting Professor of Oral Biology at the Institute of Dentistry, University of Turku, Finland. Dr. Tenovuo graduated in 1974 and received the Doctor of Odontology degree in 1976, both at the University of Turku. He has served as a Visiting Scientist at the University of Alabama in Birmingham 1980 — 1982, and 1984, and was granted the Oral Science Award by the International Association for Dental Research in 1984. Dr. Tenovuo has authored more than 100 publications dealing with various aspects of oral biology, especially the salivary defense factors. He is a member of several international scientific societies, and he has served as an Editor-in-Chief for *Proceedings of the Finnish Dental Journal* and as a reviewer for several international journals.

# CONTRIBUTORS

**Edwin A. Azen, M.D.**
Professor
Departments of Medicine and Medical
 Genetics
University of Wisconsin
Madison, Wisconsin

**Dowen Birkhed, D.D.S.**
Department of Cariology
University of Lund School of Dentistry
Malmo, Sweden

**Robert E. Cohen, Ph.D.**
Assistant Professor
Departments of Periodontology and Oral
 Biology
School of Dental Medicine
State University of New York
Buffalo, New York

**D. B. Ferguson, Ph.D.**
Senior Lecturer
Department of Physiology
University of Manchester
Manchester, England

**Donald I. Hay, Ph.D.**
Senior Member of Staff and Head
Department of Biochemistry
Forsyth Dental Center
Boston, Massachusetts

**Ulf Heintze, D.D.S.**
Department of Cariology
University of Lund School of Dentistry
Malmo, Sweden

**Michael J. Levine, Ph.D.**
Professor
Departments of Periodontology and Oral
 Biology
School of Dental Medicine
State University of New York
Buffalo, New York

**Edgard C. Moreno, Ph.D.**
Head
Department of Physical Chemistry
Forsyth Dental Center
Boston, Massachusetts

**Frank G. Oppenheim, Ph.D.**
Professor and Chairman
Department of Oral Biology
Goldman School of Graduate Dentistry
Boston University School of Medicine
Boston, Massachusetts

**Eva Soderling, Ph.D.**
Associate Professor
Department of Oral Biochemistry
Institute of Dentistry
University of Turku
Turku, Finland

**Jorma O. Tenovuo, D.Odont.**
Docent of Dental Biochemistry
Institute of Dentistry
University of Turku
Turku, Finland

# TABLE OF CONTENTS

Chapter 1

# PRACTICAL ASPECTS OF SALIVARY ANALYSES

## Eva Söderling

## TABLE OF CONTENTS

# I. INTRODUCTION

Collecting saliva for analytical studies does not normally pose particular problems though the analyses themselves may cause difficulties. Several practical aspects have to be considered before collecting saliva (Table 1). Whole saliva is a complex mixture of parotid, submandibular, sublingual, and minor salivary gland secretions mixed with bacteria, leukocytes, sloughed epithelial cells, and crevicular fluid. The use of different stimulants of saliva secretion produces samples where the secretions from the major salivary glands occur in different proportions. The concentrations of most salivary constituents depend on the flow rate of saliva. Therefore, to obtain meaningful results, the collections of saliva need to be standardized (see Tables 2 and 3 and also Chapter 2 of this volume). Table 2 lists several factors which influence the flow rate and/or the composition of saliva (see also Chapter 2). Standardization of saliva collections is especially important, since saliva varies greatly both inter- and intraindividually. Furthermore, reference values comparable to serum normal values are usually not available. The reference values published[1,2] have to be regarded mainly as a general guide. Analytical methods developed for serum are often not directly applicable to saliva without modifications. The unstandardized methodology has partly contributed to the high variability in the data published for salivary parameters. Standardization of saliva collections is important even if flow rate is the only parameter measured (see Chapter 2 of this volume). Only a few salivary analytical methods (such as the use of slide cultures for salivary microorganisms) appear to be more or less unaffected by the collection conditions. Detailed instructions for the collection of resting and stimulated whole saliva as well as parotid, submandibular, and sublingual saliva are given in Chapter 2 of this volume.

The presence of bacteria, epithelial cells, and leukocytes further complicates the analyses of whole saliva. Some salivary components, like many enzymes, may originate from both the aforementioned cells or the salivary glands, and it is often difficult to determine which components have cellular origin and which represent true salivary components. Also, as a result of bacterial action, the composition of saliva will change on standing. For most analyses, the saliva should be collected on ice to arrest the bacterial metabolism. The bacterial action can also be stopped by centrifugation of the saliva. Centrifugation removes both the cells and the turbidity, which can interfere with many analytical techniques. Clarification, however, may decrease the levels of some salivary parameters.

Thus, for these reasons it is important to plan the salivary analyses well in advance and to consider the aspects brought up in Tables 1 to 3. This chapter deals with the pretreatment and storage of saliva for various analytical purposes.

**Table 1**
**ASPECTS THAT HAVE TO BE CONSIDERED BEFORE COMMENCING SALIVA ANALYSES**

Total number of parameters to be determined and the amount of saliva needed
Type of saliva: resting or stimulated whole saliva or pure salivary gland secretions
Stimulation method
Storage properties of the salivary components to be determined (no storage, room temperature, $+4°C$, $-20°C$, or below $-20°C$)
Pretreatment of saliva before storage (centrifugation, dividing into aliquots, etc.)

**Table 2**
**SOME FACTORS INFLUENCING THE FLOW RATE AND COMPOSITION OF SALIVA**

Donor (species, sex, geographical location, diet, etc.)
Glandular source
Plasma composition
Circadian rhythm
Nature of the secretory stimulus, previous stimulation and duration of stimulation
Hormones
Exercise
Various acute and chronic diseases
Medication
Physical and chemical collection circumstances

**Table 3**
**INSTRUCTIONS FOR THE STANDARDIZATION OF WHOLE SALIVA COLLECTION WITH A STIMULANT**

The subject should not eat or drink (except water) 1 to 2 h before collection.
The subject should not have heavy physical exercise before collection.
Saliva should be collected at the same time of the day from each subject.
The saliva collection should be performed under standardized environmental conditions.
A prestimulation period (e.g., 30 s) is recommended.
A fixed collection time (e.g., 5 min) should be used, or a fixed volume should be collected.
In repeated collections, the same stimulant should be used.
All acute or chronic diseases as well as medication should be considered.
Samples containing visible blood should be discarded.

## II. COLLECTION AND TREATMENT OF THE SECRETIONS OF THE MINOR SALIVARY GLANDS

Because the collection of whole saliva samples as well as those of parotid, submandibular, and sublingual secretions is discussed in Chapter 2 of this volume, the present chapter describes only the collection of minor salivary gland (MSG) secretions. The contribution of the MSG secretions to the total volume of resting and stimulated whole saliva has been estimated to be less than 10%.[3] Provenza[4] has grouped the MSGs into sublingual, lingual, labial, buccal, palatine, and glossopalatine. The secretions of these glands are purely mucous or seromucous. The collection of MSG secretions is technically difficult. This is most probably the reason why only a few studies on these secretions have been published. The following practical aspects should be considered in the collection and analysis of MSG secretions.

1.    The secretions of the main salivary glands can easily contaminate the secretions of

the MSGs. Labial and palatine gland secretions, however, can be obtained without contaminating either the main salivary glands or the other MSG secretions.[5]

2.    Gustatory stimuli are usually applied to elicit a secretory reflex.[3,5,6] In collection of palatine gland secretions gentle mechanical stimulation of the hard palate with a round-ended instrument was effective.[7,8] An advantage of the latter method compared with gustatory stimulus is that it can be used before the collection of secretions from the main salivary glands in studies where secretions of several glands are collected sequentially. Both gustatory stimuli and mechanical stimulations can be regarded as physiological.[9] In studies in which larger amounts of MSG secretions are needed, however, pilocarpine is an effective stimulant.[5]

3.    It is difficult to obtain sufficient quantities of MSG secretions for chemical analyses. The choice of the stimulant (see item 2) may partly overcome this problem. Pooling the secretions from several subjects is often necessary.

4.    The high viscosity of the MSG secretions makes the collection complicated. Glass capillaries, which have been used in some collections,[2,3,6,7,10] may not work by capillary action only. The best results have been obtained by applying slight suction.[3,7,10,13] Quantitation of sample can also be problematic since the capillaries usually fill unevenly with saliva. Weighing of the pipettes appears to be a more accurate method than volume determination. The mucosubstances of the MSG secretions adhere to glass, which makes the emptying of the capillaries difficult, especially after freezing. The adhesion of the mucosubstances to glass can be decreased by treating the capillaries with agents such as polytetrafluoroethylene, which prevents adhesion.[11] Such a treatment has also been applied to other glass equipment used in the analyses.

•    The adhesiveness of the mucosubstances presents problems also in most other methods used to collect MSG secretions. The mucosubstances adhere to filter paper.[5,12-14] The paper can also effectively trap some water-soluble saliva components.[12-14]

•    Water treatment of paper discs used to collect palatine gland secretions (Figure 1) removes only a part of the water-soluble proteins absorbed by the discs.[13-14] The desorption of proteins from paper can be substantially improved by the use of some detergent, for example, Triton® X-100. This treatment, though, may affect enzyme stability and interfere with further analytical methods.[12] When filter papers are used, the interference of compounds eluted from the paper itself must also be considered. These problems can be avoided by using absorbent polymers to which the mucosubstances do not adhere.[141] Weighing is the most convenient way for quantitation of the secretions when an absorbent material is used for collection.

•    In addition to the methods just described, other procedures have also been proposed. The viscous secretions can simply be attached to a fine-point spatula.[15] A special collection device prepared from a pair of forceps has also been presented.[14] With such methods quantitation can be made possible using a micropipette[14] or by weighing. With these methods the saliva can easily be recovered for further studies.

5.    The mucosubstances present in the MSG secretions make the chemical analysis of these secretions difficult. These high molecular weight substances often clog gel columns in chromatographic separations. As discussed, the mucosubstances adhere to glass, paper, and cellulose acetate[5] and even trap water-soluble proteins.[12,16-18] This makes even conventional electrophoresis of MSG secretions difficult to perform. Solvent fractionation, ultracentrifugation, and equilibrium-density gradient centrifugation have been used to separate water-soluble proteins from mucosubstances.[12-14] As mentioned earlier, adherence of mucosubstances to glass can be overcome by polytetrafluoroethylene treatment of the glass. In other studies the mucosubstances have been rendered water soluble by treating with proteolytic enzymes,[19] boiling,[6,20] or with disulfide bond splitting agents.[21] These methods are, however, destructive to many biomolecules and can be used for special purposes only.

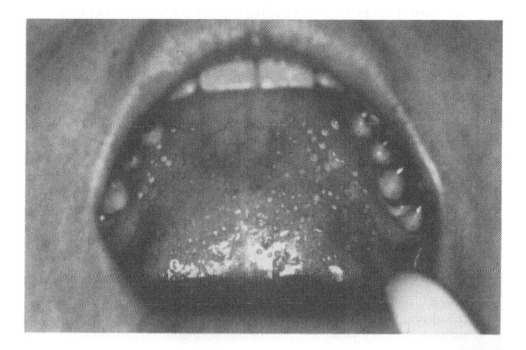

A

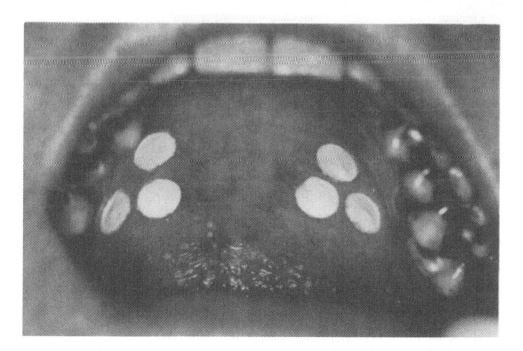

B

FIGURE 1. Collection of human palatine secretions (HPS) by filter paper method. (A) Appearance of HPS following 2-min gentle, mechanical stimulation (in the study proper, similar appearance of HPS was found following combination of stimulations); (B) filter paper discs placed for collection. Note that more HPS was secreted from the left palate than from the right palate. (From Mäkinen, K. K., Virtanen, K. K., Söderling, E., and Kotiranta, J., *Scand. J. Dent. Res.*, 93, 253, 1985.)

## III. LOW MOLECULAR WEIGHT COMPONENTS OF SALIVA

### A. Electrolytes

Various factors, both physiological and pathological, affecting the electrolyte composition of saliva are thoroughly discussed in Chapter 3 of this volume. This chapter deals with practical aspects of salivary electrolyte analyses.

Most salivary electrolytes can be determined from stored samples (e.g., after freezing). Electrolytes, which are labile or which participate in precipitate formation in saliva, have to be determined immediately after collection. Electrolyte concentrations can also be affected by the atmospheric air and/or by pH changes of saliva. Special collection conditions and equipment may be used to avoid these effects. Several electrolytes can normally be determined from the same sample. If all electrolytes cannot be immediately analyzed, it is necessary to store a part of the sample for later use. In such cases it is convenient to divide the samples into separate aliquots for each determination immediately after collection, and to make the possible dilutions at the same time to prevent evaporation losses of small samples. The disadvantageous effects of repeated thawings and freezings on samples can thereby be avoided. This recommendation concerns, of course, other salivary components as well.

### 1. Bicarbonate

Determination of the bicarbonate concentration in saliva is dealt with in Chapter 3, and that of buffer capacity in Chapter 2 of this volume. In clinical chemistry, the saliva buffer capacity tests reflect the contribution of the salivary carbonic acid/bicarbonate system (see Chapter 2). $CO_2$ diffuses out when saliva is exposed to the atmosphere, and thus the collection and storage conditions of saliva will affect the buffer capacity values. Short collection periods (for stimulated saliva) and use of collection vials with a small contact surface with air (test tubes) are recommended. Collection under liquid paraffin has been used to lower the diffusion of $CO_2$. This technique, however, evidently leads to problems in other saliva analyses. The carbonic acid/bicarbonate buffer system of saliva is also affected by individual differences in the pH of saliva, as well as by bacterial action during the storage of saliva. Thus, in principle, buffer capacity determinations of saliva should be made immediately after sample collections. Previous studies have shown that the buffer capacity of saliva changes during storage regardless of temperature.[22-24] Negligible changes, though, in the saliva buffer capacities have been observed in stimulated samples stored at room temperature for 1 h.[25] Thus, it appears that at least for clinical purposes reliable buffer capacity determinations can be made on samples after short standing.

### 2. Nitrate and Nitrite

The microorganisms of saliva reduce nitrate to nitrite and can also utilize nitrite.[26] In fresh saliva the nitrate content decreases rapidly, and the nitrite content first increases and then decreases. These changes can be prevented by collecting saliva within alkali, like NaOH.[27] The nitrate and nitrite contents of such salivas were stable at room temperature for a fortnight.[27] The nitrate determination of saliva was also affected by material eluted from some commercially available plastic containers and glassware.[27]

### 3. Thiocyanate (SCN⁻) and Hypothiocyanite (OSCN⁻/HOSCN)

$SCN^-$, $OSCN^-$, and HOSCN are usually determined from unclarified whole saliva (see Chapters 3 and 9). The turbidity of saliva may, however, disturb the spectrophotometric determinations. The $SCN^-$ can be analyzed from frozen samples. If $OSCN^-$ and HOSCN are measured, the samples should not be stored in cold for more than a few hours.[28,142] Before analyses, stored samples have to be swirled vigorously to decrease the variability of repeated measurements.[28]

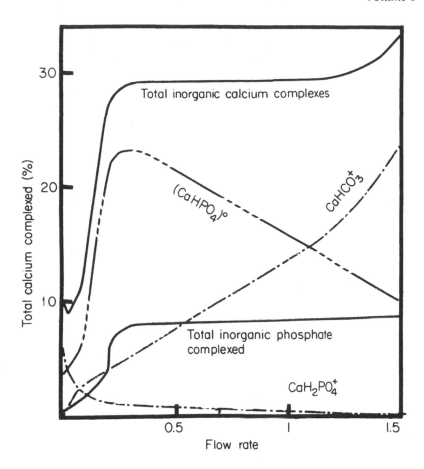

FIGURE 2. Percent of total calcium complexed by various inorganic anions in parotid saliva at various flow rates. (From McCann, H. G., in *Arts and Science of Dental Caries Research,* Harris, R. S., Ed., Academic Press, New York, 1968, 55. With permission.)

### 4. Sodium, Potassium, and Chloride

Sodium, potassium, and chloride do not need any special saliva pretreatment before analyses, but saliva is easier to handle when it is clarified before determinations. Freezing and thawing of the sample does not appreciably affect the measurement of these ions.

### 5. Calcium

In saliva, calcium is complexed with proteins, phosphate, citrate, and lactate, and only about one half of it occurs in free ionic form.[29] The degree of calcium binding depends, for example, on the pH of saliva (Figure 2).[29,30] Thus, if ionized calcium is determined, special saliva collection equipment should be used to prevent the contact between air and saliva which should be freshly collected.

Although atomic absorption spectrophotometry (using flame or furnace technique) can accurately and conveniently be used for the determination of total calcium of whole saliva, the formation of calcium-rich precipitates may interfere with the analyses. Representative samples are difficult to obtain from stored (frozen) samples; separate aliquots of freshly collected saliva should thus be obtained for calcium analyses. Clarification of the samples by centrifugation removes not only the precipitation but also a considerable portion of protein-bound calcium, which has to be taken into consideration. Centrifugation ($10,000 \times g$, 10 min) of whole salivas collected from four subjects reduced the salivary calcium concentrations with 7 to 35%.[31] With parotid saliva these problems seldom appear.

*6. Phosphate*

When salivary phosphate is determined using furnace atomic absorption spectrophotometry, the precipitate formation in saliva may make it difficult to obtain representative samples. Formation of saliva precipitates may also interfere with colorimetric phosphate measurement. In addition to standard serum phosphate methods (see Chapter 3) a simple malachite-green method has also been used for saliva analyses.[32,33] The advantages of this method include its simplicity and high sensitivity. When the phosphate of parotid saliva was analyzed by different methods, the method of Chen et al.[34] gave similar results with the malachite-green procedure, whereas the Fiske and Subbarow method[35] gave 30% higher values.[33]

In our laboratory, a comparison between the malachite-green and Lowry-Lopez methods[36] showed that the former resulted in 15% higher values with freshly collected whole saliva. Centrifugation of saliva (12,000 $\times$ $g$, 10 min) reduced the phosphate levels by 10% in both methods. Freezing ($-20°C$) of untreated or centrifuged whole saliva for 2 to 3 d resulted in 30% lower phosphate levels when measured with the malachite-green method, whereas only a 5 to 7% reduction was observed with the Lowry-Lopez method. Consequently, it appears that the malachite-green method cannot be recommended for frozen saliva samples. This may also apply to precipitated salivas which have been stored in cold.

*7. Fluoride*

Salivary fluoride is usually determined using a specific ion electrode. Salivary fluoride is not significantly bound to macromolecules or cells, but rather to low molecular weight substances.[37,38] It has been postulated that fluoride precipitates with calcium and phosphate, this reaction being affected by the pH of saliva.[38] Thus, it could be expected that storage of saliva would lead to reduced ionized fluoride levels. Experiments performed in our laboratory showed that centrifugation (12,000 $\times$ $g$, $+4°C$, 10 min) caused interindividual differences in the salivary fluoride levels, the maximal decrease being 15%. Freezing of either the centrifuged or the untreated samples, however, had no effect on the fluoride levels.

**B. Glucose**

Salivary glucose does not serve as a reliable indicator of blood sugar even though diabetic patients show elevated salivary glucose levels.[39] Microorganisms present in whole saliva utilize glucose rapidly.[40] The whole saliva glucose levels decrease even when saliva is collected on ice and kept chilled after collection. A convenient way to stop the bacterial metabolism after saliva collection appears to be acid precipitation, which is included in common blood glucose determinations.

**C. Ammonia and Urea**

The ammonia content of saliva is known to rise after standing because of the metabolism of urea and amino acids.[41] In whole saliva, the ammonia content increased about 10% even when stored at $+4°C$.[42] The increase was expectedly higher at $+20°C$.[42] The ammonia formation during storage was inhibited to some extent by diluting the sample before storage or by adding chloroform,[42,43] whereas acidification had no effect on ammonia formation.[42] The ammonia content of saliva stored at $-20°C$ was unchanged for the first 2 weeks (Figure 3).[42] Prolonged storage of saliva at $-20°C$ resulted in a decrease in the ammonia content (Figure 3),[42] while it tends to rise in frozen blood and urine.[43,44] Thus, saliva should be collected in chilled tubes and analyzed immediately after collection. If this is not possible, storage at $-20°C$ is necessary.

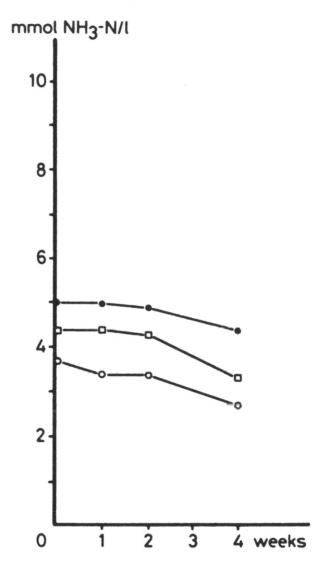

FIGURE 3. Influence of storage over 4 weeks at $-20°C$ on the saliva ammonia content. Indophenol method (●-●), enzymatic method (○-○), and electrode method (□-□). (From Huizenga, J. R. and Gips, C. H., *Clin. Chim. Acta*, 121, 399, 1982. With permission.)

## IV. PROTEINS

### A. Introduction

As shown in Table 2, several factors influence the protein composition of saliva.[45-48] Some of these factors are dealt with more thoroughly in Chapters 4 to 10 of this volume. This section discusses other important circumstances, as, for example, the effect of proteolysis and storage on salivary proteins.

### B. Sources of Salivary Proteins

The proteins present in whole saliva are derived mainly from the parotid, submandibular, sublingual, and MSG secretions. Small amounts of proteins present in whole saliva originate, however, from oral microorganisms, crevicular fluid, epithelial cells, polymorphonuclear leukocytes, and dietary constituents. Different methods for stimulation of whole saliva lead to different contribution of the preceding protein sources.[48] Thus, if whole saliva is collected by paraffin stimulation, the saliva will contain higher quantities of crevicular fluid as compared with acid stimulation. The contribution of sources other than the salivary glands to the total amount of salivary proteins will vary also depending on the type of protein. For example, most of the proteolytic activity of whole saliva originates from oral microorganisms, whereas amylase, for instance, is largely derived from the parotid glands (see Chapter 10).

## C. Flow Rate, Duration of Stimulation, Previous Stimulation, and Variation over Time

The flow rate of saliva influences both the total protein concentration as well as the proportions of the proteins secreted. Dawes[49] found that moderate stimulation of the parotid gland led to a reduction in protein concentration, while high flow rates increased the protein levels. With submandibular saliva the protein concentration increases with flow rate but is less dependent on the duration of the stimulus as compared with parotid saliva.[50] Prolonged stimulation leads to a decrease in bacterial aggregating factors.[51] This may result from a reduced glycosylation of salivary glycoproteins.[52] The effects of stimulation and prolonged stimulation on the relative proportions of various salivary gland proteins are dependent on the origin of the proteins. The proportional contribution of acinar proteins shows an increase when the flow rate increases above the unstimulated level but is thereafter relatively independent of flow rate.[53] Proteins secreted by the plasma cells (e.g., IgA) or duct cells (e.g., lysozyme) behave differently.[53] The salivary immunoglobulins are good examples of proteins which show deviating responses to stimulation. The levels of IgA in saliva are inversely correlated to the flow rate and little affected by prolonged stimulation[53,54] (cf. Chapter 8). IgG, however, is primarily derived from plasma, and the IgG concentration of saliva is rather independent of stimulation.[55] Thus, the relative proportions of salivary IgA and IgG are different in unstimulated and stimulated saliva.[55] Also, the intensity of stimulation will affect the IgA to IgG ratio. Thus, it is doubtful whether studies on salivary immunoglobulins based on different levels of stimulation are fully comparable. This stands for other salivary proteins as well.[56]

The effect of previous stimulation on saliva proteins was studied by Dawes and Chebib.[57] Sequential samples could be collected if successive collections were separated from each other by 1 to 2 h.[57] With unstimulated saliva this problem does not turn up. The effect of circadian rhythm on the salivary protein concentration has to be taken into consideration if sequential samples are collected (Figure 4).[46]

The level of total proteins in saliva of an individual seems to be maintained over time.[56-58] Also the levels of lysozyme, lactoferrin, and peroxidase in parotid saliva have shown little variation over time.[56] Contradictory reports have been published on the variation of sIgA levels.[56,59] (See also Chapter 8 of this volume.) The matter is further complicated by results which have showed that salivary IgA activities against specific bacteria may vary over time even when the total IgA levels are stable.[59]

## D. Protein Determination of Saliva

The quantitation of salivary proteins is associated with several problems. In a study[60] in which various protein determination methods were used, the total protein values for saliva varied widely and significantly depending on the method used. The UV-absorption techniques gave the highest values, and the Lowry and the biuret methods the lowest values, with Kjeldahl values being in the intermediate range. The amino acid composition as well as the high carbohydrate content of the salivary proteins lead to underestimation of the saliva protein content when the preceding methods are used. Factors such as 6.25 have been used to correct the values.[61,62]

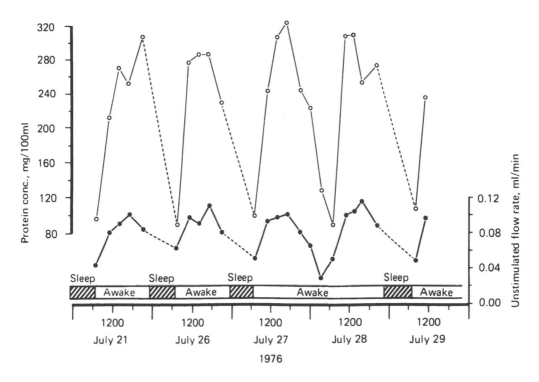

FIGURE 4. Effect of circadian rhythm and lack of sleep on the protein concentration of unstimulated parotid saliva. (From Dawes, C., *Front. Oral Physiol.*, 3, 125, 1981. With permission.)

Standard methods for serum proteins based on the presence of aromatic amino acids, for example, the method employing the Folin phenol reagent,[64] are widely used for saliva. Tyrosine is present in some salivary proteins in high amounts. More than half of the salivary proteins, however, lack aromatic amino acids: the acidic and basic proline-rich proteins as well as the proline-rich glycoproteins contain no or little aromatic amino acids.[64] Thus, the method of Lowry, as well as the determination of $A_{280}$,[65] are not very suitable techniques for the measurement of the protein content of saliva. The main reasons why the Lowry method is still used for saliva include its simplicity, sensitivity, and precision.[65] Thus, the Lowry method is about 50 to 100 times more sensitive than the UV-absorption measurement or the standard biuret assay.[65] A large number of substances interfere with the Lowry assay. EDTA, for example, may interfere if the saliva has been pretreated with EDTA to prevent precipitation of Ca-proteinates.[65]

UV-absorption methods have the advantage of being rapid and nondestructive. As stated earlier, 280 nm is not an ideal wavelength for saliva proteins. Absorbance determinations based on the wavelength of the peptide bond (206 to 220 nm) are more suitable for salivary proteins.[66,67] Wavelength pairs can be used to increase the detectability.[65] All UV-absorption methods are, however, sensitive to interfering factors, such as turbidity. The UV-absorbances of individual proteins differ, and thus the proper standard should have the same protein composition as the sample studied. With complex protein mixtures like saliva, this is naturally impossible.

The standard biuret method has also been used for protein determination of saliva.[51,68] This method is based on the reaction of the peptide bond, and it can be recommended for saliva.[65] Drawbacks of this method include its low sensitivity and the relatively large sample consumption.[65] Interfering factors can be eliminated by pretreating the saliva before analyses. Pretreatment, however, may complicate the analyses.

Protein dye binding methods developed for serum have also been used for saliva.[69,70] The most common method was introduced by Bradford, and it employs Coomassie Brilliant Blue.[71] This reagent reacts poorly with proline-rich proteins and thus underestimates the concentration of total salivary proteins. As stated for other methods, the protein dye binding procedure requires the use of standards other than serum albumin.[65] The advantage of this method is its relative intensivity to interfering factors such as EDTA.[7]

The staining properties of various salivary proteins in gels after electrophoresis or isoelectric focusing are discussed in Chapter 7 of this volume. Protein dye binding techniques are widely employed for these purposes. The poor staining of proline-rich proteins can be improved by adjusting the staining conditions (see Chapter 7). Gels have been stained also using silver-staining techniques.[72-74] A positive reaction in silver staining is obtained both for proteins and carbohydrates, which makes this staining useful in the detection of salivary glycoproteins.[73] Individual proteins stain differently in silver staining.[72,73]

## E. Changes in the Protein Composition of Saliva Due to Hydrolytic Enzymes or Storage Conditions

In nonmicrobial saliva (either whole saliva or pure salivary secretions) relatively small changes take place in the protein composition even when the saliva is incubated at 37°C (Figure 5).[75-77] In whole saliva, however, digestive enzymes originating mainly from microorganisms and degenerating host cells effectively degrade salivary proteins.[75-77] Only relatively few proteins appear to be resistant to these digestive enzymes. Such proteins include albumin and sIgA but not IgA.[78] Thus, if saliva samples are collected or stored in conditions allowing protein digestion to take place, protein fragments or peptides not originally present in saliva may be formed. Such protein degradation products may be artifacts even if they would otherwise normally occur in saliva. Glycoproteins are, in general, resistant to common proteolytic enzymes,[79] and the sulfate moieties of sulfated glycoproteins appear to be resistant to enzymatic hydrolysis in the oral cavity.[80] Hexoses, hexosamine, and sialic acid present in glycoproteins, however, are rapidly released by enzymatic hydrolysis.[75,76] The sugars released from the glycoproteins are digested by oral bacteria.[81] Thus, when studying whole saliva proteins, chilling of the saliva during the collection is important in preventing hydrolysis of proteins. For example, more than 10% of the agglutinating activity of saliva was lost when saliva was collected for 10 min without chilling the sample during collection.[76] The resistance of individual proteins to hydrolytic enzymes will be dealt with shortly.

In whole saliva, the loss of the sugar moieties of glycoproteins leads to the formation of a protein precipitate followed by a drop in the viscosity of saliva.[75] This precipitate is rich in calcium and has a low solubility. In addition to whole saliva, a precipitate is often formed in pure salivary gland secretions, for example, after storage of the samples in a freezer. EDTA treatment can be used to prevent the formation of Ca-proteinates.[82-84] EDTA, however, may interfere with analyses of saliva (e.g., protein determination, see Section IV.D). The calcium complexed by EDTA can be removed by dialysis[84] before storage of the saliva sample. EDTA treatment can also be used when concentrated or lyophilized saliva samples are reconstituted.[82] Even if the formation of Ca-proteinates has been prevented, reconstitution of saliva proteins may be difficult. The dissolving of proteins has been facilitated by use of salt solutions and/or detergents like Triton® X-100.[84,86] Practical aspects related to the reconstitution of saliva samples before electrophoresis or isoelectric focusing are discussed in Chapter 7.

Also other kinds of protein associations leading to protein precipitation may affect the protein composition of saliva. Several salivary components such as sIgA, lysozyme, and peroxidase can be precipitated with mucins (see Chapters 9 and 10). Some salivary proteins are also associated with oral bacteria (see Chapters 9 and 10), and thus the removal of the

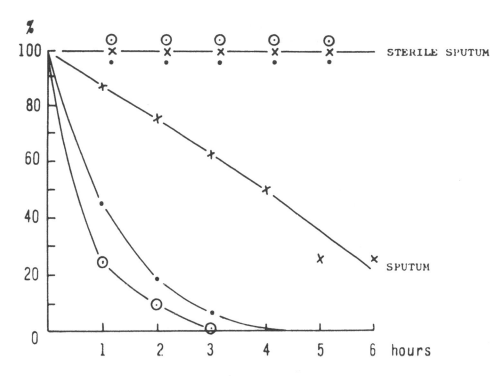

FIGURE 5.    Effect of sterilization of unstimulated whole saliva on the content of bound hexosamine (x-x) and sialic acid (●-●) as well as hemagglutination inhibition titer (⊙-⊙) during incubation at 37°C. (Rölla, G., *Acta Odontol. Scand.*, 24, 431, 1966. With permission.)

salivary sediment (by centrifugation) causes a reduction in those proteins which are "trapped" by the sediment. As a consequence, unclarified whole saliva is used for some determinations even though the use of clarified saliva would be optimal for most studies.

## F. Aspects Associated with Specific Proteins or Methods Based on Reactions of Proteins
### 1. Enzymes

The number of enzymes present in whole saliva is much higher than that of pure salivary gland secretions.[70,86] A large portion of whole saliva enzymes originate from oral microorganisms.[70] Other sources of whole saliva enzymes are the salivary glands, the crevicular fluid, polymorphonuclear leukocytes, epithelial cells, and dietary constituents.[70,86] The contribution of each source to the total amount of salivary enzymes is difficult to estimate especially when enzymes (e.g., peptidases) with similar substrate specificities are present in several of the aforementioned sources. The stimulation method used in the collection of whole saliva affects the proportion of crevicular enzymes. Thus, chewing of paraffin leads to a higher contribution of crevicular fluid enzymes as compared with collection of saliva by spitting or using a pipette. Origins of various enzymes present in saliva, as well as factors that affect the levels of salivary enzymes, are discussed in Chapter 10 of this volume.

The study of pure salivary gland secretions poses fewer problems in enzyme analyses than that of whole saliva. Since salivary enzymes are secreted by different mechanisms (see Chapter 10), the flow rate affects the enzyme and protein proportions of pure salivary secretions differently. Thus, stabilization of flow rate may be needed for optimal results. When whole saliva is used, the situation is more complex. First, the possible origin(s) of the salivary enzyme activities has to be considered. Second, a proper pretreatment of the saliva sample has to be chosen. To stop the bacterial metabolism and enzyme action, the saliva should be collected on ice. Generally, the best pretreatment for saliva with respect

**Table 4**
## PRETREATMENT AND STORAGE OF WHOLE SALIVA FOR ENZYME ANALYSES

| Enzyme | Pretreatment of saliva | Storage condition | | | |
|---|---|---|---|---|---|
| | | +4°C | | Frozen (−20°C) | |
| | | Short-term[a] | Long-term[b] | Short-term[a] | Long-term[b] |
| α-Amylase | Untreated or clarified | +[c] | −[d] | + | + |
| Lysozyme | Untreated | − | − | + | − |
| | Acidified | + | + | + | + |
| Peroxidase | Untreated or clarified[e] | + | − | + | + |
| Glycosidases | Untreated or clarified[e] | + | − | + | − |
| Esterases | Untreated or clarified[e] | + | − | + | − |
| Proteases and peptidases | Untreated or clarified[e] | + | − | + | +/− |

*Note:* For further details and references, see text.

[a]   Short-term: a few days.
[b]   Long-term: several weeks or months.
[c]   Plus (+): the enzyme is generally stable.
[d]   Minus (−): the enzyme may be unstable.
[e]   Clarification decreases enzyme activity.

to enzyme analyses is clarification by centrifugation. Clarification of saliva will render it suitable for spectrophotometric analyses. It also excludes the possible interference by oral microorganisms. The microorganisms themselves or their hydrolytic enzymes may interfere with the enzyme assay either by inactivating the enzyme in question[77,87] or by interacting with the substrate if the reaction conditions are favorable. Clarification of whole saliva also eliminates possible precipitation of salivary components during the enzyme assay. Centrifugation, however, removes a considerable part of the total enzyme activity from whole saliva where the enzymes may be bound to salivary glycoproteins, microorganisms, or other components. Such enzymes include lysozyme, and peroxidase[88] (see also Chapter 10) and α-amylase.[89] Clarification of whole saliva will substantially alter also the number and relative proportions of hydrolytic enzymes as a result of removal of microorganisms, leukocytes, and epithelial cells.[70,86] As a conclusion, pretreatment of saliva and the storage conditions will essentially affect the results of enzyme analyses (Table 4).

### a. α-Amylase

The α-amylase concentration in whole saliva and parotid saliva is high, and therefore saliva is usually diluted 1000- to 4000-fold for amylase determinations. The high salivary α-amylase concentrations, the high dilutions required for activity determinations, and the resistance of amylase to proteolytic enzymes produced by oral microorganisms[90] are probable reasons for the similar enzyme activity levels observed in clarified and untreated whole saliva.[143] The activity levels are usually similar even though α-amylase shows affinity toward oral microorganisms.[89] Both clarified[91] and untreated[92] salivas have been used for α-amylase determinations of whole saliva. The composition of the solution used for the dilution of saliva for α-amylase determination will, however, affect the results. Saliva is usually diluted with either water or saline, as proposed for dilution of serum. In tests performed in the laboratory, saline-diluted samples gave 20 to 30% higher α-amylase activities as compared with water-diluted samples. This resulted from the activation of α-amylase by $Cl^-$.[93] Dilution with solutions containing lower $Cl^-$-concentrations, corresponding the $Cl^-$-concentration of saliva, gave intermediate values. The highest α-amylase activities (about 40% higher as compared with water-diluted saliva) were found when the sample was diluted with a saline solution supplemented with 0.2% bovine serum albumin and 20 m$M$ CaCl$_2$, as suggested in the α-amylase kit instructions by Pharmacia (Uppsala, Sweden) (see also Chapter 10). Chloride ions affect the conformation and activity of many enzymes.[94] Thus the choice of the solution for dilution of saliva is important also in the determination of other enzymes.

Saliva can be stored at $-20$°C prior to α-amylase determinations.[91] To prevent massive precipitation, the saliva should be clarified before freezing.

### b. Lysozyme

Problems connected with the assay of lysozyme are discussed in Chapter 9 of this volume. For optimal results the lysozyme determination should be performed on freshly collected saliva.[95] Centrifugation of whole saliva leads to a considerable reduction in the salivary lysozyme levels due to the removal of lysozyme-mucin complexes.[95] Acidification of the samples can be used to dissociate such lysozyme complexes.[95] For pure salivary secretions such a pretreatment has been advantageous when the lysoplate technique has been used, but the pretreatment had no effect on the electroimmunodiffusion technique.[96] Acidified whole saliva and parotid saliva samples seem to retain their original lysozyme activity during storage for several days at $+20$°C, $+4$°C, or $-20$°C.[95] Untreated whole or parotid saliva may lose more than 50% of original lysozyme activity when stored in cold.[95] If whole saliva is stored at $-20$°C, the loss of enzyme activity is smaller.[142] One main factor contributing to the decrease of salivary lysozyme activities during storage at $-20$°C is the formation of insoluble lysozyme complexes.

### c. Peroxidase

The salivary peroxidase activity endures freezing and storage for several months.[97] Salivary peroxidase forms associates with various components of saliva (see Chapters 9 and 10), such as mucins.[98] Therefore, clarification of saliva leads to a decrease in the peroxidase activities. The common methods used for determination of peroxidase activity (see Chapter 9) are affected by the turbidity of saliva. Consequently, saliva is often centrifuged before enzyme activity assays even though a small part of the enzyme is lost.[99]

### d. Glycosidases

The majority of glycosidases (e.g., sucrases) are of microbial origin[70,86,100] (see also Chapter 10) and should thus be determined from whole saliva. Pure salivary gland secretions should be collected for the determination of glycosidases originating from the salivary glands. Generally, the glycosidase activities decrease during storage,[101] but short-term storage at $-20$°C resulted in relatively small activity losses.[102,103]

### e. Esterases

Centrifugation of whole saliva removes a major part of the salivary esterase activity.[70] A variety of esterases have been found in pure parotid gland secretions and in oral microorganisms.[70,86,104] Esterase activity is also present in epithelial cells.[104] Salivary esterases can be stored at $-20$°C for short time intervals without considerable loss of enzyme activity.[103,104]

### f. Proteases and Peptidases

The number of proteases of pure glandular secretions is small compared with whole saliva, which contains proteases and peptidases of oral microorganisms, leukocytes, and epithelial cells.[70,77,86,87] Proteases are generally resistant to short-term storage in cold and to long-term storage at $-20$°C. Some peptidases may, however, lose their activity during long-term storage at $-20$°C, but if the storage is restricted to a few days at $-20$°C, the activities do not decrease.[105]

### 2. Glycoproteins, Agglutinating Activity, and Blood Group Substances

As discussed previously, the salivary glycoproteins are susceptible to enzymatic hydrolysis which originates mainly from oral microorganisms.[75-77,87] The sugar moieties of the glycoproteins are rapidly released by enzymatic hydrolysis,[75,76] but the protein component is also susceptible to proteolytic activity.[77,87] The hydrolysis of glycoproteins is accompanied by a rapid reduction in the agglutinating activity of saliva.[76,87]

Blood group substances are secreted in submandibular and sublingual saliva but not in parotid saliva.[48] The blood group substance content of the MSG secretions is several-fold higher as compared with submandibular saliva.[48,81] The MSG secretions show a high content of blood group substance A, but also contain blood group substances with B, Le[a], and Le[b] specificity,[81] The blood group substances have large carbohydrate moieties and are susceptible to the hydrolytic enzyme activity of oral microorganisms. Blood group substances bind to oral microorganisms.[106] Thus, clarification reduces the levels of blood group substances in whole saliva.

If the agglutinating activity has to be determined from different types of salivas, resting saliva is always collected before stimulated saliva. The agglutinating activity of saliva is decreased by prolonged stimulation.[51] Thus, stimulated whole saliva and parotid saliva cannot be collected without a sufficient time interval (at least 1 h) between collections. For optimal results, fresh saliva should be used for agglutination tests. Storage of clarified saliva at $-20°C$ for 2 to 4 weeks led to diversified decreases in the agglutinating activities (20 to 80%).[144] The formation of varying amounts of precipitates in the samples as a result of freezing appeared to disturb the agglutination assay (see Chapter 9). Thus, if storage of saliva before the agglutination test is necessary, the samples should be clarified after thawing.

### 3. Adhesion Test

Whole saliva (either stimulated or resting saliva) is usually used in adhesion tests in which the adhesion of oral microorganisms to saliva-coated hydroxyapatite is studied.[107-112] In the method of Appelbaum et al.,[107] the saliva is clarified by centrifugation followed by heat treatment and addition of sodium azide. The saliva supernatants are used for the adhesion tests immediately or stored at $+4°C$ before use. Staat et al.[108] studied the influence of heat treatment and sodium azide addition on the adherence assay involving whole saliva and parotid saliva, and found no effect. In later studies, the samples were centrifuged, and the supernatant fluids immediately (or after a short storage at $+4°C$[108,110] or at $-20°C$[111,112]) used for the adhesion assays. Experiments performed in the laboratory showed similar results for freshly used and frozen ($-20°C$, 1 to 2 weeks) saliva supernatants even when the thawed samples had to be cleared by centrifugation before assays.

### 4. Statherin and Proline-Rich Proteins

Both statherin and proline-rich proteins (PRP) are susceptible to degradation by proteolytic enzymes of oral bacteria.[113-115] Statherin is more readily degraded than PRP.[113] Consequently, these proteins are usually studied by using pure salivary gland secretions (for references see Chapter 5 of this volume). In the absence of bacterial proteolytic enzymes, statherin and PRP appear not to be inactivated by dialysis, freezing, or lyophilization, for example.[116] Storage of parotid saliva at $+4°C$ or repeated freezing and thawing of the saliva did not decrease the activity of statherin.[117] In purified form statherin and PRP have been stored in salts or buffer solutions at $-50°C$.[116]

### 5. Histidine-Rich Polypeptides and Lactoferrin

The histidine-rich polypeptides are susceptible to hydrolysis by proteolytic enzymes present in oral bacteria[118] (see also Chapter 6). In the absence of proteolytic activity, the histidine-rich polypeptides appear not to lose their biological activity as a result of treatments such as dialysis, freezing, and lyophilization.[119]

Lactoferrin has been determined of uncentrifuged whole saliva[99] and pure saliva secretions.[99,120] Lactoferrin does not lose its biological activity after dialysis or freezing.[99,120]

### 6. *Immunoglobulins*

Salivary immunoglobulins are discussed in Chapter 8 of this volume as well as in Section IV.C of this chapter.

IgA, IgG, and IgM are susceptible to proteolytic degradation.[78,121] Thus, immediate cooling of saliva samples after the collection is important especially when studying whole saliva. Secretory IgA, however, is relatively resistant to proteolytic enzymes.[78]

As a rule, immunoglobulins should retain their biological activity for several months when stored in a freezer, especially at lower temperatures. Prolonged (1 year) freezing, however, was reported to decrease the parotid IgA levels.[53] Also short-term (10-d) freezing of saliva caused a variable decrease in IgA concentrations which was more pronounced in whole saliva than in parotid saliva.[122] Storage of the samples at $+4°C$ for 10 d resulted in unaltered IgA levels.[122] In the case of whole saliva, these findings appear to be at least partly explained by variations in precipitate formation as a result of freezing. Clarification of whole saliva before freezing and storage of saliva at different temperatures[53,122,123] also affect the recovery of salivary IgA.

### 7. *Practical Aspects Associated with Separation Techniques for Salivary Proteins*

The high molecular weight viscous proteins of saliva pose problems in most analytical or preparative separation techniques. Thus, the viscosity problems concern especially the MSG secretions (see Section II) and submandibular and whole saliva. The viscosity can be decreased by precipitating the salivary mucins with cetyltrimethylammonium bromide,[124] changing the pH of the saliva by NaOH,[125] for example, or by mechanical stirring or homogenization of the sample.[59] Cetyltrimethylammonium bromide is also widely used as one of the first steps in the purification of salivary glycoproteins.[126] High molecular weight proteins can also be elegantly removed by ultrafiltration[77] using membranes with various exclusion limits.

As can be expected, the methods for preparation of high molecular weight glycoproteins present many practical problems.[126] In chromatography the high viscosity of saliva leads to broad and overlapping peaks and tailing. Gel permeation chromatography is especially affected by the viscosity of the sample; salivary mucins tend to clog columns. In addition, the columns can be contaminated by insoluble material, for example, by Ca-proteinates present in whole saliva. To avoid these drawbacks, saliva can be filtered through 0.45-$\mu$m membranes which also sterilize the samples. Pretreatment of saliva is especially important when using high performance liquid chromatography (HPLC) techniques in which even properly filtered saliva may ruin a column. Ultrafiltration has appeared to be the most successful method to treat saliva before HPLC. Practical analytical aspects related to the electrophoresis or isoelectric focusing of salivary proteins are discussed in Chapter 7 of this volume.

Further factors interfering with the salivary protein separations include the associations between the salivary proteins and other components of saliva. The equipment used to collect or treat saliva may also cause problems. Adherence of some salivary proteins to surfaces interferes with both the collection and the analysis of saliva, particularly if glass equipment is used.[45,98] This phenomenon is especially marked with the MSG secretions (see Section II). Associations between various salivary proteins may interfere with separation techniques of saliva and give results which are difficult to interpret. Associations between various protein components of saliva are dealt with in Chapters 9 and 10 of this volume.

## V. LIPIDS

The origin of salivary lipids and technical aspects related to the isolation and analysis of lipids are dealt with in Chapter 11 of this volume. Most lipid studies stress the use of pure and freshly collected salivary gland secretions in analyses. The samples should be properly pretreated immediately after collection (for references see Chapter 11). If the samples cannot be pretreated, they should be frozen without delay and kept under nitrogen at all times to prevent oxidation, degradation, etc.[127]

## VI. MICROBIOLOGICAL ANALYSES

### A. Transport Media and Storage

For optimal results, the culturing of saliva in microbiological studies should be performed without delay after sample collection. When simple techniques such as dip-slides are used, culturing is possible even in field conditions. More time-demanding techniques which include diluting and plating of the samples are, however, often impossible to perform immediately after sample collection. Storage of the samples can be convenient also from a practical point of view: if samples for microbiological analyses are collected infrequently or at odd hours, the saliva can be stored and the culturings performed after fixed time intervals (*vide infra*).

For short-term storage, the saliva samples can be diluted with various transport media[128-134] and stored in a refrigerator or a freezer.[128,129] Anaerobic storage conditions are required for the recovery of anaerobes.[128] When the recoveries of oral microorganisms were compared after up to 2-week storage at −10°C in common transport media (reduced transport fluid [RTF], VMG II,[130] modified Stuart medium[131]), the most satisfactory medium was generally RTF.[127] These three media, however, differed in their recoveries for different bacteria.[128] Oral streptococci retained their viability in VMG II even when stored at room temperature for several days.[130] Ordinary freezing of samples (0 to −20°C) as such is not a recommended storage technique.[129] If the samples are diluted with transport media containing cryoprotective agents and stored at temperatures below −20°C (−40 to −80°C), the recoveries are good; these procedures can be used fairly successfully also for long-term storage.[129,132-134] In our laboratory, tryptic soy broth containing 10% glycerol[134] has been used for the preservation of salivary microorganisms (storage for 1 to 4 weeks at −40°C, dilution 1:10).

For long-term storage and optimal recoveries ultrafreezing is a recommended method.[129] Generally, the recoveries are better if cryoprotective agents are used.[129,132,133] The cryoprotective effect of glycerol (cell penetrating) appears to differ between different microorganisms, whereas polyvinylpyrrolidine (PVP, nonpenetrating) gives a consistent protection across microorganisms.[137] The recoveries of oral bacteria after short-term (30 min to 8 to 10 weeks) as well as long-term (1 to 2 years) storage in liquid nitrogen appear to be relatively satisfactory even when no cryoprotective agents are used.[133] The bacterial proportions of saliva samples may, however, be affected by the freezing and/or the storage procedures.[133] Thus, when plaque bacteria were suspended in a serum-based transport medium and stored in liquid nitrogen, a reduction in aerobic Gram-negative cocci was found.[138] Resistant microorganisms such as *Streptococcus mutans* retain their viability during storage at ultralow temperatures even when stored in simple salt solutions.[129,132] The effect of cryoprotective agents is of importance for the recoveries of microorganisms such as *Fusobacterium nucleatum*, which are sensitive to freezing.[132,133] Freezing the cells of *F. nucleatum* without cryoprotective agents led to a reduction of more than 95% in the number of viable microorganisms, while the use of glycerol or PVP showed no reduction in viability.[132,133]

When freezing of microorganisms is used, optimal results have been obtained by applying slow cooling rates (e.g., 1°C/min) and rapid thawing.[129]

## B. Dispersion

Dispersion of the sample is one of the main problems to overcome when culturing dental plaque. With plaque the dispersion method is always a compromise between maximum preservation and viability on the one hand and satisfactory dispersion on the other.[135] Compared with plaque, dispersion problems with whole saliva are small.

Gentle methods such as vortex mixing[136,137] or shaking with glass beads[138] give a satisfactory dispersion without loss of viability. Even when salivary sediment collected by centrifugation has been used for bacterial analyses, whirling of the sediment has been considered to be a satisfactory method.[139] The use of glass beads as compared with whirling alone gives a better dispersion especially with stored saliva samples containing aggregates. Sonication is an effective dispersion method used mainly for plaque[135] but also for whole saliva. Sonication kills Gram-negative cells and favors Gram-positive ones, especially streptococci.[140] Thus the use of sonication as a pretreatment of saliva for microbial analyses seems to be recommended for the cultivation of salivary streptococci only.

## ACKNOWLEDGMENTS

I wish to express my gratitude to Professor Kauko Mäkinen for valuable comments and to Ms. Sirpa Laakso for excellent technical assistance.

## REFERENCES

1. **Mason, D. K. and Chisholm, D. M.,** *Salivary Glands in Health and Disease,* Saunders, London, 1975.
2. **Jenkins, G. N.,** *The Physiology and Biochemistry of the Mouth,* 4th ed., Blackwell Scientific, Oxford, 1978, 284.
3. **Dawes, C. and Wood, C. M.,** The composition of human lip mucous gland secretions, *Arch. Oral Biol..,* 18, 343, 1973.
4. **Provenza, D. V.,** *Oral Histology,* Lippincott, Philadelphia, 1964.
5. **Hensten-Pettersen, A.,** Minor salivary gland secretions, in *Proceedings Saliva and Dental Caries,* Kleinberg, I., Ellison, S. A., and Mandel, I. D., Eds., Information Retrieval, New York, 1979, 81.
6. **Slomiany, B. L., Zdebska, E., Murty, V. N. L., Slomiany, A., Petropoulou, K., and Mandel, I. D.,** Lipid composition of human labial salivary gland secretions, *Arch. Oral Biol.,* 28, 711, 1983.
7. **Mäkinen, K. K., Virtanen, K. K., Söderling, E. and Kotiranta, J.,** Composition of human palatine gland secretions and evidence for the presence of specific arylamidases, *Arch. Oral Biol.,* 28, 893, 1983.
8. **Kaaber, S.,** Sodium and potassium content in human palatine gland secretion, *Arch. Oral Biol.,* 22, 529, 1977.
9. **Dawes, C.,** The composition of human saliva secreted in response to a gustatory stimulus and to pilocarpine, *J. Physiol. (London),* 183, 360, 1966.
10. **Hensten-Pettersen, A.,** Some chemical characteristics of human minor salivary gland secretions, *Acta Odontol. Scand.,* 34, 13, 1976.
11. **Hensten-Pettersen, A. and Jakobsen, N.,** *In vitro* production of sulphated mucosubstances by the labial and palatine glands of the monkey *Macaca irus, Arch. Oral Biol.,* 20, 111, 1975.
12. **Mäkinen, K. K., Söderling, E., Virtanen, K. K., and Kotiranta, J.,** Partial purification and characterization of arylamidases from human palatine gland secretions, *Arch. Oral Biol.,* 30, 513, 1985.
13. **Mäkinen, K. K., Virtanen, K. K., Söderling, E., and Kotiranta, J.,** Effect of xylitol-, sucrose-, and water-rinses on the composition of human palatine gland secretions, *Scand. J. Dent. Res.,* 93, 253, 1985.
14. **Shiba, A., Sano, K., Nakao, M., and Hayashi, T.,** A new method of collecting saliva from human palatine glands for electrophoretic study, *Arch. Oral Biol.,* 25, 503, 1980.
15. **Green, G. and Embery, D. R. J.,** The chemistry and biological properties of the minor salivary gland secretions, in *Oral Interfacial Reactions of Bone, Soft Tissue and Saliva,* Glantz, P.-O., Leach, S. A., and Ericson, T., Eds., IRL Press, Oxford, 1985, 75.
16. **Morgan, W. T. J.,** *Methods in Immunology and Immunochemistry,* Williams, C. A. and Chase, M. W., Eds., Academic Press, London, 1967, 75.

17. **Ryley, H. C. and Brogan, T. D.,** Variation in the composition of sputum in chronic chest diseases, *Br. J. Exp. Pathol.,* 49, 625, 1968.

18. **Denborough, M. A. and Creeth, J. M.,** Density gradient studies of A, B, H and Leᵃ blood group specific substances, *Clin. Chim. Acta,* 30, 447, 1970.

19. **Havez, R., Roussel, P., Degand, P., and Biserte, G.,** Etude des structures fibrillaires de la secretion bronchique humaine, *Clin. Chim. Acta,* 17, 281, 1967.

20. **Rölla, G. and Jonsen, J.,** A glycoprotein component from human sublingual-submaxillary saliva, *Caries Res.,* 2, 306, 1968.

21. **Schrager, J. and Oates, M. D. G.,** The chemical composition and some structural features of the principal salivary glycoprotein isolated from human mixed saliva, *Arch. Oral Biol.,* 19, 1215, 1974.

22. **Dewar, M. R.,** Laboratory methods for assessing susceptibility to dental caries, *J. Dent. Austr.,* 21, 509, 1949.

23. **Lilienthal, B.,** An analysis of the buffer systems in saliva, *J. Dent. Res.,* 34, 516, 1955.

24. **Ericsson, Y.,** Clinical investigations of the salivary buffering action, *Acta Odontol. Scand.,* 17, 131, 1959.

25. **Heintze, U.,** On the Secretion Rate and Buffer Effect of Whole Saliva in Adults, Acad. diss. Malmö, Sweden, 1986.

26. **Tannenbaum, S. R., Sinskey, A. J., Weisman, M., and Bishop, W.,** Nitrite in human saliva. Its possible relationship to nitrosamine formation, *J. Natl. Cancer Inst.,* 53, 79, 1974.

27. **Phizackerley, P. J. R. and Al-Dabbagh, S. A.,** The estimation of nitrate and nitrite in saliva and urine, *Anal. Biochem.,* 131, 242, 1983.

28. **Lamberts, B. L., Pruitt, K. M., Pederson, E. D., and Golding, M. P.,** Comparison of salivary peroxidase system components in caries-free and caries-active naval recruits, *Caries Res.,* 18, 488, 1984.

29. **Lagerlöf, F. and Lindqvist, L.,** A method for determining concentrations of calcium complexes in human parotid saliva by gel filtrations, *Arch. Oral Biol.,* 27, 735, 1982.

30. **McCann, H. G.,** Inorganic components of salivary secretions, in *Arts and Science of Dental Caries Research,* Harris, R. S., Ed., Academic Press, New York, 1968, 55.

31. **Grøn, P.,** The state of calcium and inorganic orthophosphate in human saliva, *Arch. Oral Biol.,* 18, 1365, 1973.

32. **Kallner, A.,** Determination of phosphate in serum and urine by a single step, malachite-green method, *Clin. Chim. Acta,* 59, 35, 1975.

33. **Lagerlöf, F.,** Determination of inorganic phosphate in human parotid saliva by the malachite green method, *Caries Res.* 16, 324, 1982.

34. **Chen, P. S., Tosibara, T. Y., and Warner, H.,** Microdetermination of phosphorous, *Anal. Chem.,* 28, 1756, 1956.

35. **Fiske, C. H., and Subbarow, Y.,** The colorimetric determination of phosphorous, *J. Biol. Chem.,* 66, 375, 1925.

36. **Leloir, C. F. and Cardini, C. E.,** Characterization of phosphorous compounds by acid lability, in *Methods in Enzymology,* Vol. 3, Colowick, S. P. and Kaplan, N. O., Eds., 1972, 840.

37. **Birkeland, J. M. and Rölla, G.,** *In vitro* affinity of fluoride to proteins, dextrans, bacteria and salivary components, *Arch. Oral Biol.,* 17, 455, 1972.

38. **Birkeland, J. M.,** The effect of pH on the interaction of fluoride and salivary ions, *Caries Res.,* 7, 11, 1973.

39. **Kjellman, O.,** The presence of glucose in gingival exudate and resting saliva of subjects with insulin-treated diabetes mellitus, *Swed. Dent. J.,* 63, 11, 1970.

40. **Sandham, H. J. and Kleinberg, I.,** Utilization of glucose and lactic acid by salivary sediment, *Arch. Oral Biol.,* 14, 597, 1969.

41. **Kopstein, J. and Wrong, O. M.,** The origin and fate of salivary urea and ammonia in man, *Clin. Sci. Mol. Med.,* 52, 9, 1977.

42. **Huizenga, J. R. and Gips, C. H.,** Preservation of saliva for ammonia determination, *Clin. Chim. Acta,* 121, 399, 1982.

43. **Gips, C. H. and Wibbens-Alberts, M.,** Ammonia determination in blood using the TCA-direct method, *Clin. Chim. Acta,* 22, 183, 1968.

44. **Gips, C. H., Reitsema, A., and Wibbens-Alberts, M.,** Preservation of urine for ammonia determination with a direct method, *Clin. Chim. Acta,* 29, 501, 1970.

45. **Ellison, S. A.,** Identification of salivary components, in *Proceedings Saliva and Dental Caries,* Kleinberg, I., Ellison, S. A., and Mandel, I. D., Eds., Information Retrieval, New York, 1979, 13.

46. **Dawes, C.,** Factors influencing protein secretion in human saliva, *Front. Oral Physiol.,* 3, 125, 1981.

47. **Mandel, I. D.,** Proteins in salivary secretions and whole saliva, in *Proteins in Body Fluids, Amino Acids, and Tumor Markers: Diagnostic and Clinical Aspects,* Ritzmann, S. E. and Killingsworth, L. M., Eds., Alan R. Liss, New York, 1983, 191.

48. **Ferguson, D. B.,** Salivary glands and saliva, in *Applied Physiology of the Mouth,* Lavelle, C. L. B., Ed., John Wright & Sons, Bristol, 1975, 145.

49. **Dawes, C.,** The effects of flow rate and duration of stimulation on the concentrations of protein and the main electrolytes in human parotid saliva, *Arch. Oral Biol.,* 14, 277, 1969.

50. **Dawes, C.,** The effects of low flow rate and duration of stimulation on the concentrations of protein and the main electrolytes in human submandibular saliva, *Arch. Oral Biol.,* 19, 887, 1974.

51. **Kashket, S., Guilmette, K. M., and Ebersole, J. L.,** The effect of prolonged stimulation of salivary flow on bacterial reactive factors, *J. Dent. Res.,* 62, 331, 1983.

52. **Levine, M. J., Ellison, S. A., and Bahl, O. P.,** The isolation from human parotid saliva and partial characterization of the protein core of a major parotid glycoprotein, *Arch. Oral Biol.,* 18, 827, 1973.

53. **Brandtzaeg, P.,** Human secretory immunoglobulins. VII. Concentrations of parotid IgA and other secretory proteins in relation to the rate of flow and duration of secretory stimulus, *Arch. Oral Biol.,* 16, 1295, 1971.

54. **Ericson, D., Bratthall, D., Björck, L., and Kronvall, G.,** $\beta_2$-Microglobulin in saliva and its relation to flow rate in different glands in man, *Arch. Oral Biol.,* 27, 679, 1982.

55. **Grönblad, E. A.,** Concentration of immunoglobulins in human whole saliva: effect of physiological stimulation, *Acta Odontol. Scand.,* 40, 87, 1982.

56. **Rudney, J. D., Kajander, K. C., and Smith, Q. T.,** Correlations between human salivary levels of lysozyme, lactoferrin, salivary peroxidase and secretory immunoglobulin A with different stimulatory states and over time, *Arch. Oral Biol.,* 30, 765, 1985.

57. **Dawes, C. and Chebib, F. S.,** The influence of previous stimulation and the day of the week on the concentrations of protein and the main electrolytes in human parotid saliva, *Arch. Oral Biol.,* 17, 1289, 1972.

58. **Ferguson, D. B.,** Physiological, pathological and pharmacologic variations in salivary composition, *Front. Oral Physiol.,* 3, 138, 1981.

59. **Bratthall, D. and Widerström, L.,** Ups and downs for salivary IgA, *Scand. J. Dent. Res.,* 93, 128, 1985.

60. **Wolf, R. O. and Taylor, L. L.,** A comparative study of saliva protein analysis, *Arch. Oral Biol.,* 9, 135, 1964.

61. **Dawes, C.,** Some characteristics of parotid and submandibular salivary proteins, *Arch. Oral Biol.,* 10, 269, 1965.

62. **Caldwell, R. C. and Pigman, W.,** Changes in protein and glycoprotein concentrations in human submaxillary saliva under various stimulatory conditions, *Arch. Oral Biol.,* 11, 437, 1966.

63. **Lowry, D. H., Rosebrough, N. J., Farr, A. L., and Randall, R. J.,** Protein measurement with the Folin phenol reagent, *J. Biol. Chem.,* 193, 265, 1951.

64. **Keller, P., Levine, M., Sreebny, L. M., and Robinovitch, M.,** Composition and properties of saliva, in *Proceedings Saliva and Dental Caries,* Kleinberg, I., Ellison, S. A., and Mandel, I. D., Eds., Information Retrieval, New York, 1979, 547.

65. **Kresze, G.-B.,** Methods for protein determination, in *Methods of Enzymatic Analysis,* 3rd ed., Bergmeyer, H. U., Ed., 1983, 84.

66. **Anderson, L. C., Lamberts, B. L., and Bruton, W. F.,** Salivary protein polymorphism in caries-free and caries-active adults, *J. Dent. Res.,* 61, 393, 1982.

67. **Anderson, L. C. and Mandel, I. D.,** Salivary protein polymorphism in caries-resistant adults, *J. Dent. Res.,* 10, 1167, 1982.

68. **Itzhaki, R. F. and Gill, D. M.,** A microbiuret method for estimating proteins, *Anal. Biochem.,* 9, 401, 1964.

69. **Suber, J. F., Boackle, R. J., Javed, T., and Vesely, J.,** Parotid saliva agglutinins for sheep erythrocytes as a measure of ongoing inflammation in periodontal disease, *J. Periodontol.,* 55, 512, 1984.

70. **Nakamura, M. and Slots, J.,** Salivary enzymes, *J. Periodontal Res.,* 18, 559, 1983.

71. **Bradford, M. M.,** A rapid and sensitive method for the quantitation of microgram quantities of protein utilizing the principle of protein-dye binding, *Anal. Biochem.,* 72, 248, 1976.

72. **Friedman, R. D.,** Comparison of four different silver-staining techniques for salivary protein detection in alkaline polyacrylamide gels, *Anal. Biochem.,* 126, 346, 1982.

73. **Deh, M. E., Dzandu, J. K., and Wise, G. E.,** Sialoglycoproteins with a high amount of o-glycosidically linked carbohydrate moieties stain yellow with silver in sodium dodecyl sulfate-polyacrylamide gels, *Anal. Biochem.,* 150, 166, 1985.

74. **Mogi, M., Hiraoka, B. Y., Fukasawa, K., Havada, M., Kage, T., and Chino, T.,** Two-dimensional electrophoresis in the analysis of a mixture of human sublingual and submandibular salivary proteins, *Arch. Oral Biol.,* 31, 119, 1986.

75. **Leach, S. A. and Chritchley, P.,** Bacterial degradation of glycoprotein sugars in human saliva, *Nature (London),* 209, 506, 1966.

76. **Rölla, G.,** Neuraminidase in human sputum, *Acta Odontol. Scand.,* 24, 431, 1966.

77. **Cowman, R. A., Fitzgerald, R. J., and Schaefer, S. J.,** Role of salivary factors in the nitrogen metabolism of plaque-forming oral streptococci, in *Proceedings Microbial Aspects of Dental Caries,* Vol. 2, Stiles, H. M., Loesche, W. J., and O'Brien, T. C., Eds., Information Retrieval, New York, 1976, 465.

78. **Mestecky, J. and Kilian, M.**, Immunoglobulin A (IgA), in *Methods in Enzymology*, Vol. 116, Colowick, S. P., and Kaplan, N. O., Eds., 1985, 37.

79. **Hashimoto, Y., Tsuiki, S., Nisizawa, K., and Pigman, W.**, Action of proteolytic enzymes on purified bovine submaxillary mucin, *Ann. N.Y. Acad. Sci.*, 106, 233, 1963.

80. **Embery, G.**, The role of anionic glyco-conjugates, particularly sulphated glycoproteins in relation to the oral cavity, in *Proceedings Saliva and Dental Caries*, Kleinberg, I., Ellison, S. A., and Mandel, I. D., Eds., Information Retrieval, New York, 1979, 105.

81. **Amir, S. M., Barker, S. A., and Woodsbury, S. A.**, N-Acetylmannosamine digestion by human oral bacteria, *Nature (London)*, 207, 979, 1965.

82. **Dawes, C.**, Disodium ethylene-diaminetetraacetate as an aid for the reconstitution of lyophilized human salivary proteins before paper electrophoresis, *Arch. Oral Biol.*, 8, 653, 1963.

83. **Cowman, R. A., Baron, S. S., Glassman, A. H., Davis, M. E., and Strosberg, A. M.**, Changes in protein composition of saliva from radiation-induced xerostomia patients and its effect on growth of oral streptococci, *J. Dent. Res.*, 62, 336, 1983.

84. **Cowman, R. A., Baron, S. S., Fitzgerald, R. J., Stuchell, R. E., and Mandel, I. D.**, Comparative growth responses of oral streptococci on mixed saliva or the separate submandibular and parotid secretions from caries-active and caries-free individuals, *J. Dent. Res.*, 62, 946, 1983.

85. **Smith, Q. T., Runchey, C. D., and Shapiro, B. L.**, Polyacrylamide gel slab electrophoresis of human salivary proteins, *Arch. Oral Biol.*, 19, 407, 1974.

86. **Chauncey, H. H.**, Salivary enzymes, *J. Am. Dent. Assoc.*, 63, 360, 1961.

87. **Sato, S., Koga, T., and Inoue, M.**, Degradation of the microbial and salivary components participating in human dental plaque formation by proteases elaborated by plaque bacteria, *Arch. Oral Biol.*, 28, 211, 1983.

88. **Iacono, V. J., MacKay, B. J., Grossbard, B. L., DiRienzo, S., and Pollock, J. J.**, Lysozyme binding by a polyglycerol phosphate polymer of the oral bacterium *Streptococcus mutans* BHT, *Arch. Oral Biol.*, 27, 347, 1982.

89. **Douglas, C. W I.**, The binding of human salivary α-amylase by oral strains of streptococcal bacteria, *Arch. Oral Biol.*, 28, 567, 1983.

90. **Jacobsen, N., Melvaer, K. L., and Hensten-Pettersen, A.**, Some properties of salivary amylase: a survey of the literature and some observations, *J. Dent. Res.*, 5, 381, 1972.

91. **Hafkenscheid, J. C. M. and Hessels, M.**, Measurement of pancreatic and salivary alpha-amylase in serum: comparison of methods with five different substrates, *Enzyme*, 33, 128, 1985.

92. **Fiehn, N.-E., Oram, V., and Moe, D.**, Streptococci and activities of sucrases and α-amylases in supra-gingival dental plaque and saliva in three caries activity groups, *Acta Odontol. Scand.*, 44, 1, 1986.

93. **Rauscher, E., Neumann, U., Schaich, E., von Bülow, S., and Wahlfeld, A. W.**, Optimized conditions for determining activity concentration of α-amylase in serum, with 1,4-α-D-4-nitrophenylmaltoheptaoside as substrate, *Clin. Chem.*, 31, 14, 1985.

94. **Timasheff, S. N.**, Thermodynamics of protein interactions, in *Protides of the Biological Fluids*, Vol. 20, Peeters, H., Ed., Pergamon Press, Oxford, 1972, 511.

95. **Virella, G. and Goudswaard, J.**, Measurement of salivary lysozyme, *J. Dent. Res.*, 57, 326, 1978.

96. **Stuchell, R. N., Herrera, M. S., and Mandel, I. D.**, Immunochemical quantification of human sub-mandibular-sublingual lysozyme, *J. Immunol. Methods*, 44, 15, 1981.

97. **Tenovuo, J.**, Different molecular forms of human salivary lactoperoxidase, *Arch. Oral Biol.*, 26, 1051, 1981.

98. **Ericson, T. and Arwin, H.**, Lactoperoxidase and a salivary agglutinin at liquid-solid interfaces: adsorption and interaction, in *Oral Interfacial Reactions of Bone, Soft Tissue and Saliva*, Glantz, P.-O., Leach, S. A., and Ericson, T., Eds., IRL Press, Oxford, 1985, 33.

99. **Tenovuo, J., Lehtonen, O.-P. J., Aaltonen, A. S., Vilja, P., and Tuohimaa, P.**, Antimicrobial factors in whole saliva of human infants, *Infect. Immn.*, 51, 49, 1986.

100. **Menguy, R., Masters, Y. F., and Desbaillets, L.**, Human salivary glycosidases, *Proc. Soc. Exp. Biol. Med.*, 134, 1020, 1970.

101. **Fiehn, N.-E. and Moe, D.**, Method for determination of invertase activity in homogenates of human dental plaque, *Scand. J. Dent. Res.*, 89, 450, 1981.

102. **Den Tandt, W. R. and Jaeken, J.**, Determination of lysosomal enzymes in saliva, *Clin. Chim. Acta*, 97, 19, 1979.

103. **Den Tandt, W. R., and Jaeken, J.**, Saliva, in *Methods of Enzymatic Analysis*, Vol. 3, Bergenmeyer, H. U., Ed., 1983, 35.

104. **Lindqvist, L., Nord, C.-E., and Söder, P.-Ö.**, Origin of esterases of human whole saliva, *Enzyme*, 22, 166, 1977.

105. **McDonald, J. K. and Schwabe, C.**, in *Proteinases in Mammalian Cells and Tissues*, Barrett, A. J., Ed., North-Holland, Amsterdam, 1977, 311.

106. **Gibbons, R. J. and Qureshi, J. B.,** Selective binding of blood group reactive salivary mucins by *Streptococcus mutans* and other oral organisms, *Infect. Immun.,* 22, 665, 1978.

107. **Appelbaum, B., Golub, E., Holt, S. C., and Rosen, B.,** *In vitro* studies of dental plaque formation: adsorption of oral streptococci to hydroxyapatite, *Infect. Immun.,* 25, 717, 1979.

108. **Staat, R. H., Langley, S. D., and Doyle, R. J.,** *Streptococcus mutans* adherence: presumptive evidence for protein-mediated attachment followed by glucan-dependent cellular accumulation, *Infect. Immun.,* 27, 675, 1980.

109. **Köhler, B., Krasse, B., and Carlén, A.,** Adherence and *Streptococcus mutans* infection: *in vitro* study with saliva from noninfected and infected preschool children, *Infect. Immun.,* 34, 633, 1981.

110. **Douglas, C. W. I. and Russell, R. R. B.,** The adsorption of human salivary components to strains of the bacterium *Streptococcus mutans, Arch. Oral Biol.,* 29, 751, 1984.

111. **Rosan, R. E. and Golub, E.,** Optimization of an hydroxyapatite adhesion assay for *Streptococcus sanguis, Infect. Immun.,* 44, 287, 1984.

112. **Hoppenbrouwers, P. M. M., Borggrevan, J. M. P. M., and van der Hoeven, J. S.,** Adherence of oral bacteria to chemically modified hydroxyapatite, *Caries Res.,* 18, 1, 1984.

113. **Hay, D. I. and Grøn, P.,** Inhibitors of calcium phosphate precipitation in human whole saliva, in *Proceedings Microbial Aspects of Dental Caries,* Vol. 1, Stiles, H. M., Loesche, W. J., and O'Brien, T. C., Eds., Information Retrieval, New York, 1976, 143.

114. **Kousvelari, E. E., Baratz, R. S., Burke, B., and Oppenheim, F. G.,** Immunochemical identification and determination of proline-rich proteins in salivary secretions, enamel pellicle and glandular tissue specimens, *J. Dent. Res.,* 59, 1430, 1980.

115. **Hay, D. I.,** Some observations on human saliva proteins and their role in the formation of the acquired enamel pellicle, *J. Dent. Res.,* 48, 806, 1969.

116. **Moreno, E. C., Varughese, K., and Hay, D. I.,** Effect of human salivary proteins on the precipitation kinetics of calcium phosphate, *Calcif. Tissue Int.,* 28, 7, 1979.

117. **Hay, D. I., Smith, D. J., Schluckebier, S. K., and Moreno, E. C.,** Relationship between concentration of human salivary statherin and inhibition of calcium phosphate precipitation in stimulated human parotid saliva, *J. Dent. Res.,* 63, 857, 1984.

118. **Baum, B. J., Bird, J. L., Millar, D. B., and Longton, R. W.,** Studies on histidine-rich polypeptides from human parotid saliva, *Arch. Biochem. Biophys.,* 177, 427, 1976.

119. **MacKay, B. J., Pollock, J. J., Iacono, V. J., and Baum, B. J.,** Isolation of milligram quantities of a group of histidine-rich polypeptides from human parotid saliva, *Infect. Immun.,* 44, 688, 1984.

120. **Arnold, R. R., Russell, J. E., Devine, S. M., Adamson, M., and Pruitt, K. M.,** Antimicrobial activity of the secretory innate defense factors lactoferrin, lactoperoxidase and lysozyme, in *Cariology Today,* Guggenheim, B., Ed., S. Karger, Basel, 1984, 75.

121. **Lindler, L. E. and Stutzenberger, F. J.,** Inactivation and stabilization of IgA protease from the human oral bacterium *Streptococcus sanguis, Arch. Oral Biol.,* 28, 977, 1983.

122. **Ben-Aryeh, H., Naon, H., Szargel, R., Horowitz, G., and Gutman, D.,** The concentration of salivary IgA in whole and parotid saliva and the effect of stimulation, *Int. J. Oral Maxillofacial Surg.,* 15, 81, 1986.

123. **Bolton, R. W. and Hlava, G. L.,** Evaluation of salivary IgA antibodies to cariogenic microorganisms in children: correlation with dental caries activity, *J. Dent. Res.,* 61, 1225, 1982.

124. **Mansoor Baig, M., Winzler, R. J., and Rennert, O. M.,** Isolation of mucin from human submaxillary secretions, *J. Immunol.,* 111, 1826, 1973.

125. **Nordbö, H., Darwish, S., and Bhatnagar, R. S.,** Salivary viscosity and lubrication-influence of pH and calcium, *Scand. J. Dent. Res.,* 92, 306, 1984.

126. **Roukema, P. A. and Nieuw Amerongen, A. V.,** Sulphated glycoproteins in human saliva, in *Proceedings Saliva and Dental Caries,* Kleinberg, I., Ellison, S. A., and Mandel, I. D., Eds., Information Retrieval, New York, 1979, 67.

127. **Rabinowitz, J. L. and Shannon, I. L.,** Lipid changes in human male parotid saliva by stimulation, *Arch. Oral Biol.,* 20, 403, 1975.

128. **Syed, S. A. and Loesche, W. J.,** Survival of human dental plaque flora in various transport media, *Appl. Microbiol.,* 24, 638, 1972.

129. **Gherna, R. L.,** Preservation, in *Manual Methods for General Bacteriology,* Gerhardt, P., Murrey, R. G. E., Costilow, R. N., Nester, E., Wood, W. A., Krieg, N. R., and Phillips, G. B., Eds., ASM, Washington, D.C., 1981, 208.

130. **Jordan, H. V., Krasse, B., and Möller, A.,** A method of sampling human dental plaque for certain caries inducing streptococci, *Arch. Oral Biol.,* 13, 919, 1968.

131. **Gästrin, B., Kallings, L. O., and Marcetic, A.,** The survival time for different bacteria in various transport media, *Acta Pathol. Microbiol. Scand.,* 74, 371, 1968.

132. **Gilmour, M. N., Turner, G., Berman, R. G., and Kreuzer, A. K.,** Compact liquid nitrogen system yielding high recoveries of Gram-negative anaerobes, *Appl. Environ. Microbiol.,* 35, 84, 1978.

133. **Wilson, R. F., Woods, A., and Ashley, F. P.,** The effect of storage in liquid nitrogen on the recovery of human dental plaque bacteria, *Arch. Oral Biol.,* 29, 941, 1984.

134. **Aaltonen, A. S., Tenovuo, J., Lehtonen. O.-P., Saksala, R., and Meurman, O.,** Serum antibodies against oral *Streptococcus mutans* in young children in relation to dental caries and maternal close-contacts, *Arch. Oral Biol.,* 30, 331, 1985.

135. **Hardie, J. M. and Bowden, G. H.,** The microbial flora of dental plaque: bacterial succession and isolation considerations, in *Proceedings Microbial Aspects of Dental Caries,* Vol. 1, Stiles, H. M., Loesche, W. J., and O'Brien, T. C. O., Eds., Information Retrieval, New York, 1976, 63.

136. **Westergren, G. and Krasse, B.,** Evaluation of a micromethod for determination of *Streptococcus mutans* and *Lactobacillus* infection, *J. Clin. Microbiol.,* 7, 82, 1978.

137. **Kalfas, S., Edwardsson, S., and Birkhed, D.,** Determination of salivary *Streptococcus mutans* level in a stable sucrose-sulphasomide-containing broth, *Caries Res.,* 19, 320, 1985.

138. **Birkhed, D., Edwardsson, S., and Andersson, H.,** Comparison among a dip-slide test (Dentocult®), plate count, and Snyder test for estimating number of lactobacilli in human saliva, *J. Dent. Res.,* 60, 1832, 1981.

139. **Denepitiya, L. and Kleinberg, I.,** A comparison of the microbial compositions of pooled human dental plaque and salivary sediment, *Arch. Oral Biol.,* 27, 739, 1982.

140. **Robrish, S. A., Grove, S. B., Bernstein, R. S., Marucha, P. T., Socransky, S. S., and Amdur, B.,** Differential breakage of oral microorganisms during sonic plaque dispersion, *J. Dent. Res.,* 54, Abstr. No. 236, 1975.

141. **Virtanen, K. K.,** personal communication.

142. **Tenovuo, J.,** personal communication.

143. **Söderling, E.,** unpublished results.

144. **Tenovuo, J.,** unpublished results.

Chapter 2

# SALIVARY SECRETION RATE, BUFFER CAPACITY, AND pH

**Dowen Birkhed and Ulf Heintze**

## TABLE OF CONTENTS

## I. INTRODUCTION

Saliva has an important role in maintaining oral health. The mucous membranes are lubricated and protected by the salivary glycoproteins and mucoids. Furthermore, saliva keeps the mouth moist, and softens the food, thereby facilitating chewing and swallowing. Saliva accomplishes its mechanical cleansing and protective functions through various physical and biochemical mechanisms. According to McNamara et al.,[1] the constant interaction with oral tissues establishes saliva as a major determinant of the environment within the oral cavity.

Low salivary secretion rate increases the risk for various diseases in the mouth, especially dental caries.[2] It has been speculated that a reduced salivary flow also affects infections of the oral mucosa, plaque accumulation on the teeth, and periodontitis.[3-6] Without doubt, the relationship between low salivary secretion and dental caries is the best documented. If the secretion rate is reduced to extremely low values, called dry mouth or xerostomia, normal physiological activities of the mouth, like talking, chewing, and swallowing, may be difficult.[3-6] Dry mouth patients with dentures may also present many problems.

The protective effects of saliva with respect to dental caries may be accomplished by means of several clearly defined processes, such as the secretion rate, buffer capacity, calcium and phosphate concentrations, as well as various antibacterial systems.[1,2,7] This multifactorial line of defense makes saliva an essential endogenous and modifying resistance factor against the caries disease. Among the salivary factors, the secretion rate and buffer capacity seem to show the best clinically documented inverse correlation with caries frequency.[8-10]

This chapter focuses on the relationship between salivary secretion rate, buffer capacity, pH and dental caries, on various clinical methods for analyzing the secretion rate and buffer effect, and on various factors influencing these two salivary parameters. Since xerostomia is an important clinical problem, the symptoms related to dry mouth and its treatment will also be discussed.

## II. SALIVARY SECRETION RATE

### A. Measurement of Salivary Flow Rate

Saliva can be collected under both resting and stimulated conditions. It is important, however, to remember that it is more or less impossible to obtain true "resting" saliva, since saliva flow is always influenced by some kind of stimulation.[11]

Flow rate is usually calculated by dividing the volume (milliliters) of saliva per minute. It is also possible to weigh the amount of saliva and express the secretion rate in gram saliva per minute. In a great majority of cases, a single saliva test must be considered as fully adequate.[12,13] At a very low flow rate, however, repeated sampling reduces the risk of obtaining a misleading extreme value due to individual variation.[13]

The duration of the collection period is important, since the flow rate can vary with time. Kerr[11] has shown that many factors, such as chewing and swallowing during saliva collection, influence the secretion rate. Therefore, if saliva is collected, for example, during 5 min and 5 ml is obtained, the mean flow rate will be 1.0 ml/min, but the rate might have been different minute for minute. Thus it is important to standardize the collection procedure during the whole sampling period, to keep the secretion rate as constant as possible, and not to use too short collection periods.

It must be remembered that many factors related directly to the test situation can modify salivary flow rate and that all these factors must be kept in mind when interpreting the objective findings. Examples of such factors are (1) emotional status, (2) acute illness, and (3) masticatory dysfunction.

**1. Emotional Status** — If a patient is nervous at the test, this can result in reduced flow.

Moreover, stress also affects the flow. Therefore, it is recommended that patients relax at least 5 min before the saliva test.

**2. Acute illness** — If the patient does not feel very well at the salivary test, for example, has a fever, sore throat, etc., the salivary values may be lower than normal.

**3. Masticatory dysfunction** — Painful teeth, occlusal disharmonies, and temporal mandibular joint diseases can temporarily reduce chewing efficiency and thereby the saliva production rate. Moreover, patients with dentures may have difficulty in chewing the test piece, which may influence the flow rate.

It is important to standardize the collection procedures as much as possible. One trained person should be responsible for the collection. The patient must be informed about the purpose of the test and also about practical problems, such as not swallowing during the collection period. The patient should be instructed to avoid any oral intake and smoking at least 1 h preceding the test. Collection can be performed at a certain time of the day, for instance, between 9:00 a.m. and 11:00 a.m.

Techniques for assessing salivation and salivary secretion rate have been reviewed and evaluated by many authors, among them Kerr,[11] Mason and Chisholm,[3] White,[14] Navazesh and Christensen.[15] Accurate measures of salivary flow rate are required for a variety of clinical and experimental situations. Two methods are the most commonly used: (1) measurement of whole saliva and (2) measurement of parotid gland secretion rate. Assessment of the flow rate of other major salivary glands — that is, the sublingual and submandibular — cannot routinely be performed because of practical problems.

*1. Whole Saliva*

Measurement of whole saliva may be superior and more relevant than measurement of individual gland secretion.[15] Several methods have been suggested to collect resting and stimulated whole saliva flow rate.[3,11,14] The most commonly used techniques for measuring unstimulated ("resting") salivary flow rate are (1) the draining method (i.e., saliva is allowed to drain into a vessel for weight or volume determination), (2) the spitting method (i.e., saliva is collected in the oral cavity and then spit out into a vessel), (3) the suction method (i.e., a suction tube is used to draw saliva from the mouth into a vessel), and (4) the swab method (i.e., preweighed dental cotton rolls or swabs are placed in the mouth in order to absorb saliva).[14]

**1. Draining method** — After swallowing, the patient is told to allow saliva to drain out between open lips into a test tube with a funnel held near the mouth. At the end of the collection time, for example, 5 min, the patient is told to collect all remaining saliva and expectorate it.

**2. Spitting method** — This is similar to the draining method, but the saliva is collected with closed lips, and all saliva is expectorated, for example, one to two times per minute during the whole collection period.

**3. Suction method** — A plastic dental saliva ejector tip connected to a vacuum pump, is placed under the tongue. The saliva is led by a plastic tube into a test tube. At the end of the collection, the ejector tip is moved around in the mouth, in a standardized way, to collect the remaining saliva.

**4. Swab method** — Three preweighed dental cotton rolls are placed in the mouth, one under the tongue close to the sublingual and submaxillary gland orifices, and two in the upper vestibulum close to the parotid gland duct. At the end of the collection session, the cotton rolls are removed and immediately weighed.

When resting saliva secretion rate is determined, the patient is asked to sit in a forward position with the elbows resting on the knees. The tongue, cheeks, and jaw should not be moved. If the spitting method is used, the patient should be told only to drool passively and not to spit actively.

**Table 1**
**CLASSIFICATION OF SALIVARY SECRETION
RATE ACCORDING TO THE REFERENCE
INTERVALS OF ERICSSON AND HARDWICK[9] FOR
RESTING AND PARAFFIN-STIMULATED WHOLE
SALIVA**

| Secretion rate (ml/min) | Very low | Low | Normal |
|---|---|---|---|
| Resting saliva | <0.1 | 0.1—0.25 | 0.25—0.35 (mean: 0.30) |
| Stimulated | <0.7 | 0.7—1 | 1—3 (mean: 1.5) |

If stimulated salivary flow rate is to be determined, the following two collection methods can be used: (1) masticatory method and (2) gustatory method. If both resting and stimulated saliva are collected at the same visit, it is important to remember that the former test should always be carried out first. Otherwise the secretion rate of unstimulated saliva will be too high because of the former stimulation.

**1. Masticatory method** — The patient is given a standardized piece (weighing approximately 1 to 2 g) of paraffin (melting point 42 to 44°C) or a piece of gum base. After initial chewing for 2 min in order to soften the paraffin and remove saliva from the mouth, the saliva produced is swallowed. During the subsequent 5 min, stimulated saliva is collected while the patient is chewing on the same bolus of paraffin. Some authors recommend that number of strokes per minute should be standardized, for instance, by a metronome.[16] The patient is expectorating intermittently during the whole collection period. Foam can be avoided or reduced by using an ice-chilled beaker or by the addition of a drop of octanol.[16]

**2. Gustatory method** — Saliva is stimulated by 1 to 6% citric acid. A standardized amount of the solution is applied on the anterior dorsal part of the tongue every 30 s or every minute. Before new acid is applied again, the patient is asked to expectorate. This is repeated up to 3 to 5 min. Instead of the citric acid solution, filter paper disks containing a standardized amount of acid can be placed on the tongue.

Any of the methods here described may be useful, but it is important to standardize the procedure as much as possible. The spitting method for estimating resting salivary flow rate, and the masticatory method with paraffin chewing for stimulated salivary flow rate are reliable and useful in many situations.[12] The normal values of secretion for these two methods, as well as the borderline values for low and very low secretion rates, are given in Table 1.

The reliability, validity, and correlation between different methods for measuring the flow rate of whole saliva have been studied. Kerr[11] found that the resting saliva volume differed in the draining, spitting, and suction methods. White[14] found a significant correlation between the swab and spitting methods with respect to resting flow rate. White[14] also compared chewing stimulated and resting salivary flow rate and found that they correlated significantly. This is somewhat in contrast to observations by Becks and Wainwright.[17]

Heintze et al.[12] studied secretion rate of both resting and stimulated whole saliva in duplicate determinations of 629 adults. They concluded that the secretion rates of resting and stimulated saliva were highly correlated. Because of the wide range of stimulated secretion rates, however, as estimated from individual values of resting secretion rates (Figure 1), predicting the level of stimulated secretion rate from that of the resting one is not possible. Some kind of relationship between the secretion rate of resting and stimulated saliva is, however, to be expected and has been confirmed in studies in both children[18] and the elderly.[19]

Navazesh and Christensen[15] compared whole mouth resting and stimulated salivary measurement procedures. Resting salivary flow values were roughly equivalent for draining, spitting, suction, and swab collection technique, but the swab technique was less reliable

**STIMULATED
SALIVA**

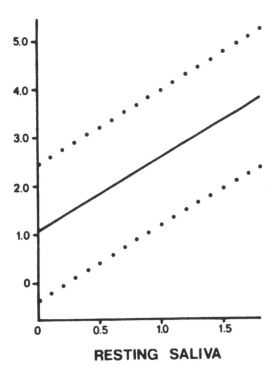

**RESTING SALIVA**

FIGURE 1.   Regression of paraffin-stimulated secretion rate on that of resting secretion rate for whole saliva
expressed as ml/min. Dotted lines = 95% prediction
belt. Number of subjects: 629. (From Heintze, U.,
Birkhed, D., and Björn, H., *Swed. Dent. J.,* 7, 227,
1983. With permission.)

**Table 2**
**RESTING WHOLE MOUTH SALIVARY FLOW
PARAMETERS FOR DIFFERENT COLLECTION
METHODS[15]**

| Collection method | Flow rate (g/min)[a] | Test-retest reliability (r) | Within-subject variance |
|---|---|---|---|
| Draining | 0.47 | 0.75 | 0.11 |
| Spitting | 0.47 | 0.79 | 0.10 |
| Suction | 0.54 | 0.93 | 0.14 |
| Swab | 0.52 | 0.68 | 0.19 |

[a]   Mean values (n = 17).

(Table 2). As expected, gustatory and masticatory stimuli induced a significantly higher
salivary flow rate compared with resting levels, but the between- and within-subject variances
were higher (Table 3). The authors concluded that methods for determining resting salivary
flow rate will better differentiate individual secretion rates because the measures are less
variable. Nevertheless, it is often suitable to use both methods for characterizing a patient's
salivary flow level.

**Table 3**

**WHOLE MOUTH SALIVARY FLOW PARAMETERS FOR DIFFERENT METHODS OF SALIVARY STIMULATION**[15]

| Stimulation method | Flow rate (g/min)[a] | Test-retest reliability (r) | Within-subject variance |
|---|---|---|---|
| Chewing (gum base) | 2.38 | 0.95 | 0.11 |
| Drops (citric acid) | 2.64 | 0.76 | 0.49 |
| Filter paper (citric acid) | 1.51 | 0.79 | 0.29 |

[a]   Mean values (n = 12).

**Table 4**

**MEAN PAROTID SALIVARY FLOW RATES (ml/min) IN NORMAL SUBJECTS ACCORDING TO MASON AND CHISHOLM**[3]

| Age range (years) | Resting | | Lemon juice-stimulated | |
|---|---|---|---|---|
| | Male | Female | Male | Female |
| < 20 | 0.06 | 0.083 | 1.49 | 1.99 |
| 21—40 | 0.104 | 0.09 | 1.73 | 1.76 |
| 41—60 | 0.078 | 0.064 | 1.68 | 1.36 |
| > 60 | 0.084 | 0.06 | 1.58 | 1.15 |

*2. Parotid Saliva*

Determining the secretion rate of parotid saliva is from a practical point of view more complicated than determining that of whole saliva. Nevertheless, there are situations when clinical tests of parotid flow rate are indicated.

Both resting and stimulated parotid salivary secretion rates may be determined. The salivary output of parotid glands is usually collected in a two-chambered type of suction and collection cup according to Lashley.[20,21] Different types of stimulation, both gustatory and cholinergic, have been described in the literature.[3,14,22-25] The most commonly used stimuli is citric acid, usually of 5% strength. The following clinical test according to Mason and Chisholm[3] may be useful.

1.    The subject is seated comfortably in a dental chair.
2.    The collection device is applied. Five drops of 5% citric acid solution are dropped on the tongue to flush out stagnant secretion for approximately 15 min.
3.    Saliva is then collected under ''resting'' conditions for 30 min, and after 5% citric acid stimulation for 2 min. The citric acid is applied for at least 1 min before beginning the collection of the stimulated sample.

Normal values for resting and stimulated saliva have been defined (Table 4) using this method. The importance of age and sex on normal values is apparent, and it is important that these parameters should be considered when interpreting salivary flow rates.

It is worthy of note, as Ericson[25] has pointed out, that the results obtained from different sialometric methods are not comparable because individuals with a high secretory response to one stimulus do not necessarily have the same response to another.

*3. Sublingual and Submandibular Saliva*

Some authors have described appliances for collecting both sublingual and submandibular saliva.[26-30] There are difficulties, however, in using these methods to determine the rate of secretion. Enfors[22] reported successful submandibular cannulation using finely drawn polyethylene tubing for determination of salivary flow rate, expressed as drops of saliva per milliliter (volume of each drop ~0.05 ml). In 95% of the subjects, aged 20 to 60 years, with healthy salivary glands, the resting secretion from the cannulated submandibular glands was 0 to 28 drops per 5 min — that is, 0 to 0.28 ml/min. The corresponding value for resting secretion rate from the parotid glands, collected with a sialometric and without concurrent recording from submandibular glands, ranged from 0 to 11 drops per 5 min — that is, 0 to 0.11 ml/min.[22]

## B. Local Stimulants

The most important factor which influences both the secretion rate and the proportion of the various types of gland saliva is the degree of stimulation. The rate of secretion of individual salivary glands ranges from no activity during sleep[31] to approximately 4 to 8 ml/min on stimulation with citric acid.[11,22] During minimal stimulation, the proportion of submandibular saliva flow compared with parotid flow is approximately 2:1, while the reverse proportion is found at maximal stimulation.[11]

Kerr[11] described three different types of stimulation on production of salivary secretion: (1) extraoral stimuli, such as thought, sight, and smell of food and other products, (2) chewing of insoluble substances, such as paraffin wax, and (3) gustatory stimulation, for example, with sucrose, sodium chloride, and citric acid.

1.    The inhalation of some odors, such as orange essence, produced a substantial increase in the rate of flow of whole saliva.[11] This was regarded as evidence for a direct olfactory-salivary reflex rather than a conditional response.
2.    The secretion rate of parotid saliva during chewing of paraffin wax was not affected by chewing frequency within physiological limits.[11] The flow rate was greatly influenced by other factors such as site of chewing and by the plasticity of the bolus as well as the weight of the paraffin wax piece.[11]
3.    The highest salivary secretion responses were obtained by dissolving a crystallized mixture of sugars and citric acid in the mouth.[11] The gustatory-salivary reflex showed no evidence of fatigue after repeated applications of this stimulus up to 3 h.

Regarding chewing effects on secretion rate, Lourides et al.[32] found that high and low chewing rates, either below or above the normal range of 40 to 80 strokes per minute, can significantly influence secretion rate of whole saliva. Thus, according to these authors, the chewing rate is an additional factor that should be considered for saliva secretion measurements, which is in contrast to the observations by Kerr.[11]

Ericson[25] studied the parotid saliva secretion rate in response to different types of stimulation, both gustatory with citric acid and cholinergic with injection with acetyl-beta-methylcholine (Table 5). He concluded that the correlation coefficient between parotid flow rate at rest and with various types of stimulation is either very low or even negative. This stresses the importance of measuring both resting and stimulated salivary flow rate in individual cases.

Many studies have been conducted on the gustatory stimulus on the flow rates of parotid, submandibular, and whole saliva.[11,22,25,33-39] There seems to be a curvilinear response of at least parotid salivary flow rate with ascorbic acid and sodium chloride, whereas a linear response is found with sucrose as the stimulus[38] (Figure 2). Acid acts as a better saliva stimulant than salts and especially sugars.[36,38] Lagerlöf and Dawes[40] found in contrast to Speirs,[38] however, a significant stimulation of salivary flow at relatively low concentrations of sucrose solutions.

**Table 5**
**MEAN VALUES OF PAROTID**
**FLOW RATE FROM BOTH**
**LEFT AND RIGHT GLAND ON**
**DIFFERENT STIMULATIONS**
**ACCORDING TO ERICSON[25]**

| Stimulus | No. of drops/5 min |
|---|---|
| Resting secretion | 6.6 |
| Citric acid 1% | 105.0 |
| Citric acid 6% | 119.4 |
| Betacholyl 0.2 mg | 121.8 |
| Betacholyl 0.3 mg | 199.9 |

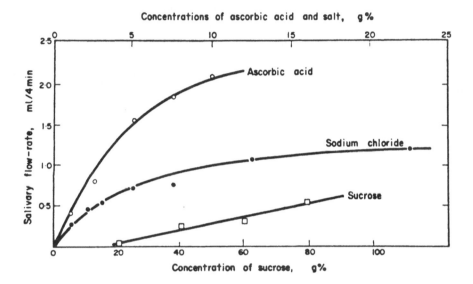

FIGURE 2.   Parotid salivary flow rate in response to the application (during 4 min) of solutions of various concentrations of ascorbic acid, sodium chloride, and sucrose on the front of the tongue. One subject was studied. (From Speirs, E. L., *Arch. Oral Biol.*, 16, 351, 1971. With permission.)

The influence of previous stimulation, for example, of a meal, before salivary flow measurement may have some clinical importance. Krasse[41] and Heintze and Birkhed[42] reported a tendency to an increased amount of saliva immediately after a meal. Dawes and Chebib[43] drew the following conclusions from a series of experiments of parotid saliva. The flow rate of unstimulated saliva is unaffected by gustatory stimulation carried out 1 h or more previously. If multiple samples of stimulated saliva are to be collected on 1 d, collections should be separated by at least 1 or 2 h.

## C. Diet and Malnutrition

Several studies have been conducted on the effects of diet on salivary secretion (for review, see Dawes[44] and Johansson[45]). The main criticism that could be raised against many of these studies is that the experimental design does not control the nondietary variables that also can influence the salivary secretion rate, for example, the method of collection, stress factors in relation to the diet regime, and the liquid intake.[44]

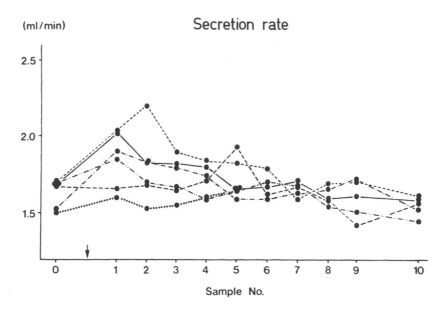

FIGURE 3. Influence of five different test meals (- - - = fat; ——— = water; -·-·- = vegetable juice; -··-·· = protein; ——— = glucose) and of fasting (······) on paraffin-stimulated whole saliva secretion rate (ml/min) during a 4-h period. Mean values of 9 subjects. Saliva samples were collected before (no. 0) and after (no. 1 to 10) ingestion (marked with an arrow). Sampling intervals: 0 to 1 and 9 to 10, 30 min, otherwise 15 min. (After Heintze, U. and Birkhed, D., *Caries Res.*, 18, 265, 1984. With permission.)

It is very important to distinguish between local effects of the diet in the oral cavity and systemic effects. Foods that require chewing or are flavored will increase the salivary flow rate. Systemic effects of the diet, though, require that the diet first be metabolized before they reach the salivary glands.

Of practical and ethical reasons, relatively few controlled studies of the diet have been conducted in humans. In a recent study, Heintze and Birkhed[42] measured the flow rate after a single intake of various test meals in nine female dental hygienists. The following meals were used: glucose, powdered hens' egg white, peanut oil, vegetable juice, and water (control). All test meals were served as 400-ml liquid portions. Samples of paraffin-stimulated whole saliva were collected before and on 10 occasions during a 4-h period after the intake. No obvious differences were found between the various products (Figure 3). Thus the results of this study did not indicate a dietary influence on secretion rate of stimulated whole saliva.

Hall et al.[46] showed a marked reduction (approximately 30%) of parotid flow rate, stimulated with pilocarpine, when young adult men were maintained for 7 d on a diet consisting exclusively of a special mode liquid diet (Metrecal®) containing 900 kcal/d. Water was the only other substance ingested. No effect was seen, however, on submandibular flow rate. This study may indicate that the defective functional status of the parotid gland is attributed to a reduction in mastication and eventually also to a reduced caloric intake. The latter statement is supported by Johansson et al.,[47] who studied the effect of fasting for 8 d on saliva of 8 female subjects. Samples of resting whole saliva and whole saliva stimulated by chewing on paraffin were collected before, during, and after the fasting (300 kcal/d including at least 3 l of liquid). The effect of fasting varied greatly among the individuals. However, a significant decrease in secretion rate of stimulated whole saliva was found (Table 6). After the fasting period, the salivary flow almost reached the baseline value again. The secretion rate could not be calculated for resting saliva because of the extremely long collection times required for some individuals, which made standardized collection impossible. Anyway,

**Table 6**
**EFFECT OF 8 d OF FASTING ON SECRETION RATE**
**OF PARAFFIN-STIMULATED WHOLE SALIVA[47]**

| Secretion rate | Before fasting | At the end of fasting | Postexperimental |
|---|---|---|---|
| ml/min[a] | 1.6 ± 0.6 | 1.1 ± 0.6[b] | 1.4 ± 0.6 |

[a]  Mean ± SD for eight subjects.
[b]  All eight subjects showed a decrease compared with the prefasting value.

this study clearly indicates that a short period of fasting reduces the salivary secretion rate, but that the effect is reversible.

It must be remembered that during fasting the individuals are subjected to psychological and physiological reactions to starvation, involving stress and behavioral changes.[47] These factors may also influence the salivary flow rate. Another factor of interest is whether or not the lower secretion rate during fasting is an effect of absence of masticatory stimulation. In a follow-up study, Johansson and Ericson[48] found that fasting in combination with a chewing program still led to a decrease in secretion rate of paraffin-stimulated whole saliva. Thus, our present knowledge is that the nutritional status of an individual is important for the secretion rate and that stimulation by chewing cannot compensate this effect.

Contrary to Johansson et al.,[47] Birkhed et al.[49] did not find any effect of short-term fasting and lactovegetarian diet on the secretion rate of whole saliva (the saliva had been stimulated with paraffin some time before collection). Many participants, however, complained about a dry mouth.

There are other indications that diet and diet composition may have an effect on salivary flow rate. De Muñiz et al.[50] followed 66 healthy boys, aged 6 to 12, during a 45-d experimental period. Before the study, the children had a lower daily energy and a higher carbohydrate intake. There were no quantitative differences in protein intake. More than half of the proteins used in the experimental diet, however, were of animal origin, whereas the proteins in the habitual diet were mostly of vegetable origin. The fat intake was higher in the experimental diet. The flow rate of citric-acid-stimulated saliva increased approximately 40%. It is of course difficult to determine which dietary factors of the experimental period were responsible for the salivary changes. It is probable that both local and systemic effects may have been involved.

Salivary factors have been studied in groups of people eating a lactovegetarian diet.[51-53] There are no indications from these studies that lactovegetarians have a higher salivary flow rate than nonlactovegetarians, even if they eat food that requires more chewing. In a recently completed study of 20 healthy, nonsmoking individuals, who changed from a mixed to a lactovegetarian diet during 12 months, a significant increase of paraffin-stimulated whole salivary secretion rate was found.[54] No corresponding effect was seen on citric-acid-stimulated parotid saliva.

Thus there are indications that diet and the nutritional status of a person can influence the salivary secretion rate to a certain extent. It seems likely, however, that these changes are relatively small unless the dietary deficiencies are very severe, as, for example, during long-term malnutrition. As regards the possibility of systemic effects of the diet increasing the salivary flow rate, the evidence from the literature is very vague. It is more probable that the changes in flow rate which have been reported are related more to local effects of the diet than to systemic effects.

**D. Sex and Age**
Many studies have shown a higher flow rate for men than for women, although this sex

**Table 7**
**MEDIAN SECRETION RATE (ml/min) OF**
**RESTING AND PARAFFIN-STIMULATED**
**WHOLE SALIVA IN MALES AND FEMALES OF**
**FOUR DIFFERENT AGE GROUPS ACCORDING**
**TO HEINTZE ET AL.[12]**

| Age-group[a] (years) | Resting saliva | | Stimulated saliva | |
|---|---|---|---|---|
| | Males | Females | Males | Females |
| 15—29 | 0.34 | 0.25 | 1.60 | 1.45 |
| 30—44 | 0.44 | 0.31 | 1.89 | 1.65 |
| 45—59 | 0.33 | 0.22 | 1.80 | 1.30 |
| 60—74 | 0.30 | 0.20 | 1.84 | 1.20 |
| All groups | 0.36 | 0.26 | 1.80 | 1.40 |

[a]   Total number of subjects 629.

**Table 8**
**MEAN SECRETION RATE**
**OF PARAFFIN-STIMULATED**
**WHOLE SALIVA (ml/min) IN**
**BOYS AND GIRLS OF SEVEN**
**DIFFERENT AGE GROUPS**
**ACCORDING TO**
**ANDERSSON ET AL.[18] AND**
**CROSSNER[13]**

| Age group (years) | Boys[a] | Girls[b] |
|---|---|---|
| 5 | 0.67 | 0.52 |
| 6 | 0.91 | 0.77 |
| 7 | 1.09 | 0.79 |
| 8 | 1.17 | 0.87 |
| 10 | 1.23 | 1.01 |
| 13 | 1.90 | 1.59 |
| 15 | 2.24 | 1.92 |

[a]   Total number of boys 473.
[b]   Total number of girls 468.

difference is not always statistically significant.[12,19,55-59] This holds true for both resting and stimulated saliva as well as for various age groups[12] (Table 7). Data from children and adolescents also show that boys consistently have higher salivary flow rates than girls[13,18,60,61] (Table 8). This sex difference may be due to smaller size of the salivary glands in females.[24,62,63] As a consequence of the lower secretion rate in females, the use of a fixed reference value common to both sexes according to Ericsson and Hardwick[9] might in females unnecessarily characterize many secretion rates of unstimulated as well as paraffin-stimulated whole saliva as being low or very low.[12]

In children, there is an increased salivary flow rate with age both for boys and for girls[13,18] (Table 8). As far as flow rate is concerned, the salivary glands seem to be fully developed at the age of 15.[13]

Regarding age-related salivary gland changes in adults, some contradictionary results have been published. The glandular parenchymal volume is reduced and replaced by fatty deposits

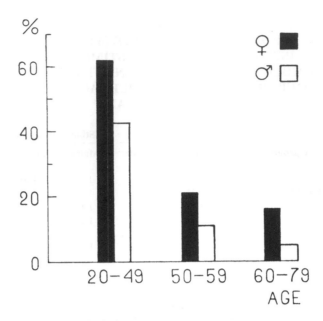

FIGURE 4.    Frequency distribution of individuals with pronounced secretion rate of palatine gland according to age and sex. Number of subjects: 110 men and 146 women. (From G:son Östlund, S., *Odontol. Tidskr.*, 62 [Suppl.], 1953. With permission.)

and connective tissue with increasing age.[64-67] Scott[68] measured the volumes of dissected submandibular glands from both men and women and found a reduction in gland size, especially among women, in old age. These glandular changes would be expected also to have functional manifestations. Many recent studies, however, have failed to find significant effects of age on unstimulated or stimulated parotid as well as whole saliva flow rate.[12,56,58,60,70] In the study by Heintze et al.,[12] resting secretion rate was negatively correlated with age only for women (Table 7). Ben-Aryeh et al.[57] found that both old females and males had a significantly lower resting flow rate compared with the rates in the young. A similar trend was found by Bertram.[71] Significant age-related decrease has also been reported in stimulated whole saliva rate.[72] Ericson[24] found that the resting parotid secretion rate diminished with increasing age, but that the stimulated flow rates were independent of age.

The explanation for the inconsistency regarding age and salivary flow rate may lie in the difficulties associated with measuring resting saliva, since most data suggest that aging does not affect stimulated salivary flow. This conclusion is, however, not supported by observations by Pederson et al.,[59] who used a standardized method for collection of both resting and poststimulated submandibular gland flow rates. They found that both resting and post-stimulated flow decreased with age.

Age-related changes in structure of the minor salivary glands have also been reported.[73,74] This is in accordance with earlier observations by Östlund,[75] who found that the secretion rate of the palatine glands decreases with age in both man and woman (Figure 4). This may be one explanation of the fact that many old people feel subjective dryness in the mouth,[19] even when the secretion rate of whole saliva shows normal values.

## E. Sex Hormones

In an investigation of the rate of secretion, water content, and crystalline pattern of submandibular saliva, Kullander and Sonesson[76] found that the flow rate of stimulated saliva was highest during the secretory phase of the menstrual cycle. They also found that the

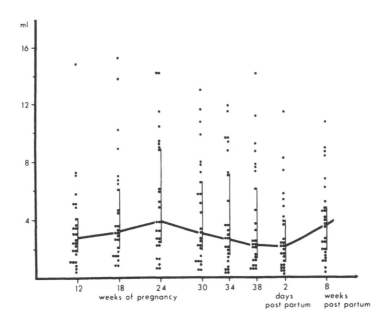

FIGURE 5. Original and medium values surrounded by 95% confidence intervals of citric-acid-stimulated parotid flow rate during 5 min of collection at various weeks of pregnancy and days/weeks post partum, from 26 women, 19 to 20 years of age. (From Hugoson, A., *Acta Odontol Scand.*, 30, 49, 1972. With permission.)

salivary secretion rate was lower during pregnancy than otherwise and also after the menopause than during the reproductive years.

In a longitudinal study of salivary secretion during pregnancy and 8 weeks after parturition, Hugoson[77] studied the parotid saliva flow rate in 26 women. During pregnancy, there was a decrease of both resting and citric-acid-stimulated parotid saliva. After delivery, the flow rate increased again. Large intra- and interindividual differences were found (Figure 5), however. Laine et al.[78] reported recently an analysis of flow rate and other variables of whole saliva during and after the pregnancy of 16 women. Significantly, changes were observed in the buffer capacity and pH but not in the flow rates.

Samples of stimulated whole saliva, as well as individual parotid and submandibular gland secretion, were collected repeatedly from 12 23- to 26-year-old women during 1 or 2 menstrual cycles before administration of oral contraceptives and for about 2 months after the start of the hormone administration.[79] Large intra- and interindividual variations were found in the secretion rates. However, the flow rates for both parotid and submandibular secretions increased somewhat during the hormone treatment, but the differences were not statistically significant.

Several studies have shown that postmenopausal women have a lower salivary flow rate than women during the reproductive years.[12,76] Such postmenopausal variations in secretion rate have, however, not been found by Ericson,[24] Baum,[69] and Parvinen and Larmas.[56] Furthermore, Baum[69] stressed that diminished secretion rates were observed only in medicated postmenopausal women.

## F. Drugs

Since the neural control of salivation is very complex and regulated by at least the parasympathetic and sympathetic nerves,[80] it is not surprising that a variety of drugs affect salivary flow. Some authors have tried to list representative drugs that cause a decrease (and

**Table 9**
**MEAN VALUES (AND SD) FOR STIMULATED SALIVARY
FLOW RATE IN WOMEN BY DRUG CATEGORY IN
DESCENDING ORDER OF MAGNITUDE ACCORDING TO
PARVINEN ET AL.[84]**

| Medicated with | n | x̄ | SD | Significance |
|---|---|---|---|---|
| Diuretics (alone or with digitalis glycosides) | 19 | 10.5 | 3.74 | $p < 0.05$ |
| Nitrates | 6 | 10.5 | 2.67 | NS |
| Other drugs | 34 | 8.7 | 3.87 | NS |
| No drugs | 316 | 8.6 | 3.76 | |
| Corticosteroids | 7 | 8.4 | 2.84 | NS |
| Drugs supplementing the diet | 13 | 8.3 | 2.87 | NS |
| Estrogens (alone and in combination) | 20 | 8.1 | 2.90 | NS |
| Diuretics as a part of multimedication | 20 | 8.1 | 2.82 | NS |
| One analgesic drug | 22 | 7.8 | 2.45 | NS |
| Other antihypertensive drugs | 15 | 7.5 | 2.96 | NS |
| Beta blocking agents together with a diuretic | 15 | 7.5 | 2.66 | NS |
| Digitalis glycosides and vasodilators | 7 | 7.4 | 3.44 | NS |
| Two or more analgesics or analgesics with minor tranquilizers | 15 | 7.4 | 2.07 | NS |
| Antidiabetic drugs | 12 | 7.3 | 2.82 | NS |
| Other anticholinergics | 25 | 7.3 | 2.85 | NS |
| Chlonidine chloride | 7 | 7.1 | 2.78 | NS |
| Alpha methyldopa | 22 | 6.5 | 2.43 | $p < 0.05$ |
| Neuroleptics and tricyclic antidepressants | 23 | 5.8 | 3.98 | $p < 0.01$ |
| Beta blocking agents | 5 | 5.5 | 1.54 | $p < 0.05$ |
| Medicated women | 287 | 7.8 | 3.20 | $p < 0.01$ |

*Note:* The significance of the difference compared with mean value for unmedicated
subjects is indicated.

in few cases also an increase) in salivary flow rate.[81-83] It must be remembered, however,
that relatively few controlled studies have been conducted on the effect of various pharmaceutical substances on secretion rate of saliva.

Hyposalivation and xerostomia is one of the most common side effects of drugs and must
be taken seriously. Since the use of drugs is very widespread in industrial countries, it is
probably the most common reason that many old patients have a low salivary flow rate.[19]

In a study of 463 medicated persons, Parvinen et al.[84] monitored the flow rate of paraffin-
stimulated saliva and compared the obtained data with that for a group of 642 unmedicated
subjects. The criterion for classification as "medicated" was permanent use of the drug(s)
concerned for 3 months before the examination, or in a few cases the use of drugs of an
acute character. The results are shown in Tables 9 and 10. Only a few groups of drugs were
found to decrease salivation to such an extent that it could be shown by a salivary test.
These groups were neuroleptics, tricyclic antidepressants, antihypertensives, and diuretics.

In a study of 1148 70-year-olds, intake of drugs from the groups of anticholinergics,
antihistamines, sedatives, hypnotics, or phenothiazines seemed to have the highest predictive
value for subjective feelings of dryness in the mouth.[19]

Johnson et al.[85] determined the salivary flow rate and the prevalence of mouth dryness
among 154 patients in somatic long-term hospitals. Background factors with a significant
effect on salivary flow rate could be found among men taking tricyclic antidepressants,
especially in combination with diuretics.

**Table 10**
## MEAN VALUES (AND SD) FOR STIMULATED SALIVARY FLOW RATE IN MEN BY DRUG CATEGORY IN DESCENDING ORDER OF MAGNITUDE ACCORDING TO PARVINEN ET AL.[84]

| Medicated with | n | x̄ | SD | Significance |
|---|---|---|---|---|
| Other drugs | 23 | 13.5 | 6.98 | $p < 0.05$ |
| Other anticholinergics | 11 | 12.7 | 6.36 | NS |
| Nitrates | 14 | 11.9 | 3.83 | NS |
| One analgesic drug | 20 | 10.6 | 5.58 | NS |
| No drugs | 326 | 10.1 | 4.32 | |
| Digitalis glycosides and vasodilators | 7 | 9.1 | 3.79 | NS |
| Beta blocking agents | 9 | 8.6 | 5.31 | NS |
| Chlonidine chloride | 5 | 8.3 | 3.90 | NS |
| Beta blocking agents together with a diuretic | 16 | 8.3 | 4.20 | $p < 0.05$ |
| Other antihypertensive drugs | 8 | 8.2 | 2.40 | NS |
| Diuretics (alone or with digitalis glycosides) | 10 | 8.2 | 3.31 | NS |
| Two or more analgesics or analgesics with minor tranquilizers | 6 | 7.9 | 1.24 | NS |
| Antidiabetic drugs | 4 | 7.5 | 4.14 | NS |
| Alpha methyldopa | 11 | 7.2 | 2.33 | $p < 0.05$ |
| Diuretics as a part of multimedication | 6 | 6.9 | 2.44 | NS |
| Neuroleptics and tricyclic antidepressants | 23 | 6.6 | 3.33 | $p < 0.001$ |
| Drugs supplementing the dict | 1 | 6.5 | 0 | NS |
| Corticosteroids | 2 | 6.3 | 1.77 | NS |
| Medicated men | 176 | 9.4 | 5.03 | NS |

*Note:* The significance of the difference compared with mean value for unmedicated subjects is indicated.

Salivary flow rate was studied in 32 patients who had received long-term treatment (median 5.5 years) with cyclic antidepressant drugs.[86] Although a normal secretion rate for stimulated saliva was recorded in about 50% of the patients, all but 4 complained of dry mouth. Thus, the patient's subjective experience of dry mouth did not agree well with the secretion rates recorded, suggesting that the stimulation used to produce secretion overruled at least some of the anticholinergic effect.

Low production of saliva in medicated populations has been confirmed in several cross-sectional population studies. Besides the studies cited previously, Baum[69] compared stimulated parotid saliva flow rate in medicated and nonmedicated adults of various ages. Of subjects taking medication, postmenopausal women but not older men produced stimulated saliva at rates significantly lower than their nonmedicated counterparts.

Since treatment with anticholinergic drugs reduces salivary secretion rate, there is a strong need for the development of new antidepressants with reduced anticholinergic side effects. With this approach, Molander and Birkhed,[87] Rafaelsen et al.,[88] Mikkelsen et al.,[89] and Clemensen et al.[90] compared the effect of single oral doses of various neuroleptic drugs or antidepressants by a crossover design in healthy volunteers. The results of one of these studies is presented in Figure 6. All tested drugs reduced salivary flow rate, but there were statistically significant differences between them. Caution should be exercised, however, in extrapolating the results of a single-dose experiment in healthy subjects to prolonged treatment in patients.

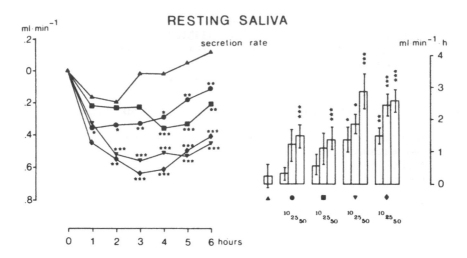

FIGURE 6. The effect of placebo (▲), melperone (●), thioridazine (■), levomepromazine (▼), and chlorprotixene (◆) on resting salivary secretion rate (ml/min). To the left is shown the temporal changes after treatment with the highest dosage of the drugs (change from predrug) and to the right is shown the total effect (mean ± SEM of 8 subjects) (AACO-6 h) after administration of 10, 25, and 50 mg of the drugs. All statistical comparisons made with placebo. *$p < 0.05$; **$p < 0.01$; ***$p < 0.005$. (From Molander, L. and Birkhed, D., *Psychopharmacologia*, 75, 114, 1981. With permission.)

Salivary secretion rate following short- and long-term antidepressant treatment has also been studied.[91-93] Both quantitative and qualitative changes seem to occur in saliva. There are indications, however, that these changes are reversible when the plasma level of active components decreases.

Saliva secretion rate in a group of drug addicts has been studied.[94,95] Amphetamines may have a certain reducing effect on salivary flow, contrary to marijuana and opiates. The methodological problems in studying these groups of people are obvious. For example, it is difficult to measure the drug intake and to control the time of the intake.

### G. Nicotine

There is an overwhelming evidence that cigarette smoking is a significant health risk. Several conflicting reports, though, have been published concerning the influence of smoking on salivary secretion rate. Increased parotid salivary secretion in eight smokers was reported by Panghorn and Sharon,[96] while Winsor[97] and Korting and Kleinschmidt[98] found the opposite. Normal cigarette smoking has been found to increase the salivary flow among habitual smokers.[96,97,99]

Heintze[100] and Parvinen[101] have recently published two similar but separate studies comparing a group of nonsmokers with a group of smokers. Their conclusions were very much the same — that is, that regular smoking is not associated with any significant changes in secretion rate of paraffin-stimulated whole saliva. Heintze's study[100] also included determination of the flow rate of resting whole saliva (Figure 7). In a complementary study, immediate smoking of two cigarettes did not influence the secretion rate of stimulated saliva in either smokers or nonsmokers.[100]

Nicotine-containing chewing gums are used to aid in quit-smoking efforts. In an attempt to compare various salivary parameters of smokers and nonsmokers, a nicotine gum was used for 15 weeks and compared with a placebo gum.[102] At the baseline, the flow rate of paraffin-stimulated saliva did not differ between the smokers and nonsmokers, and no effect was seen from the period of use of the nicotine gum. This is in agreement with observations

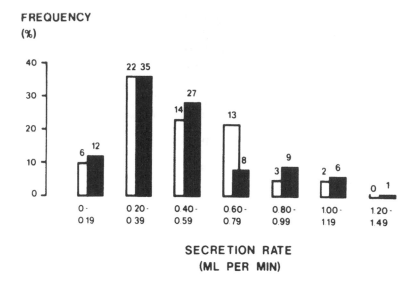

FIGURE 7. Frequency distribution of secretion rate of resting whole saliva (ml/min) for smokers (■) and nonsmokers (□). Figures above columns represent number of subjects: 182 patients participated, 109 smokers (44 men and 65 women), and 73 nonsmokers (38 men and 35 women). (From Heintze, U., *Scand. J. Dent. Res.*, 92, 294, 1984. With permission.)

by Dunér-Engström et al.,[103] who conducted a study with a single intake of a nicotine-containing chewing gum on healthy volunteers. It was concluded that the addition of nicotine to a chewing gum does not provide an additional stimulus for salivation.

## H. General Health and Various Diseases

State of health and various salivary gland disorders may be important for the salivary secretion rate.[3,4,16,63,104] Consequently, the finding of low salivary secretion values of resting and stimulated saliva might reflect a disease state, possibly on a subclinical level.[105]

There are relatively few controlled studies relating a specific disease and the salivary secretion rate. However, there are reasons to believe that any disease that dramatically affects the general health also affects the salivary flow rate.

Bertram[71] studied 58 patients who had been referred to a dental clinic on account of feelings of dryness in the mouth. The results are presented in Table 11. A suction method was used for determining resting salivary flow rate, since a large proportion of the patients were old, feeble, and demented persons. He concluded that xerostomia is most often a symptom of a systemic disease. The most frequent cause of xerostomia was Sjögren's syndrome and collagen diseases.

Österberg et al.[19] studied a population of more than 1000 70-year-olds and found that besides a correlation between number of drugs and subjective dryness of the mouth, there was also a significant correlation between subjective dryness and number of definiable diseases in both men and women.

The most widely known disease that affects salivary gland function is Sjögren's syndrome.[106] Several authors have reported reduced salivary flow rate in these patients.[71,107,108] Stuchell et al.[109] found no measurable parotid flow in the absence of a gustatory stimulant in a group of 15 subjects with Sjögren's syndrome. The flow rate of citric-acid-stimulated parotid saliva was, however, within normal range in six of these patients. They concluded that the subjective complaints of dry mouth usually reflect the lack of flow at rest.[109] Patients with systemic lupus erythematosus also show signs of xerostomia and has been found to

**Table 11**
**THE OCCURRENCE OF XEROSTOMIA AND**
**HYPOSALIVATION IN 50 INDIVIDUALS WITH DRY**
**MOUTH SYMPTOMS ACCORDING TO BERTRAM[71]**

| Diagnosis | No. | Salivary secretion | | |
|---|---|---|---|---|
| | | Xerostomia | Hyposalivation | Normal |
| Sjögren's syndrome | 20 | 18 | 2 | |
| Polyarthritis | 2 | 1 | — | 1 |
| Cirrhosis of the liver | 1 | 1 | — | — |
| Scleroderma | 1 | — | 1 | — |
| Diabetes mellitus | 2 | 2 | — | — |
| Collagen disease | 9 | 3 | 3 | 3 |
| Pernicious anemia | 2 | 1 | 1 | — |
| Psychoneurosis | 2 | — | 1 | 1 |
| Myxoedema | 1 | — | 1 | — |
| Medical xerostomia | 2 | 1 | 1 | — |
| Menopause | 2 | — | 1 | — |
| Idiopathic | 6 | 4 | 2 | — |
| Total | 50 | 31 | 13 | 6 |

have reduced values of salivary flow rate.[110] Individuals with rheumatoid arthritis showing radiographic signs of distinct inflammation also have a reduced salivary flow rate.[111,112]

Diabetes mellitus can manifest in many oral symptoms like thirst and a feeling of dry mouth. In studies of 35 adult diabetic patients by Tenovuo et al.,[113,114] measurements of flow rate of paraffin-stimulated whole saliva were included. No significant difference was found between the diabetic patients and a sex- and age-matched control group. This is in agreement with studies by Marder et al.[115] and Sharon et al.,[116] but somewhat in contrast to observations by Conner et al.[117] and Kjellman.[118] Thus, there are contradictionary results regarding diabetes and salivary flow rate. This may depend on how well the control group has been matched to the studied population. Nevertheless, flow rate of saliva in diabetic patients seems to fall within the normal biological range of variation and is not likely to contribute to caries development among diabetic patients.[113]

Thyroid diseases probably affect salivary secretion rate.[83] There are, however, minimal data in humans, although there are number of studies in experimental animals.[119] A report of dental erosions indicate a reduced salivary flow rate in hyperthyroid patients.[120] Doses of radioiodine for thyrotoxicosis exhibited a marked reduction in salivary flow.[121] This has been discussed in a review article by Mason et al.[122]

Since secretion from the salivary glands is primarily regulated by the nervous system,[80] one can expect that endogenous depression, symptomatic depression, and mania affect salivation. Investigations concerning salivary flow rate were introduced in psychiatry already in the beginning of this century.[20,21] A more detailed review of secretion rate in depressed patients has been given by Brown[123] and Bolwig and Rafaelsen.[124] Salivation rate is decreased, for example, in individuals with endogenous depression and mania. After treatment without using drugs, flow rate tended to increase toward normal values again. There is also a clear relationship between the diurnal mood and the salivary flow rate.[125]

The salivary flow rate has been examined in patients with hypertension before treatment with drugs.[126-128] A minor reduction of salivary secretion rate was noted compared with a control group. Other diseases that have been studied with respect to salivary flow rate are salivary gland disorders, for example, chronic parotitis and sialoadenosis,[3,83,105,129] duodenal ulcer diseases,[120] chronic pancreatitis and other pancreatic disorders,[131-134] alcoholic cirrhosis,[135] oral lichen planus,[136,137] cystic fibrosis,[138,139] and various neurological diseases, such as Parkinsonism,[140] Bell's palsy,[141] and cerebral palsy.[142] Most of these studies do not show any or only small differences in salivary flow rate compared with healthy controls.

Conclusively, there are many diseases that may have an influence on salivary flow rate, but relatively little evidence is available in the literature, except for Sjögren's syndrome. Excellent reviews of saliva in relation to health and disease have been written by Mason and Chisholm,[3] Wotman and Mandel,[104] Mandel,[83] and Mandel and Wotman.[4]

## I. Radiotherapy

Many tumors of the head and neck are radiosensitive, and therefore irradiation is often a part of the pre- and postsurgical treatment. There is always some degree of side effects to normal tissues, and the salivary glands, including the major as well as the minor ones, are especially sensitive to radiation. Many studies have focused on this problem, especially since the radiotherapy often results in severe xerostomia and dental caries.[143-145]

Ben-Aryeh et al.,[146] Dreizen et al.,[147] and Shannon et al.[148] examined the salivary flow rate before, during, and after radiation therapy. At 6 weeks after treatment, for example, the glands can still generate some saliva in response to strong stimulus, but are virtually not functioning at rest. There are also data indicating that the parotid gland is more sensitive to irradition than the other major and minor salivary glands.[149-151]

In an extensive study of 29 patients treated with external irradiation to the head and neck areas, Mira et al.[152] studied various factors influencing the salivary function. Resting saliva samples were collected before and during the radiotherapy course and followup. They found that more than 50% of the parotids have to be outside the therapy fields to prevent severe dryness. Neck fields which do not encompass salivary glands do not decrease salivary secretion. There is some relation between initial flow rate and the dose necessary to produce dryness, patients with high initial salivary flow rate requiring higher doses.[152,153]

Objective recovery of the flow rate has not been observed after treatment in spite of the subjective improvement in the sensation of dryness of some patients.[152] Statements from the literature about recovery of flow rate after a full course of radiotherapy are, however, contradictory. It may be that many patients adjust to the low salivary flow, and thus there is a discrepancy between subjective and objective findings.

As mentioned previously in Section H, there are also some indications that radioactive iodine used for the treatment of thyrotoxicosis and thyroid carcinoma may result in salivary gland dysfunction.[154] Iodine, which is actively taken up by the salivary glands, can damage the secretory cells. It must be remembered, however, that patients with thyroid diseases may also have disturbed salivary production as a result of hormonal effects.[83,120,123]

## J. Circannual and Circadian Rhythms

The importance of rhythm in salivary flow rate has been reviewed by Dawes.[155] The best example in this respect is the circannual one described by Shannon[156] for unstimulated parotid saliva. He studied nearly 4000 recruits in Texas and found a maximum flow rate in the winter months and a minimum in the summer. The lower secretion rate in the hot summer months was attributed to the fact that the subjects may have been more dehydrated at that time of the year. Even if the differences in secretion rate were highly statistically significant, it must be remembered that the variations of the calculated mean values were rather small. Nevertheless, they may have some implication for long-term studies of saliva and salivary flow rate.

Some studies have been focused on the circadian rhythm of salivary flow.[157-160] The data are, however, rather contradictary, even if most studies indicate that there is some kind of circadian rhythm, with the salivary flow rate peaking at noon or in the middle of the afternoon. Therefore, by standardizing the time of day of salivary collection it is possible to diminish the influence of the circadian rhythm.

## K. Gland Size

Another factor which also may influence the salivary flow rate is the size of the gland. Ericson[24,161] has shown that differences in the secretion rate of the parotid glands of healthy subjects may be ascribed at least partly to differences in salivary gland size. This holds true also for the submandibular flow rate.[162] These results are in agreement with Dawes et al.,[163] who found that the maximum flow rate of parotid saliva is proportional to the gland size. Thus the degree of interindividual variation in the flow rate can in many cases be explained by differences in the salivary gland size. For practical reasons, however, it is difficult to measure the size of the glands, and therefore it seems reasonable to use salivary tests without assessment of the gland size. It has been speculated that body weight could have an effect on the size of the salivary glands and thereby on the salivary flow rate. No such correlation seems, however, to exist.[163,164]

## L. Dentition

The status of dentition has been shown to have some effect on salivation when the flow rate is measured by chewing stimulation.[165-169] Number of teeth[168] and masticatory dysfunction[169] may, for example, affect secretion rate, as well as the time when saliva is collected in relation to wearing new complete dentures. This stresses the importance of not extracting teeth or making new dentures during a period of salivary tests. Gabay[167] found that subjects with either a small number of remaining natural teeth mostly out of occlusion, or following their extraction, had a remarkably reduced flow rate. As expected, salivary secretion rate seems to be faster in persons wearing complete dentures in both jaws as compared with edentulous persons not wearing dentures.[166] This holds true only for paraffin-stimulated whole saliva but not for resting whole saliva.[166]

## M. Dry Mouth

Dry mouth (xerostomia) is a clinical condition which is characterized by a desiccation of the intraoral tissues. The most common reason is a reduced saliva production (sialopenia). Exceptionally, dry mouth can also be caused by increased evaporation from the oral mucosa, for example, through mouth breathing. The clinical conception is often connected to reduced physiological values of saliva production.[19] Dry mouth can be present, however, even if the salivary flow rate shows normal values. Some patients with a reduced secretion rate do not complain at all.

### 1. Etiology

The etiology of dry mouth is multifactorial.[5,6,71,170,171] The most frequent cause seems to be side effects from drugs.[19] Numerous products, representing many various groups of pharmaceutical preparations — for example, antidepressants, tranquilizers, sedatives, and diuretics (see Section F) — depress the saliva production.

A critical review of available data from both human and animal studies on salivary gland function during aging has recently been presented.[172] It was concluded that there is no generalized diminution with age in salivary gland performance. Thus, in substantially healthy older persons, one should not expect to hear complaints about dry mouth[172] (see also Section D).

Nutritional deficiencies or various diseases are sometimes accompanied by a reduced salivary flow rate. It should be emphasized, however, that the relationship between these two factors and dry mouth is poorly documented in the literature, except for Sjögren's syndrome (see Sections C and H, respectively).

Destruction of glandular tissues is one of the main problems after irradiation of tumors in the head and neck regions. Thus such treatment is often accompanied by a condition of dry mouth (see Section I).

## 2. *Symptoms*

Saliva is important for the remineralization of the teeth. It also keeps the pH at a constant level in the mouth. Therefore, when the saliva flow is reduced, the risk for dental caries is obvious. Thus many patients with xerostomia have high caries activity (see Section N).

One of the most important components involved in the protection of the oral mucosa is a covering salivary layer (pellicle). The maintenance and function of this pellicle are highly dependent on a sufficient production of saliva. The pellicle is important for protection against infections and for mechanical damage to the mucosa. In addition, saliva contains various systems of defense against microorganisms. Thus dry mouth might lead not only to an increased risk of bacterial and candidal infection but also to an increased risk of ulcerations. The oral mucosa of a patient with dry mouth often shows redness, and the patient has a severe pain.

Patients with dentures may present many problems.[174] The retention of the dentures is based on physical mechanisms, in which the saliva plays an important role comprising a layer of adhesion. The mucosa of a patient with dry mouth has lost most of this property, and the dentures show a tendency to loosen. Frequently, the dentures can also cause ulcerations of the mucosa, which in connection with dry mouth is more easily damaged by mechanical stress.

Patients with dry mouth often find normal physiological activities of the mouth disagreeable. For many patients, talking can be so difficult that it becomes a social problem. This may also be applied to eating. Chewing might be difficult, since the friction against the mucosa is increased, which also makes swallowing hard. The food may not taste "normal", since xerostomia might entail a disturbance of taste physiology.

## 3. *Treatment*

Patients with a chronic or temporary sensation of dry mouth need some kind of treatment to relieve the symptoms.[175] These patients are often advised to drink water *ad libitum* and to try either a saliva stimulant or a saliva substitute.[176-188] These products may be of great help for the patient, even if they only relieve the symptoms temporarily. With present knowledge, the following recommendations can be given to patients with dry mouth: (1) First, try a saliva stimulating sucking pastille or a chewing gum and, second, a saliva substitute. Use only products which can be considered as safe for teeth. (2) Drink water and chew food products which stimulate the saliva production and which have a high water content. (3) In order to reduce the risk of dental caries, avoid sugar-containing foods between meals, use fluoridated toothpaste or other fluoride-containing preparations, and clean the teeth carefully, even after meals. For further information regarding treatment of dry mouth patients, see reviews by Navazesh and Ship,[170] Glass et al.,[171] and Imfeld.[175]

## N. Secretion Rate and Dental Caries

Various attempts to establish a direct relationship between caries and secretion rates within normal variations have not been too successful.[2,10,189] This might depend on the influence of other variables in the caries process such as the oral microorganisms, dietary habits, fluoride prophylaxis, and oral hygiene. Because of the multifactorial background of caries, one cannot expect any strong correlation between the amount of saliva secreted and tooth decay. There is a tendency, though, for persons with very low caries activity to show a higher salivary flow rate than caries-active persons,[190-195] but only a few studies have shown statistically significant differences between these groups. An interesting observation is that a lack of saliva secretion from a single gland is reported to be connected with local rampant caries over the corresponding area.[196,197]

In healthy children, a significant correlation between the salivary secretion rate and caries frequency has been reported only in primary teeth.[198,199] Hyposalivation is very uncommon

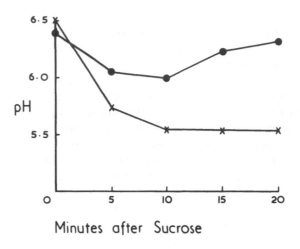

6.5

pH   6.0

5.5

0        5        10       15       20

Minutes after Sucrose

● WITHOUT SALIVARY RESTRICTION
X WITH SALIVARY RESTRICTION

FIGURE 8.   Changes in plaque pH following a sugar rinse with and without access of saliva. (Redrawn by Jenkins, G. N., in *Proceedings Saliva and Dental Caries,* Kleinberg, I., Ellison, S. A., and Mandel, I. D., Eds., Information Retrieval, New York, 1979, 307, from Englander, H. R., Carter, W. J., and Fosdick, L. S., *J. Dent. Res.,* 35, 792, 1956. With permission.)

in children, but when present — for example, following treatment with antidepressive drugs or after surgical treatment of drooling — it increases caries activities even in children.[200,201]

The importance of saliva as a resistance factor against the caries disease is clearly demonstrated when the secretion is severely impaired. In cases of xerostomia, a well-known consequence is a marked increase in caries activity.[3,5,71,170,171,175] Xerostomia patients often show increased number of aciduric and acidogenic microorganisms, for example, *Streptococcus mutans* and lactobacilli.[144,145] Furthermore, many salivary properties essential for caries are actually connected with flow rate. The diluting effect of the saliva naturally depends on the volume secreted. Plaque pH levels are regulated by the salivary flow rate.[7,202-204] The pH and buffer capacity of the saliva are also strongly dependent on the flow rate[12,18,19,35,55,56,60,61] as well as the oral sugar clearance from saliva.[205-207] Thus, low salivary flow rate means impaired cleaning of the oral cavity, prolonged duration of low plaque pH (Figure 8), as well as insufficient remineralization of the teeth. Therefore, reduced salivary flow, especially in severe cases of xerostomia, should always be considered as a risk factor for dental caries.

## III. BUFFER CAPACITY AND pH

### A. Buffer Systems

Solutions containing both weak acids and their salts are referred to as buffer solutions. These solutions have the capacity of resisting changes of pH when either acids or alkalies are added to them. For the buffering properties of saliva, the two terms "buffer capacity" and "buffer effect" are frequently used synonymously. The buffer capacity expresses the resistance to pH changes at an arbitrary point. The term "buffer effect" refers to the amount of acid required to change the pH of the saliva sample from one value to another. In reality, each of these two terms merely relates to a different manner of describing the same property.[208] In the present text, the term "buffer capacity" will be used throughout.

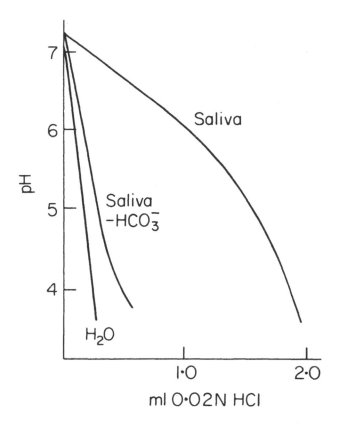

FIGURE 9. Buffer titration curve of paraffin-stimulated saliva compared with that of distilled water and saliva from which bicarbonate has been removed. These curves show that bicarbonate is the most important buffer in saliva. (After Lilienthal, B. and Jenkins, G. N., in *The Physiology and Biochemistry of the Mouth*, 4th ed., Blackwell Scientific, Oxford, 1978. With permission.)

The buffer capacity of human saliva is regulated by three buffer systems — the carbonic acid/bicarbonate system, the phosphate system, and the proteins. The carbonic acid/bicarbonate system is the most important one.[209-214] It is based on the equilibrium

$$H_2CO_3 \rightleftharpoons HCO_3^- + H^+ \qquad (1)$$

When an acid is added, the bicarbonates release the weak carbonic acid. Carbonic acid is rapidly decomposed into water and $CO_2$, which leaves the solution. In contrast to most buffers, the net result is therefore not an accumulation of a weaker acid but a complete removal of acid. This change of phase for $CO_2$ from dissolved state to gas phase, for which the term "phase buffering" is used, is essential for the buffer action of the bicarbonate system. The importance of bicarbonate may be demonstrated as in Figure 9, which shows how the removal of bicarbonate from a saliva sample greatly reduces the buffer capacity to a level not far from that of distilled water.

The phosphate buffer system in saliva functions basically by the same general principle as the $HCO_3^-$ system except for the fact that no phase change is involved. At physiological pH, the system operates according to the following equilibrium

$$H_2PO_4^- \rightleftharpoons HPO_4^{2-} + H^+ \qquad (2)$$

This system has a pK of 6.8 to 7.0.[16] Thus the two buffer systems described act together to keep the salivary pH above 6.

The salivary proteins are usually not considered to have any significant buffer capacity at the pH values involved in the oral cavity.[212] It is possible, however, that carbamino compounds or carbamates will contribute to the acid buffering of saliva. Leung[215] reported the presence of carbamino compounds in saliva, but his conclusion was disputed by Grøn and Messer.[216] Later, Izutsu and Madden[217] presented data which suggest that there are significant amounts of carbamino compounds in saliva.

In resting saliva, the bicarbonate concentration is much lower than in stimulated saliva. Consequently, also the buffer capacity and pH are reduced. *In vitro,* the bicarbonate-dependent salivary buffering accounts for approximately 25% and 70% of the total buffer capacity of resting and stimulated whole saliva.[212,213] In an open system which may resemble mouth conditions, however, the corresponding percentages are about 60% and 90%.[213] About one half of the nonbicarbonate salivary buffer capacity in resting and stimulated whole saliva is due to the phosphate content. The protein presumably contributes the remainder.[213]

## B. pH

At a given secretion rate, the salivary pH is mainly regulated by the ratio between carbonic acid and bicarbonate as expressed by the Henderson-Hasselbalch equation

$$pH = pK + \log\left[\frac{HCO_3^-}{H_2CO_3}\right] \tag{3}$$

Reported figures for pK, which is the negative log for the apparent dissociation constant for the acid, vary between approximately 6.1[216] and 6.3[215] while $H_2CO_3 = 0.03 \times P_{CO_2}$. The factor 0.03 is derived on the assumption of a value of 0.51 for the carbon dioxide absorption coefficient. The partial pressure of carbon dioxide in saliva is relatively constant and independent of secretion rate[218] (Figure 10). Consequently, the pH will vary according to variations in the bicarbonate concentration of saliva.

## C. Regulation of Salivary Bicarbonate and Phosphate Levels

The bicarbonate concentration is strongly dependent on secretion rate.[218-221] This explains why saliva may be slightly acidic at unstimulated secretion rates and may reach about pH 8 when stimulated.[35,221,222] As expected, since bicarbonate is the chief determinant also of the salivary buffer capacity, there is an interrelationship between pH, buffer capacity and secretion rate.[12,18,19,35,55,56,60,61,218,221,223-226]

The regulation of bicarbonate is far from clear. The salivary bicarbonate can be derived from both glandular metabolic activity and plasma.[218,227,228] Rapid formation of bicarbonate by the gland probably requires the action of carbonic anhydrase (CA) for hydration of dissolved $CO_2$.

$$CO_2 + H_2O \overset{\overset{\displaystyle CA}{\displaystyle\downarrow}}{\rightleftharpoons} H_2CO_3 \rightleftharpoons H^+ + HCO_3^- \tag{4}$$

The use of inhibitors of carbonic anhydrase such as acetazolamide (Diamox) has not strengthened this hypothesis.[229,230] Therefore, although several reports have indicated the presence of carbonic anhydrase activity in salivary glands of both man and mammals,[231-233] the effect on bicarbonate formation is not established. Carbonic anhydrase has been found also in saliva, but Maren[233] could find none in human samples. The possibility remains either that

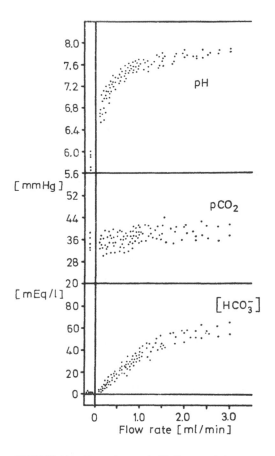

FIGURE 10. Dependence of pH, $P_{CO_2}$, and the concentration of $HCO_3^-$ on the salivary flow rate. With increasing secretion rate there is a rapid rise of pH and $HCO_3^-$ while $P_{CO_2}$ is relatively constant. The values obtained during the resting state are given before zero flow rate. (After Kreusser, W., Heidland, A., Hennemann, H., Wigand, M. E., and Knauf, H., *Eur. J. Clin. Invest.*, 2, 398, 1971. With permission.)

the enzyme is refractory to acetazolamide or that it is not accessible to the inhibitor in the intact gland.

The relationship between salivary bicarbonate and the plasma is not simple. Results of experimental metabolic acidosis and alkalosis have been inconsistent.[8,227,234] It has been found, though, that after a respiratory acidosis is induced by inhalation of 4% $CO_2$, the parotid bicarbonate and pH increased markedly. These changes were influenced primarily by the $P_{CO_2}$ increase of the blood. It has also been demonstrated in the dog that the saliva-to-plasma ratio for bicarbonate and the absolute level of salivary bicarbonate are directly related to the arterial $CO_2$ tension.[228] This effect on saliva of an increased $P_{CO_2}$ has been confirmed in human subjects.[221]

The salivary phosphate content is considerably higher than in plasma. Up to 80% is present in the inorganic form.[228] The inorganic phosphate exists as both the monovalent and the divalent ion, and the relative proportions of the two forms change with the salivary pH. The orthophosphate concentration is inversely related to secretion rate, while the concentration of $HPO_4^{2-}$ is relatively independent.[35,218,221,225,235,236] These variations are illustrated in Figure 11, where the phosphate content and pH of parotid saliva are plotted as a function of secretion rate.

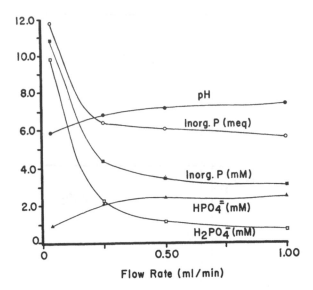

FIGURE 11.    The effect of flow rate on the concentrations of
the different types of inorganic orthophosphate in human parotid
saliva. (After Dawes, C., *Arch. Oral Biol.*, 14, 277, 1969.
With permission.)

## D. Clinical Tests of Buffer Capacity and pH

Various procedures have been used to measure the salivary buffer capacity. These include
titration under oil, titration while open to air, and titration with $CO_2$.[8,210,212,229,237-239] Due
to the variety of methods, the values for buffer capacity presented in different studies are
not comparable. To solve this problem, Izutsu[213] has proposed that the *slyke* should be used
as the unit of buffer value. The slyke is defined as the negative of the slope of the titration
curve, its units are the amount of acid added per liter divided by the resulting change in pH
(millimole per liter per pH change).

Even with a carefully performed microtitration method, the error is about 6%.[237] Simplified
methods[8,209,240] may therefore be used with little or no loss of accuracy. In Sweden the
method of Ericsson[8] is routinely used at the departments of cariology and in the Public
Dental Health Service. The buffer capacity is usually assessed immediately after the collection
of saliva. After mixing of the sample by twice inverting the collection tube, 1.0 ml of saliva
is transferred to 3.0 ml of HCl (0.0033 mol/l for resting saliva and 0.005 mol/l for stimulated
saliva). One drop of 2-octanol is added to prevent foaming when a stream of air is passed
through the mixture for 20 min to remove $CO_2$. The combination of aeration and addition
of HCl completes the removal of $CO_2$. The final pH of the solution, which to a large extent
is related to the original concentration of $HCO_3^-$, is assessed electrometrically (Figure 12)
and taken as an expression of the buffer capacity of the saliva sample.

The stronger acid used for stimulated saliva results in a better differentiation between
samples at the higher final pH levels, that is, the most strongly buffered samples. A comparison between buffer capacity values of samples of resting and stimulated saliva is not
possible, however, because of the difference in acid concentration. Within the final pH
range 3.0 to 8.0 there is a linear relationship between the results obtained with this method
and those of standard titration procedures.[8]

With this method[8] special laboratory equipment is required. A simplified colorimetric test
was therefore described by Bratthall and Hager.[241] Using the same volumes as before, a
sample of stimulated saliva is left for 2 min. after the addition of acid (0.005 mol/l).
Thereafter, the pH of the sample is determined with pH indicator sticks. This modification

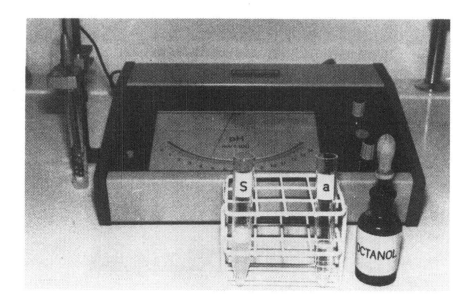

FIGURE 12.    Assessment of the salivary buffer capacity (final pH) according to the method of Ericsson.[8] First, 1.0 ml of saliva (S) is transferred to 3.0 ml HCl (a). Then 2-octanol is added to prevent foaming. The final pH of the solution is assessed electrometrically. For further details, see text. (With permission.)

of Ericsson's[8] method — that is, without the elimination of carbon dioxide with air bubbling — results in a higher pH in the lower buffer capacity regions. The situation is reversed at the other end of the scale.

A further development has been made by Frostell[242] with the Dentobuff® kit system (Figure 13). A sample of saliva is injected with a disposable syringe through a plastic stopper into a Dentobuff® ampule which contains hydrochloric acid and an indicator system. With this method a sample volume of 1.0 ml is used for stimulated saliva and 1.5 ml for resting saliva. The ampule is then shaken vigorously for 10 s. The stopper is removed, and the carbon dioxide is allowed to evaporate for 2 to 5 min. Based on the color change of the solution in the ampule, the buffer capacity is assessed in comparison with a color chart. There is a general tendency to underestimate values in the higher final pH regions with the Dentobuff® system. When compared with Ericsson's method,[8] however, the difference between the two methods is usually small in the lower final pH regions.[242,243] It is therefore possible to sort out subjects with an impaired salivary buffer capacity with this simplified technique.

From a practical point of view, a further simplification has been presented by Linder et al.[244] With the Cario-Test method a sample of stimulated saliva is transported to a commercial laboratory where secretion rate, buffer capacity, and number of lactobacilli and *Streptococcus mutans* are assessed. According to this study,[244] the time needed for transport does not seem to influence appreciably the buffer capacity of the sample. A rather good correlation ($r \sim 0.8$) was reported between test results obtained immediately and up to 48 h after collection of the saliva sample. Previous studies indicate that storage of saliva samples, however, may markedly increase the buffer capacity regardless if at room temperature or at $-18°C$.[8,93,212,245]

The pH is usually assessed electrometrically. If a very great precision is required, the saliva should be collected under oil and tested for pH within a few minutes of collection.[246] Otherwise, if exposed to the air, the $CO_2$ will diffuse out and pH will rise. According to Parvinen,[222] a continuous loss of $CO_2$ from the saliva sample causes a corresponding change in the second decimal during the measurement with an electrical pH meter. This was illus-

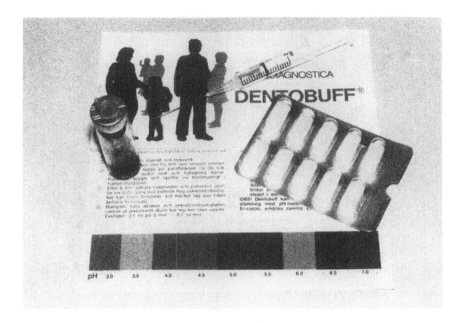

FIGURE 13.   The Dentobuff® kit system for assessing the salivary buffer capacity. Paraffin-stimulated saliva (1.0 ml) is injected with a disposable syringe through a plastic stopper into an ampul containing HCl and an indicator system. Based on the color change of the solution, the buffer capacity is assessed when comparing with a color chart. For further details, see text. (With permission.)

trated with the mean pH values for stimulated whole saliva in males and females which differed statistically only if the pH was assessed with two decimals. The accuracy of the measured pH value therefore depends on the method of saliva collection and on the time interval between collection and measurement.

### E. Normal Values and Reference Intervals

The results of these clinical tests[8,242] of the salivary buffer capacity are generally judged according to the normal values reported by Ericsson and Hardwick,[9] which are shown in Table 12. A very low buffer capacity is considered to represent a pathological condition. The results[9] from other studies do, however, indicate that the normal values[9] are rather high especially as regards the buffer capacity of stimulated saliva (Table 12). For this variable, mean or median final pH values varying from 4.6 to 5.3 have been reported.[12,247,248] Krasse,[249] for example, has also recently recommended somewhat different reference values. Thus, for stimulated saliva a final pH <5.0 is considered as low and >7.0 as normal or high.

The salivary buffer capacity is generally most pronounced from pH 7.5 down to about pH 6, while a weaker buffer capacity is found between pH 6 and 4 (Figure 14). A frequency diagram of the results from buffer capacity test[8,242] might therefore be expected to have two peaks, one with a maximum over pH 6 and another with a maximum below pH 4.[242] This type of bimodal frequency distribution has also been shown by Ericson[247] (Figure 15) and others[100,243] for the buffer capacity of stimulated whole saliva but does not seem to be a regular finding. As illustrated by the results from another study,[12] the expected distribution was found for resting saliva and in females only (Figures 16 and 17). According to Söderling et al.,[250] the two-maxima distributions observed with these methods[8,242] are only to a minor degree caused by the properties of the methods used. Possibly, such distributions also reflect individual habits or qualities of various subgroups forming the total population studied.

**Table 12**
**BUFFER CAPACITY AND pH OF WHOLE
SALIVA FROM SUBJECTS AGED 15 TO 55
YEARS, NORMAL AND VERY LOW
VALUES ACCORDING TO ERICSSON AND
HARDWICK[9]**

|  | Resting saliva | Stimulated saliva |
|---|---|---|
| Buffer capacity |  |  |
|   Normal final pH | 4.25—4.75 | 5.75—6.50 |
|   Very low final pH | <3.5 | <4.0 |
| pH |  |  |
|   Normal | 6.5—6.9 | 7.0—7.5 |
|   Very low | <6.3 | <6.8 |

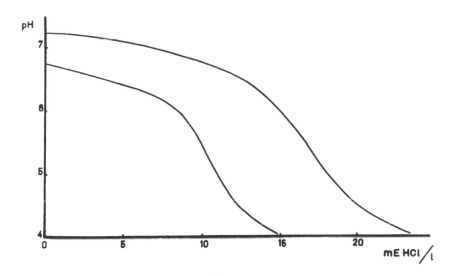

FIGURE 14.    Buffer titration curves for salivary samples taken from the same patient. The lower curve represents resting saliva, and the higher curve stimulated saliva. Note the low buffer capacity between pH 6 and pH 4. (After Ericsson, Y., *Nordisk lärobok i cariologi,* Sveriges Tandläkarförbunds förlagsförening u p a, Stockholm, 1976. With permission.)

When duplicate saliva samples are collected with an interval of approximately 2 weeks, there is a highly significant correlation between test 1 and test 2.[12] Furthermore, no seasonal variation is observed for the buffer capacity of stimulated saliva during 1 year with saliva being collected monthly. These findings indicate that the intraindividual variation in buffer capacity is rather small. As described previously for secretion rate, although the buffer capacity of resting and stimulated saliva is significantly correlated, it must be determined for both types of saliva.

According to Ericsson,[8] the buffer capacity is higher immediately on rising than after breakfast. During the day a general trend toward increasing buffer capacity with a downward tendency in the evening may be observed.

For the pH of whole saliva, normal and very low values are shown in Table 12. Parvinen[222] reports a range of pH 6.30 to 8.08 for stimulated saliva. In Table 13[251] the means and ranges for means of several other studies are given. The pH of resting or unstimulated saliva is lower than in whole saliva. Submandibular saliva has a higher resting pH than that from the parotid gland.

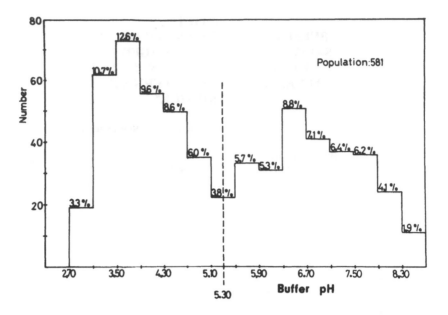

FIGURE 15.   Frequency distribution of buffer capacity of stimulated whole saliva from 581 subjects. (After Ericson, T., in *Oral Physiology*, Pergamon Press, Oxford, 1972. With permission.)

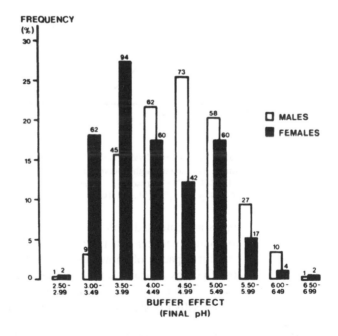

FIGURE 16.   Frequency distribution of buffer capacity of resting whole saliva for 629 male and female subjects. (After Heintze, U., Birkhed, D., and Björn, H., *Swed. Dent. J.*, 7, 227, 1983. With permission.)

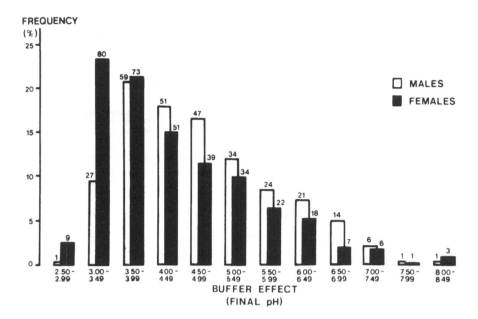

FIGURE 17. Frequency distribution of buffer capacity of stimulated whole saliva for 629 male and female subjects. (After Heintze, U., Birkhed, D., and Björn, H., *Swed. Dent. J.*, 7, 227, 1983. With permission.)

**Table 13**
**pH OF UNSTIMULATED AND**
**STIMULATED GLANDULAR AND**
**WHOLE SALIVA ACCORDING TO**
**SUDDICK ET AL.[251]**

|  | Parotid | | Subman-dibular | | Whole | |
|---|---|---|---|---|---|---|
|  | U | S | U | S | U | S |
| pH | 5.8 | 7.7 | 6.5 | 7.4 | 6.7 | 6.8—7.5 |

*Note:* Means or ranges for means are given. Values are for unstimulated (U) or stimulated (S) flow rates approximately 1.0 ml/min for pure secretions, usually exceeding 1.0 ml/min for whole saliva.

The salivary pH varies throughout the day, which is probably controlled by variations in secretion rate.[246]

**F. Sex and Age**

Data on sex- and age-related variations as regards the salivary buffer capacity in adults are rather sparse. The buffer capacity of both resting and stimulated whole saliva is significantly lower for females than for males.[12,248] The frequency distributions also show a female predominance among subjects with final pH values <4.0 (Figures 16 and 17). A diminished buffer capacity might therefore be considered to be normal for females. These findings might in part be explained by the generally lower secretion rate in females, since the salivary buffer capacity and secretion rate are considered interrelated as described previously. Similarly,

**Table 14**

**MEDIAN BUFFER CAPACITY OF RESTING AND STIMULATED WHOLE SALIVA (FINAL pH ACCORDING TO THE METHOD OF ERICSSON; MEAN OF TWO TESTS) IN MALES AND FEMALES OF VARIOUS AGE GROUPS[8]**

| Age groups (years) | Resting saliva | | | Stimulated saliva | | |
|---|---|---|---|---|---|---|
| | Males | | Females | Males | | Females |
| 1 (15—29) | 4.53 | *** | 3.95 | 4.35 | *** | 3.85 |
| (n = 179) | NS | | NS | NS | | NS |
| 2 (30—44) | 4.55 | *** | 3.80 | 4.44 | *** | 3.95 |
| (n = 237) | NS | | *** | NS | | * |
| 3 (45—59) | 4.71 | NS | 4.40 | 4.60 | NS | 4.45 |
| (n = 128) | NS | | NS | * | | NS |
| 4 (60—74) | 4.91 | NS | 5.05 | 5.23 | NS | 4.70 |
| (n = 85) | | | | | | |
| All groups (1—4) | 4.65 | *** | 4.10 | 4.55 | *** | 4.05 |
| (n = 629) | | | | | | |

$* = n < 0.05$, $** = p < 0.01$, $*** = p < 0.001$.

sex differences with regard to buffer capacity have been observed also for children, adolescents, and 70-year-old subjects.[18,19,60,61]

When analyzed for separate age groups, the difference between sexes persists only within age groups 1 and 2, that is, 15 to 44 years of age. No significant differences are found between males and females in the two older age groups (Table 14). Therefore, the buffer capacity of females is positively correlated with age. Reasons for these age-related variations in the buffer capacity of both resting and stimulated saliva of females are unknown but might be of postmenopausal character.

For stimulated saliva, the mean pH of unmedicated subjects is significantly lower for females than for males.[222] In these subjects, age had no significant influence on the pH of stimulated whole saliva.[56] For stimulated parotid saliva, Chauncey et al.,[70] however, have reported a significant decline in the pH with age in healthy males.

## G. Diet

A question of interest is whether the salivary secretion rate and buffer capacity may be influenced by individual dietary regimens. There are previous indications that diets high in protein, vegetables, or fat and low in carbohydrates might increase the buffer capacity or pH of both resting and stimulated saliva.[8,252-255] If so, suitable dietary changes might be recommended in order to improve the buffer capacity when necessary. According to Wills and Forbes,[253] for example, a negative influence on the salivary buffer capacity might be observed already after a single carbohydrate meal. In these studies, however, the salivary secretion rate was not assessed, and therefore it is not known whether the buffer capacity was affected per se or indirectly via an altered secretion rate.

The results obtained in a study[42] of the effect on saliva during a 4-h period after a single intake of various liquid test meals do not indicate an endogenous influence on the salivary buffer capacity. One reason is that the use of liquid test meals eliminated differences in chewing resistance. Masticatory stimuli could therefore not be interpreted as being a possible systemic effect. The water content of the various meals was not considered to have any influence, since Shannon and Chauncey[256] found that ingestion of similar volumes of water did not affect the secretion rate.

Since only single intakes of foods were allowed, it might be argued that the volumes given were insufficient or that the effect on saliva was followed for too short a time. However, food begins to leave the stomach within 2 to 3 min after ingestion.[257] Depending on the type of test meal, after 60 to 90 min most of the gastric contents were presumably emptied into the duodenum. Therefore, during the time period studied, complex digestion and absorption processes were stimulated also from parts further down the gastrointestinal system. In this context, the so-called postprandial alkaline tide in urine[258] and the rise and fall of, for example, alveolar carbon dioxide pressure,[259] which appear within an hour after eating, might be mentioned. Nevertheless, no parallel changes were found for the salivary buffer capacity, which mainly depends on the salivary $HCO_3^-$ concentration in saliva.[209-214] Nor was an increased buffer capacity[8,41] or pH[41] after a meal confirmed.

It is possible that more marked dietary changes may be required for a longer period of time. After a transition from an ordinary mixed diet to an initial fasting period for 6 d,[47-49] no dietary influence on the buffer capacity of whole saliva was found. The diet used before the various dietary periods just mentioned may possibly have influenced the results obtained. An examination of the published figures from the study of Ericsson[8] shows that the stimulating influence on the salivary buffer capacity was found mostly when the results from the experimental dietary periods were compared. No significant difference was observed between, for example, the periods with vegetables and customary diet.

According to Dawes,[44] there is little evidence that different diets can exert different systemic effects on the salivary buffer capacity. The findings mentioned previously might support this conclusion. Nor do available data on possible dietary endogenous influences on saliva suggest that a vegetable-dominated diet per se should be superior in this respect. On a group basis, when vegetarians and subjects on ordinary diets are compared, no differences are found regarding the salivary buffer effect.[52,53,237] If a trend is inferred from most of these studies, it would seem to indicate (1) a transition to a carbohydrate-dominated diet might decrease the buffer capacity, (2) a very marked reduction of the dietary carbohydrate content might increase the buffer capacity, and (3) such changes may require a relatively long time before they become noticeable.

Therefore, it might be promising that Johansson et al.[54] have recently demonstrated that following a transition from ordinary food to a strict lactovegetarian diet, both secretion rate and buffer capacity of whole saliva increased significantly after 6 and 12 months. The notable length of the experimental periods indicates that dietary influences on saliva might take some time to develop. Presumably, the positive buffer capacity changes were related to the simultaneous increase in secretion rate, which is a factor that has not been studied in many of the previous investigations.

## H. General Health

As described previously, the salivary secretion rate may be influenced by various diseases, drugs, and emotional disorders. The relationship between general health and other salivary variables such as buffer capacity and pH have not been comprehensively studied. Consequently, it is not known whether, for instance, disease-related changes in buffer capacity and pH are specific effects or occur secondarily because of the well-known relationship with secretion rate.

The evidence concerning a direct effect on the salivary buffer capacity and pH per se are scarce or contradictory. In cystic fibrosis patients, the buffer capacity is higher than in controls.[260] Possibly, this finding is related to the higher phosphorus levels in the saliva of these patients.[261,262] During pregnancy the buffer capacity and pH, though not the secretion rate, may increase,[78] while Flodhammar[263] reported a lower buffer capacity for pregnant subjects. The salivary pH is lower during pregnancy.[264] For insulin-dependent diabetics the buffer capacity may be higher than for controls according to Kjellman,[118] which was not confirmed by Tenovuo et al.[113] At least in pathological conditions the $HCO_3^-$ concentration and thereby the buffer capacity[209-214] may be influenced by aldosterone,[265] a mineralocorticoid hormone physiologically regulated by renin. No differences in this respect were found, however, in a comparison between healthy subjects with high and low salivary buffer capacity.[266]

Kakizaki et al.[267] have reported a series of experimental and clinical studies concerning the interrelationship between the parotid gland and the pancreas. A screening test for pancreatic disorders, based on the salivary output (ml/kg), maximum bicarbonate concentration, and amylase content of parotid saliva, was developed. Also in whole saliva the bicarbonate concentration is lower for subjects with chronic pancreatitis.[131] Lankisch et al.[268] and Dobrilla et al.,[134] however, could not recommend the parotid saliva test[267] as a screening test for chronic pancreatitis. Further studies are needed to clarify whether the reduced bicarbonate concentration was the result of a pancreatic disorder or a reduced secretion rate.

Many common anticholinergic drugs reduce the salivary secretion rate. Consequently, the buffer capacity and pH may also be reduced.[86,87,93] In medicated subjects, a significantly lower salivary pH was related to the use of beta blocking agents, nitrates and analgesics with minor tranquilizers in males, and analgesics and diuretics in females.[84] The pH changes were mostly explained by the changes in secretion rate.

Emotional and psychic variables may be of great importance. Anxiety and shrewdness are related to the pH and bicarbonate levels in parotid saliva, while introversion is related to bicarbonate.[269] To a varying extent psychological factors may also be connected with a temporal mandibular joint (TMJ) dysfunction. Le Bell et al.[169] have reported a significant increase in the buffer capacity of stimulated saliva after treatment of the TMJ dysfunction. However, this effect was only found in those patients who had low starting values. The improvement in buffer capacity was related to an increase in secretion rate. Thus the treatment did not affect the bicarbonate content per se. As regards stimulated saliva, also the number of teeth may be of importance. With increasing tooth loss, the mean buffer capacity decreases. The same relationship has been found for pH.[19,165]

Thus, general health may in many cases influence the salivary gland function in various ways.[71,83,270] A reduction in buffer capacity and pH might therefore be assumed to reflect a disease state, possibly on a subclinical level. A recent study[105] examined both dental patients with a very low buffer capacity according to the reference values of Ericsson and Hardwick[9] (Table 12) and reference subjects. Blood and urine analyses were included. Despite the extensive medical examination, no direct explanations for the salivary insufficiencies were obtained. Rather, it appeared quite "normal", with medical findings being made for about 30 to 40% of both patients and reference subjects. Such a frequency of medical findings might seem high, but it has been shown that 30 to 35% of middle-aged attendees in medical screenings do show some findings.[271] Nevertheless, the fact remains that the finding of one or more very low salivary values as judged by the reference values[9] do not necessarily indicate impaired health, at least not when defined by the present diagnostic criteria.

## I. Smoking Habits

It is possible that cigarette smoking may influence the salivary buffer capacity. In a comparison of smokers and nonsmokers, the buffer capacity of both resting and stimulated whole saliva was significantly lower in smokers.[100] When judged by the reference intervals of Ericsson and Hardwick,[9] the median buffer capacity of stimulated saliva was for the smokers (final pH 4.2) close to what is considered to be very low. In contrast, for nonsmokers (final pH 6.2) it was within the normal range. The frequency of very low values was about four times higher for the smokers. In a complementary study,[100] smoking two cigarettes did not significantly influence the buffer capacity of stimulated saliva. Also for these smokers the salivary buffer capacity was significantly lower than for nonsmokers (final pH 4.6 vs. 7.0).

Reasons for an impaired salivary buffer capacity in cigarette smokers are not readily apparent. Possibly also covariating factors might have some influence. As was shown by Janzon et al.,[272] among subjects attending health screening the frequency of certain medical findings is higher in smokers. A systemic action on the salivary buffer capacity may not be excluded, however. Since bicarbonate is the most important buffer constituent of saliva,[209-214] the lower buffer capacity of smokers' saliva most probably reflected a lower concentration of $HCO_3^-$. An interesting parallel to the present findings may therefore be drawn from several studies on pancreatic juice, for which a significantly lower bicarbonate concentration has been reported in smokers.[273,274] A systemic influence on the salivary buffer capacity seemed further implicated, since no differences between smokers and nonsmokers as regards secretion rate were observed.

The aforementioned salivary findings were not confirmed in a later study of a population of smokers with an expressed desire to stop smoking.[102] In an unmedicated population, however, Parvinen[101] has observed also a significantly lower pH in stimulated saliva of smokers. Furthermore, there is a negative correlation between the salivary pH and nicotine concentration.[275] In addition to the lower buffer capacity[100] and pH,[101] the number of lactobacilli and *S. mutans* was significantly higher in stimulated saliva of smokers.[100] With regard to the number of lactobacilli, similar findings were recently reported by Parvinen.[101] Further studies are therefore needed. If the present findings are confirmed, the caries risk must be considered to be higher for cigarette smokers than for nonsmokers.

## J. Buffer Capacity, pH, and Dental Caries

The importance of saliva as a resistance factor against the caries disease is most obvious when the secretion is severely impaired. According to Dawes,[276] a reduction in bicarbonate concentration and thereby the buffer capacity is considered to be the most important consequence of a reduced secretion rate. Since the diffusion of bicarbonate into plaque is reduced, the possibility for saliva to counteract a fall in plaque pH after carbohydrate consumption will be reduced.[204,205,277,278] Recently, Lagerlöf et al.[205] have demonstrated the pronounced influence of the salivary buffer capacity on bacterial pH changes *in vitro*.

The pH of early plaque tends to reflect salivary pH and buffer capacity.[279] A low salivary pH seems to favor the growth of aciduric microorganisms, such as lactobacilli,[55,56,264,280] streptococci,[280] and yeasts.[55,56,281,282] Because of the salivary influence, plaque pH varies between different parts of the mouth. Mandibular plaque pH values are, for example, higher than maxillary values. As a consequence, regional plaque pH levels show a distribution pattern very similar to the patterns previously reported for the intraoral incidence of caries.[203] Furthermore, a sufficiently alkaline salivary pH is necessary for the remineralization of teeth to occur.[283]

An inverse relationship between buffer capacity and caries experience is well established according to Ericsson,[8] who evaluated the results of 21 reports published up to 1956. In addition, the Vipeholm study showed that caries-active subjects had a lower buffer capacity than caries-inactive subjects.[254] This finding was especially notable for the so-called 24-toffee group, which also demonstrated the highest caries activity. More recently, Marlay[284] in a longitudinal study of adolescents has demonstrated a fall in buffer capacity of saliva about 9 months before a rising of sustained caries increments. Also in children there may be a negative correlation between caries frequency and buffer capacity.[198,199] Agus and Schamschula[226] reported a consistent inverse trend between buffer capacity and various expressions of caries experience. The finding of higher mean buffer capacity and pH values in the saliva of cystic fibrosis patients is worthy of note. These patients also appear to have a lower caries experience than the unaffected controls.[260]

The pH of saliva has been regarded as one of the environmental factors which might influence the initiation of caries. In his review of the older literature, Afonsky[286] concluded that many studies have been devoted to correlating the hydrogen ion concentration of saliva with incidence of caries. The findings made were not too successful, as is often the case when trying to implicate one single factor in the etiology of caries. Caries-active subjects, however, have often had a lower salivary pH than caries-inactive subjects.[195,237,255,260,285]

## IV. PREDICTIVE AND PROGNOSTIC VALUE OF SALIVARY TESTS

The caries incidence may be of some value when calculating the caries risk — that is, the risk for a given individual of getting new caries lesions. In modern practice, however, diagnostic salivary measurements (secretion rate and buffer capacity) should be used in order to supplement the anamnestic information and clinical findings with regard to prevention of dental caries.[9,249] The salivary secretion rate and buffer capacity are considered to be important endogenous resistance factors which may modify the intensity and progression of the caries disease. Since the caries lesion is the result of a multifactorial disease, the assessment of two separate salivary factors is not sufficient unless they are of overriding importance, which may occur in an individual patient. Therefore, in the Swedish dental health program for adults the Swedish National Board of Health and Welfare has provided further criteria for evaluating the caries risk[287] (Table 15).

Taken together, the combination of these anamnestic, clinical, and laboratory findings constitutes an important test battery for the prediction of prognosis of dental caries. Some test results may not always coincide with the clinical picture, which may depend on the fact that caries lesions take some time to develop. Another reason which Ravald et al.[288] reported in a study on root surface caries is that no single variable was found to be discriminative for development of the disease in all subjects. This is illustrated in Figure 18, which is an individual graphic illustration of 8 variables including salivary secretion rate and salivary buffer capacity in 4 patients. One of them who developed 13 new DFS% had both a low secretion rate and a low buffer capacity, and another one who developed 23 DFS% during a 4-year observation period had a low buffer capacity. However, there were no clear-cut differences compared with the 2 patients who were caries free during the same observation period. These results support the generally adopted opinion that the more risk variables, the more risk for dental caries.[289-292]

For clinical use, the secretion rate and buffer capacity are generally determined for paraffin-stimulated whole saliva. Possibly, this is not always the relevant type of saliva to analyze, since stimulation tends to reduce interindividual differences in secretion rate.[15,17,57] The caries process occurs during and immediately following the intake of cariogenic foods. During this period, the secretion is stimulated, and it might therefore be argued that stimulated rather than resting saliva should be studied. This line of reasoning may be illustrated by the findings of Imfeld,[293] who showed that resting saliva was unable to stop the continuous decrease in plaque pH during a 15-min control period after a sucrose rinse (Figure 19). In contrast, a relatively quick rise in plaque pH was achieved by the chewing of neutral paraffin, which increased the salivary secretion rate and consequently the buffer capacity and sucrose clearance (Figure 20).

In cases of suspected xerostomia both resting and stimulated whole saliva should preferably be studied. Although a significant correlation has been found between the secretion rates of resting and stimulated saliva, the secretion rate of one type could not readily be predicted from the other because of the large variations.[12] Consequently, in the individual case, for example, impaired secretion of resting saliva may be found together with a normal secretion of stimulated saliva. The subjective feeling of dryness for these patients, however, may not always be related to objective findings obtained in salivary tests.

When an impaired secretion has been confirmed, it can be recommended to go one step further. In order to analyze whether the low secretion rate is general or might be ascribed

**Table 15**

**EVALUATION OF THE CARIES RISK ACCORDING TO THE SWEDISH DENTAL HEALTH PROGRAM FOR ADULTS[287]**

| Evaluation | Anamnestic evaluation | Data to be considered | | Clinical appearance of cavities or lesions |
| | | Resistance of enamel | Previous caries activity | |
|---|---|---|---|---|
| Low caries risk (good prognosis) | No indication of caries-accelerating factors such as systemic diseases, medications with saliva-affecting drugs, etc. | Increased resistance through earlier and/or present fluoride supplementation | No or only a small number of new cavities during the immediate past | Carious lesions only on surfaces normally at risk. Arrested lesions |
| High caries risk (unfavorable prognosis) | Medications, social situations, which can be regarded as caries accelerating | Decreased resistance through low earlier and present fluoride supplementation | Several new cavities during the immediate past | Lesions also on surfaces not normally affected by caries. Soft, whitish appearance |

| Evaluation | Oral hygiene | Data to be considered | | Saliva |
| | | Dietary record | Composition of oral microflora | |
|---|---|---|---|---|
| Low caries risk (good prognosis) | Good | Low intake of sucrose, especially in the form of between-meal snacks | Low numbers of *Streptococcus mutans* and lactobacilli | Normal secretion rate and buffering capacity |
| High caries risk (unfavorable prognosis) | Plaque present | Frequent intake of sucrose in the form of caries-accelerating snacks | High numbers of *Streptococcus mutans* and lactobacilli | Low secretion rate and buffering capacity |

*Note:* The caries risk indicates the caries activity at the time of the examination and for the coming period. It is based on the evaluation of anamnestic, clinical, and laboratory data. The caries risk is expressed as high, low, or levels in between.

From Nyman, S., Bratthall, D., and Böhlin, E., The Swedish dental health programme for adults, *Int. Dent. J.*, 34, 130, 1984.

to dysfunctions of separate salivary glands, glandular saliva may be studied. Concerning dental caries, separate glandular analyses are perhaps not quite that important, since most of the relationship between secretion rate and caries has been observed for whole saliva.[10] With the exception of the study of Shannon and Terry,[190] no relationship with caries has been found for parotid and submandibular saliva.[10]

In conclusion, standardized salivary tests may be recommended for prediction of the caries risk when the number of new lesions tends to increase, or when a high caries risk may be expected because of, for example, certain diseases and substantial changes of various habits. In addition, salivary tests should be performed and analyzed before planning an extensive and expensive restorative therapy.

## V. CONCLUSIONS

The salivary secretion rate is affected by many different factors. Gustatory stimulation with a sour product is the best example among the local stimulants. Drugs with an anti-cholinergic effect and diuretics may reduce the salivary flow significantly, as well as ra-

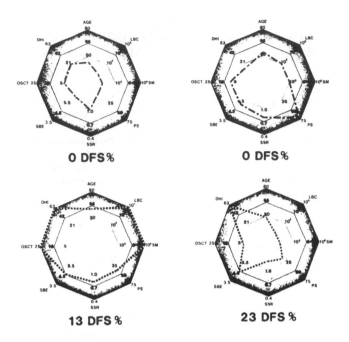

FIGURE 18.  Graphic illustration of various factors considered to be related to the dental caries risk. The following 8 variables were examined at the end of a 4-year observation period: age of the patient (AGE, years), number of lactobacilli (LBC, log CFU/ml) and *Streptococcus mutans* (SM, log CFU/ml) in saliva, plaque score (PS, %), salivary secretion rate of paraffin-stimulated whole saliva (SSR, ml/min), salivary buffer effect (SBE, pH), oral sugar clearance time (OSCT, min), and dietary habit index (DHI, score). (After Ravald, N., Hamp, S.-E., and Birkhed, D., *J. Clin. Periodontol.*, 13, 758, 1986. With permission.)

diotherapy of the head and neck region. Among diseases, Sjögren's syndrome is the best documented for having a negative effect on salivary flow rate. Regarding the relationship between age and salivary flow in adults, the available data are rather conflicting. Some studies show a reduced secretion rate with increasing age, others not. In children, however, there is an increased salivary flow rate with age up to the age of 15. Many studies have shown a higher flow rate for men than for women, which probably depends on variation in the gland size. The nutritional status of a person can influence the salivary secretion rate to a certain extent. It seems likely, however, that these changes are relatively small unless the dietary deficiencies are very severe, as, for example, during long-term malnutrition. Other factors discussed in this chapter, like sex hormones, circannual and circadian rhythms, and the use of nicotine, seem to have no or only minor effect on the salivary flow rate.

The salivary buffer capacity and pH are mainly regulated by the carbonic acid/bicarbonate system. Both bicarbonate concentration and pH are strongly dependent on secretion rate. As a consequence, most variables that may influence the secretion rate negatively will also affect the buffer capacity and pH. In adults, the buffer capacity of both resting and stimulated whole saliva is significantly lower for females than for males. Similar sex differences have been observed also for children, adolescents, and 70-year-old subjects. The salivary buffer capacity is positively correlated with age but in females only. Also, pH may show the same trend. Possibly, diet may influence the buffer capacity, but such changes seem to require a relatively long time to become detectable. It is not known whether disease-related alterations in the buffer capacity and pH are caused by the disease per se or occur secondarily due to a changed salivary secretion rate. Low values, however, do not necessarily indicate impaired

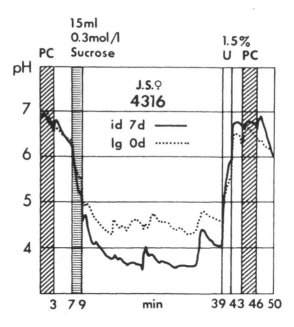

FIGURE 19. Continuous recording of interdental plaque pH (full line) during and 15 min after rinses with 10% sucrose solutions. Resting saliva is unable to stop the decrease in plaque pH during this period. (After Imfeld, T., in *Monographs in Oral Science,* Vol. 11, Howard, M. Myers, Eds., Philadelphia, 1983. With permission.)

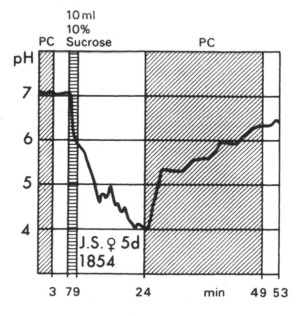

FIGURE 20. Continuous recordings of interdental plaque pH during and 15 min after rinses with 10% sucrose solutions. A quick rise in plaque pH is achieved by the chewing of neutral paraffin, which increases the salivary secretion rate and buffer capacity. (After Imfeld, T., in *Monographs in Oral Science,* Vol. 11, Howard, M. Meyers, Ed., Philadelphia, 1983. With permission.)

health. Cigarette smoking may also influence the buffer capacity and pH negatively. These changes appear to be unrelated to the secretion rate.

The relationship between salivary secretion rate, buffer capacity, and pH on one side and dental caries on the other is well known. In caries-active patients or in patients with a questionable caries risk, use of these salivary tests must be recommended, especially those measuring salivary flow rate and buffer capacity, for a better prediction of the caries risk. In addition, the tests should always be performed before planning an extensive and expensive restorative therapy.

# REFERENCES

1. **McNamara, T. F., Friedman, B. K., and Roth, P.,** Salivary access as an ecological determinant, in *Proceedings Saliva and Dental Caries,* Kleinberg, I., Ellison, S. A., and Mandel, I. D., Eds., Information Retrieval, New York, 1979, 211.
2. **Sweeney, E. A.,** Salivary flow and composition in relation to dental caries — methods and problems in studying this relationship in humans and animals, in *Proceedings Saliva and Dental Caries,* Kleinberg, I., Ellison, S. A., and Mandel, I. D., Eds., Information Retrieval, New York, 1979, 183.
3. **Mason, D. K. and Chisholm, D. M.,** *Salivary Glands in Health and Disease,* W. B. Saunders, London, 1975.
4. **Mandel, I. D. and Wotman, S.,** The salivary secretions in health and disease, *Oral Sci. Rev.,* 8, 25, 1976.
5. **Imfeld, T.,** Oligosialie und Xerostomie I: Grundlagen, Epidemiologie, Ätiologie, Pathologie, *Schweiz. Mschr. Zahnmed.,* 94, 741, 1984.
6. **Fox, P. C., van der Ven, P. F., Sonies, B. C., Weiffenbach, J. M., and Baum, J. B.,** Xerostomia: evaluation of a symptom with increasing significance, *J. Am. Dent. Assoc.,* 110, 519, 1985.
7. **Jenkins, G. N.,** Salivary effects on plaque pH, in *Proceedings Saliva and Dental Caries,* Kleinberg, I., Ellison, S. A., and Mandel, I. D., Eds., Information Retrieval, New York, 1979, 307.
8. **Ericsson, Y.,** Clinical investigations of the salivary buffering action, *Acta Odontol. Scand.,* 17, 131, 1959.
9. **Ericsson, Y. and Hardwick, L.,** Individual diagnosis, prognosis and counselling for caries prevention, *Caries Res.,* 12 (Suppl. 1), 94, 1978.
10. **Sreebny, L. M.,** Salivary flow and dental caries, in *Cariology Today,* Guggenheim, B., Ed., Karger, Basel, 1984, 56.
11. **Kerr, A. C.,** The physiological regulation of salivary secretions in man. A study of the response of human salivary glands to reflex stimulation, *International Series of Monographs on Oral Biology,* Vol. I, 1961.
12. **Heintze, U., Birkhed, D., and Björn, H.,** Secretion rate and buffer effect of resting and stimulated whole saliva as a function of age and sex, *Swed. Dent. J.,* 7, 227, 1983.
13. **Crossner, C.-G.,** Salivary flow rate in children and adolescents, *Swed. Dent. J.,* 8, 271, 1984.
14. **White, K. D.,** Salivation: a review and experimental investigation of major techniques, *Physiology,* 14, 203, 1977.
15. **Navazesh, M. and Christensen, C. M.,** A comparison of whole mouth resting and stimulated salivary measurement procedures, *J. Dent. Res.,* 61, 1158, 1982.
16. **Ericson, T. and Mäkinen, K. K.,** Saliva — formation, composition and possible role, in *Textbook of Cariology,* Thylstrup, A. and Fejerskov, O., Eds., Munksgaard, Copenhagen, 1986, chap. 3.
17. **Becks, H. and Wainwright, W. W.,** Human saliva. IX. The effect of activation on salivary flow, *J. Dent. Res.,* 18, 447, 1939.
18. **Andersson, R., Arvidsson, E., Crossner, C.-G., Holm, A.-K., Månsson, B., and Grahnén, H.,** The flow rate, pH and buffer effect of mixed saliva in children, *J. Int. Assoc. Dent. Child.,* 5, 5, 1974.
19. **Österberg, T., Landahl, S., and Hedegård, B.,** Salivary flow, saliva, pH and buffering capacity in 70-year-old men and women. Correlation to dental health, dryness in the mouth, disease and drug treatment, *J. Oral Rehab.,* 11, 157, 1984.
20. **Lashley, K. S.,** The human salivary reflex and its use in psychology, *Psychol. Rev.,* 23, 446, 1916.
21. **Lashley, K. S.,** Reflex secretion of the human parotid gland, *J. Exp. Psychol.,* 1, 461, 1916.
22. **Enfors, B.,** The parotid and submandibular secretion in man. Quantitative recordings of the normal and pathological activity, *Acta Oto-Laryngol., Suppl.,* 172, 1962.
23. **Dawes, C.,** The composition of human saliva secreted in response to a gustatory stimulus and to pilocarpine, *J. Physiol. (London),* 183, 360, 1966.

24. **Ericson, S.,** The parotid gland in subjects with and without rheumatoid arthritis. A sialographic and physiologic study, *Acta Radiol., Suppl.* 275, 1968.

25. **Ericson, S.,** An investigation of human parotid saliva secretion rate in response to different types of stimulation, *Arch. Oral Biol.,* 14, 591, 1969.

26. **Schneyer, L. H.,** Method for the collection of separate submaxillary and sublingual salivas in man, *J. Dent. Res.,* 32, 257, 1953.

27. **Henriques, B. L. and Chauncey, H. H.,** A modified method for the collection of human submaxillary and sublingual saliva, *Oral Surg.,* 9, 1124, 1961.

28. **Wolf, R. O.,** Regulated vacuum system for collecting submaxillary and sublingual saliva, *J. Dent. Res.,* 43, 303, 1964.

29. **Stephen, K. W., Lamb, A. B., and McCrossan, J.,** A modified appliance for the collection of human submandibular and sublingual salivas, *Arch. Oral Biol.,* 23, 835, 1978.

30. **Coudert, J. L., Lissac, M., and Parret, J.,** A new appliance for the collection of human submandibular saliva, *Arch. Oral Biol.,* 31, 411, 1986.

31. **Schneyer, L. H., Pigman, W., Hanahan, L., and Gilmore, R. W.,** Rate of flow of human parotid sublingual and submaxillary secretions during sleep, *J. Dent. Res.,* 35, 109, 1956.

32. **Louridis, O., Demetriou, N., and Bazopoulou-Kyrkanides, E.,** Chewing effects on secretion rate of stimulated human mixed saliva, *J. Dent. Res.,* 49, 1132, 1970.

33. **Schneyer, L. H. and Levin, L. K.,** Rate of secretion by exogenously stimulated salivary gland pairs of man, *J. Appl. Physiol.,* 7, 609, 1955.

34. **Chauncey, H. H. and Shannon, I. L.,** Parotid gland secretion rate as method for measuring response to gustatory stimuli in humans, *Proc. Soc. Exp. Biol. Med.,* 103, 459, 1960.

35. **Dawes, C. and Jenkins, G. N.,** The effects of different stimuli on the composition of saliva in man, *J. Physiol. (London),* 170, 86, 1964.

36. **Feller, R. P., Sharon, I. M., Chauncey, H. H., and Shannon, I. L.,** Gustatory perception of sour, sweet, and salt mixtures using parotid gland flow rate, *J. Appl. Physiol.,* 20, 1341, 1965.

37. **Ericson, S.,** The variability of the human parotid flow rate on stimulation with citric acid, with special reference to taste, *Arch. Oral Biol.,* 16, 9, 1971.

38. **Speirs, R. L.,** The effects of interactions between gustatory stimuli on the reflex flow-rate of human parotid saliva, *Arch. Oral Biol.,* 16, 351, 1971.

39. **Shannon, I. L.,** Reference table for human parotid saliva collected at varying levels of exogenous stimulation, *J. Dent. Res.,* 52, 1157, 1973.

40. **Lagerlöf, F. and Dawes, C.,** Effect of sucrose as a gustatory stimulus on the flow rates of parotid and whole saliva, *Caries Res.,* 19, 206, 1985.

41. **Krasse, B.,** Amount, pH, buffer effect, and amylolytic activity of parotid saliva between and immediately following meals, *J. Dent. Res.,* 40, 433, 1961.

42. **Heintze, U. and Birkhed, D.,** Influence of a single intake of various test meals on secretion rate, buffer effect, and electrolytes of human stimulated whole saliva, *Caries Res.,* 18, 265, 1984.

43. **Dawes, C. and Chebib, F. S.,** The influence of previous stimulation and the day of the week on the concentrations of protein and the main electrolytes in human parotid saliva, *Arch. Oral Biol.,* 17, 1289, 1972.

44. **Dawes, C.,** Effects of diet on salivary secretion and composition, *J. Dent. Res.,* 49, 1263, 1970.

45. **Johansson, I.,** The Effect of Malnutrition on Saliva Composition and Caries Development, Umeå University Odontological Dissertations, 1986.

46. **Hall, D. H., Merig, J. J., Jr., and Schneyer, C. A.,** Metrecal-induced changes in human saliva, *Proc. Soc. Exp. Biol. Med.,* 124, 532, 1967.

47. **Johansson, I., Ericson, T., and Steen, L.,** Studies on the effect of diet on saliva secretion and caries development: the effect of fasting on saliva composition of female subjects, *J. Nutr.,* 114, 2010, 1984.

48. **Johansson, I. and Ericson, T.,** Effect of chewing on the secretion of salivary components during fasting, *Caries Res.,* 20, 141, 1986.

49. **Birkhed, D., Heintze, U., Edwardsson, S., and Aly, K.-O.,** Short term fasting and lactovegetarian diet does not affect human saliva, *Scand. J. Dent. Res.,* 92, 408, 1984.

50. **de Muñiz, B. R., Maresca, B. M., Tumilasci, O. R., and Perec, C. J.,** Effects of an experimental diet on parotid saliva and dental plaque pH in institutionalized children, *Arch. Oral Biol.,* 28, 575, 1983.

51. **Smeds, M.,** A Survey of Some Salivary Characteristics of Vegetarians. Determination of Flow Rate, Buffer Capacity and Calcium Concentration. Unpublished.

52. **Ravald, N. and Lindström, G.,** Salivegenskaper och tandstatus hos vegetarianer, *Tandlaekartidningen,* 74, 576, 1982.

53. **Linkosalo, E., Ohtonen, S., Markkanen, H., Karinpää, A., and Kumpusalo, E.,** Caries, periodontal status and some salivary factors in lactovegetarians, *Scand. J. Dent. Res.,* 93, 304, 1985.

54. **Johansson, G., Heintze, U., and Birkhed, D.,** Long term effects of a change from a mixed to a lacto-vegetarian diet on human saliva, Abstr. from 1st Int. Congr. on Vegetarian Nutrition, Loma Linda, 1987.

55. **Parvinen, T. and Larmas, M.,** The relation of stimulated salivary flow rate and pH to lactobacillus and yeast concentrations in saliva, *J. Dent. Res.,* 60, 1929, 1981.
56. **Parvinen, T. and Larmas, M.,** Age dependency of stimulated salivary flow rate, pH, and lactobacillus and yeast concentrations, *J. Dent. Res.,* 61, 1052, 1982.
57. **Ben-Aryeh, H., Miron, D., Szargel, R., and Gutman, D.,** Whole-saliva secretion rates in old and young healthy subjects, *J. Dent. Res.,* 63, 1147, 1984.
58. **Heft, M. W. and Baum, B. J.,** Unstimulated and stimulated parotid salivary flow rate in individuals in different ages, *J. Dent. Res.,* 63, 1182, 1984.
59. **Pedersen, W., Schubert, M., Izutsu, K., Mersai, T., and Truelove, E.,** Age-dependent decreases in human submandibular gland flow rates as measured under resting and post-stimulation conditions, *J. Dent. Res.,* 64, 822, 1985.
60. **Andersson, R.,** The flow rate, pH and buffer effect of mixed saliva in schoolchildren, *Odontol. Revy,* 23, 421, 1972.
61. **Klock, B. and Krasse, B.,** Microbial and salivary conditions in 9- to 12-year-old children, *Scand. J. Dent. Res.,* 85, 56, 1977.
62. **Scott, J.,** Age, sex and contralateral differences in the volumes of human submandibular salivary glands, *Arch. Oral Biol.,* 20, 885, 1975.
63. **Dawes, C., Cross, H. G., Baker, C. G., and Chebib, F. S.,** The influence of gland size on the flow rate and composition of human parotid saliva, *Dent. J.,* 44, 21, 1973.
64. **Andrew, W.,** A comparison of age changes in salivary glands of man and of the rat, *J. Gerontol.,* 7, 178, 1952.
65. **Scott, J.,** Quantitative age changes in the histological structure of human submandibular salivary glands, *Arch. Oral Biol.,* 22, 221, 1977.
66. **Scott, J.,** A morphometric study of age changes in the histology of the ducts of human submandibular glands, *Arch. Oral Biol.,* 22, 243, 1977.
67. **Scott, J.,** The proportional volume of mucous acinar cells in normal human submandibular salivary glands, *Arch. Oral Biol.,* 24, 479, 1979.
68. **Scott, J.,** Age, sex and contralateral differences in the volumes of human submandibular salivary glands, *Arch. Oral Biol.,* 20, 885, 1975.
69. **Baum, B. J.,** Evaluation of stimulated parotid saliva flow rate in different age groups, *J. Dent. Res.,* 60, 1292, 1981.
70. **Chauncey, H. H., Borkan, G. A., Wayler, A. H., Feller, R. P., and Kapur, K. K.,** Parotid fluid composition in healthy aging males, *Adv. Physiol. Sci.,* 28, 323, 1981.
71. **Bertram, U.,** Xerostomia. Clinical aspects, pathology and pathogenesis, *Acta Odontol. Scand.,* 25 (Suppl. 49), 1967.
72. **Meyer, J., Golden, J. S., Steiner, N., and Necheles, H.,** The ptyalin content of human saliva in old age, *Am. J. Physiol.,* 119, 600, 1937.
73. **Drummond, J. R. and Chisholm, D. M.,** A qualitative and quantitative study of the ageing human labial salivary glands, *Arch. Oral Biol.,* 29, 151, 1984.
74. **Syrjänen, S.,** Age-related changes in structure of labial minor salivary glands, *Age Ageing,* 13, 159, 1984.
75. **Östlund, G:son, S.,** Palatine glands and mucin factors influencing the retention of complete dentures, *Odontol. Tidskr.,* 62, 1, 1953.
76. **Kullander, S. and Sonesson, B.,** Studies on saliva in menstruating, pregnant and post-menopausal women, *Acta Endocrinol. (Copenhagen),* 48, 329, 1965.
77. **Hugoson, A.,** Salivary secretion in pregnancy. A longitudinal study of flow rate, total protein, sodium, potassium and calcium concentration in parotid saliva from pregnant women, *Acta Odontol. Scand.,* 30, 49, 1972.
78. **Laine, M., Tenovuo, J., Lehtonen, O.-P., Ojanotko-Harri, A., Vilja, P., and Tuohimaa, P.,** Pregnancy-related changes in human whole saliva, *Arch. Oral Biol.,* in press, 1988.
79. **Magnusson, I., Ericson, T., and Hugoson, A.,** The effect of oral contraceptives on the concentration of some salivary substances in women, *Arch. Oral Biol.,* 20, 119, 1975.
80. **Emmelin, N.,** Control of salivary glands, *Oral Physiol.,* 20, 1, 1972.
81. **Bahn, S. L.,** Drug-related dental destruction, *Oral Surg.,* 33, 49, 1972.
82. **Rydgren, K.-O.,** Side-effects of odontological interest of psychopharmaco-therapy, *Swed. Dent. J.,* 69, 85, 1976.
83. **Mandel, I. D.,** Sialochemistry in diseases and clinical situations affecting salivary glands, *Clin. Lab. Sci.,* 12, 321, 1980.
84. **Parvinen, T., Parvinen, I., and Larmas, M.,** Stimulated salivary flow rate, pH and lactobacillus and yeast concentrations in medicated persons, *Scand. J. Dent. Res.,* 92, 524, 1984.
85. **Johnson, G., Barenthin, I., and Westphal, P.,** Mouthdryness among patients in longterm hospitals, *Gerodontology,* 3, 197, 1984.

86. **Rundegren, J., van Dijken, J., Mörnstad, H., and von Knorring, L.,** Oral conditions in patients receiving long-term treatment with cyclic antidepressant drugs, *Swed. Dent. J.,* 9, 55, 1985.

87. **Molander, L. and Birkhed, D.,** Effect of single oral doses of various neuroleptic drugs on salivary secretion rate, pH, and buffer capacity in healthy subjects, *Psychopharmacology,* 75, 114, 1981.

88. **Rafaelsen, O. J., Clemmesen, L., Lund, H., Mikkelsen, P. L., and Bolwig, T. G.,** Comparison of peripheral anticholinergic effects of antidepressants: dry mouth, *Acta Psychiatr. Scand.,* 63, 364, 1981.

89. **Mikkelsen, P. L., Clemmesen, L., Lund, H., Bolwig, T. G., and Rafaelsen, O. J.,** Hyposalivation after single doses of antidepressants, *Int. Pharmacopsychiat.* 17 (Suppl. 1), 35, 1982.

90. **Clemmesen, L., Mikkelsen, P. L., Lund, H., Bolwig, T. G., and Rafaelsen, O. J.,** Assessment of the anticholinergic effects of antidepressant in a single-dose cross-over study of salivation and plasma levels, *Psychopharmacology,* 82, 348, 1984.

91. **Bertram, U., Kragh-Sørensen, P., Rafaelson, O. J., and Larsen, N.-E.,** Saliva secretion following long-term antidepressant treatment with nortriptyline controlled by plasma levels, *Scand. J. Dent. Res.,* 87, 58, 1979.

92. **von Knorring, L.,** Changes in saliva secretion and accommodation width during short-term administration of imipramine and zimelidine in healthy volunteers, *Int. Pharmacopsychiat.,* 16, 69, 1981.

93. **von Knorring, L. and Mörnstad, H.,** Qualitative changes in saliva composition after short-term administration of imipramine and zimelidine in healthy volunteers, *Scand. J. Dent. Res.,* 89, 313, 1981.

94. **Di Cugno, F., Perec, C. J., and Tocci, A. A.,** Salivary secretion and dental caries experience in drug addicts, *Arch. Oral Biol.,* 26, 363, 1981.

95. **Scheutz, F.,** Saliva secretion rate in a group of drug addicts, *Scand. J. Dent. Res.,* 92, 496, 1984.

96. **Pangborn, R. M. and Sharon, I. M.,** Visual deprivation and parotid response to cigarette smoking, *Physiol. Behav.,* 6, 559, 1971.

97. **Winsor, A. L.,** The effect of cigarette smoking on secretion, *J. Gen. Psychol.,* 6, 190, 1932.

98. **Korting, G. W. and Kleinschmidt, W.,** Veränderungen der Speichelsekretion bei Hautkrankheiten, *Dermatol. Wochenschr.,* 128, 772, 1953.

99. **Barylko-Pikielna, N., Pangborn, R. M., and Shannon, I. L.,** Effect of cigarette smoking on parotid secretion, *Arch. Environ. Health,* 17, 731, 1968.

100. **Heintze, U.,** Secretion rate, buffer effect and number of lactobacilli and *Streptococcus mutans* of whole saliva of cigarette smokers and non-smokers, *Scand. J. Dent. Res.,* 92, 294, 1984.

101. **Parvinen, T.,** Stimulated salivary flow rate, pH and lactobacillus and yeast concentrations in non-smokers and smokers, *Scand. J. Dent. Res.,* 92, 315, 1984.

102. **Olson, B. L., McDonald, J. L., Gleason, M. J., Jr., Stookey, G. K., Schemehorn, B. R., Drook, C. A., Beiswanger, B. B., and Christen, A. G.,** Comparisons of various salivary parameters in smokers before and after the use of a nicotine-containing chewing gum, *J. Dent. Res.,* 64, 826, 1985.

103. **Dunér-Engström, M., Larsson, O., Lundberg, J., and Fredholm, B. B.,** Effect of nicotine chewing gum on salivary secretion, *Swed. Dent. J.,* 10, 93, 1986.

104. **Wotman, S. and Mandel, I. D.,** The salivary secretion in health and disease, in *Diseases of the Salivary Glands,* Rankow, R. M. and Polayes, I. M., Eds., W. B. Saunders, Philadelphia, 1976, chap. 3.

105. **Heintze, U., Frostell, G., Lindgärde, F., and Trell, E.,** Secretion rate and buffer effect of resting and stimulated whole saliva in relation to general health, *Swed. Dent. J.,* 10, 213, 1986.

106. **Chisholm, D. M. and Mason, D. K.,** Salivary gland function in Sjögren's syndrome, *Br. Dent. J.,* 135, 393, 1973.

107. **Mandel, I. D. and Baurmash, H.,** Sialochemistry in Sjögren's syndrome, *Oral Surg.,* 41, 182, 1976.

108. **Ben-Aryeh, H., Spielman, A., Szargel, R., Gutman, D., Scharf, J., Nahir, M., and Scharf, Y.,** Sialochemistry for diagnosis of Sjögren's syndrome in xerostomic patients, *Oral Surg.,* 52, 487, 1981.

109. **Stuchell, R. N., Mandel, I. D., and Baurmash, H.,** Clinical utilization of sialochemistry in Sjögren's syndrome, *J. Oral Pathol.,* 13, 303, 1984.

110. **Jonsson, R., Bratthall, D., and Nyberg, G.,** Histologic and sialochemical findings indicating sicca syndrome in patients with systemic lupus erythematosus, *Oral Surg.,* 54, 635, 1982.

111. **Ericson, S.,** The prevalance of hyposalivation in rheumatoid arthritis and its relation to the sialographic appearance of the parotid glands, *Oral Surg.,* 38, 315, 1974.

112. **Syrjänen, S.,** Salivary glands in rheumatoid arthritis, *Proc. Finn. Dent. Soc.,* 78 (Suppl. 3), 1982.

113. **Tenovuo, J., Alanen, P., Larjava, H., Viikari, J., and Lehtonen, O.-P.,** Oral health of patients with insulin-dependent diabetes mellitus, *Scand. J. Dent. Res.,* 94, 338, 1986.

114. **Tenovuo, J., Lehtonen, O.-P., Viikari, J., Larjava, H., Vilja, P., and Tuohimaa, P.,** Immunoglobulins and innate antimicrobial factors in whole saliva of patients with insulin-dependent diabetes mellitus, *J. Dent. Res.,* 65, 62, 1986.

115. **Marder, M. Z., Abelson, D. C., and Mandel, I. D.,** Salivary alterations in diabetes mellitus, *J. Periodontol.,* 46, 567, 1975.

116. **Sharon, A., Ben-Aryeh, H., Itzhak, B., Yoran, K., Szarger, R., and Gutman, O.,** Salivary composition in diabetic patients, *J. Oral Med.,* 40, 23, 1985.

117. **Conner, S., Iranpour, B., and Mills, J.,** Alteration in parotid salivary flow in diabetes mellitus, *Oral Surg.*, 30, 55, 1970.

118. **Kjellman, O.,** Secretion rate and buffering action of whole mixed saliva in subjects with insulin-treated diabetes mellitus, *Odontol. Revy*, 21, 159, 1970.

119. **Shafer, W. G. and Muhler, J. C.,** Endocrine influence upon the salivary glands, *Ann. N.Y. Acad. Sci.*, 85, 215, 1960.

120. **Xhonga, F. A. and VanHerle, A.,** The influence of hyperthyroidism on dental erosions, *Oral Surg.*, 36, 349, 1973.

121. **Schneyer, L. H. and Tanchester, D.,** Some oral aspects of radioactive iodine therapy for thyroid disease, *N.Y. J. Dent.*, 24, 308, 1954.

122. **Mason, D. K., Harden, McG., R., and Alexander, W. D.,** The salivary and thyroid glands, *Br. Dent. J.*, 122, 485, 1967.

123. **Brown, C. C.,** The parotid puzzle: a review of the literature on human salivation and its applications to psychophysiology, *Psychophysiology*, 7, 66, 1970.

124. **Bolwig, T. G. and Rafaelsen, O. J.,** Salivation in affective disorders, *Psychol. Med.*, 2, 232, 1972.

125. **Palmai, G., Blackwell, B., Maxwell, A. E., and Morgenstern, F.,** Patterns of salivary flow in depressive illness and during treatment, *Br. J. Psychiatry*, 113, 1297, 1967.

126. **Wotman, S., Mandel, I. D., Thompson, R. H., Jr., and Laragh, J. H.,** Salivary electrolytes, urea nitrogen, uric acid and salt taste thresholds in hypertension, *J. Oral Ther. Pharmacol.*, 3, 239, 1967.

127. **Ben-Aryeh, H., Schiller, M., Shasha, S., Szargel, R., and Gutman, D.,** Salivary composition in patients with essential hypertension and the effect of pindolol, *J. Oral Med.*, 36, 76, 1981.

128. **van Hooff, M., van Baak, M. A., Schols, M., and Rahn, K. H.,** Studies of salivary flow in borderline hypertension: effects of drugs acting on structures innervated by the autonomic nervous system, *Clin. Sci.*, 66, 599, 1984.

129. **Skurk, A., Krebs, S., and Rehberg, J.,** Flow rate, protein, amylase, lysozyme and kallikrein of human parotid saliva in health and disease, *Arch. Oral Biol.*, 24, 739, 1979.

130. **Blum, A. L.,** Salivary secretion in duodenal ulcer disease, *Gut*, 13, 713, 1972.

131. **Descos, L., Lambert, R., and Minaire, Y.,** Comparison of human salivary secretion in health and chronic pancreatitis, *Digestion*, 9, 76, 1973.

132. **Kakizaki, G., Noto, N., Saito, T., Fujiwara, Y., Ohizumi, T., Soeno, T., and Ishidate, T.,** Laboratory diagnosis test for pancreatic disorders by examination of parotid saliva, *Tohoku J. Exp. Med.*, 109, 121, 1973.

133. **Dobrilla, G., Valentini, M., Fillipini, M., Bonoldi, M. C., Felder, M., and Moroder, E.,** The study of parotid and mixed saliva in the diagnosis of chronic pancreatitis, *Ir. J. Med. Sci.*, 146 (Suppl. 13), 1977.

134. **Dobrilla, G., Valentini, M., Fillipini, M., Bonoldi, M., Felder, M. C., Moroder, E., Schnabl, D., and Gaspa, U.,** Study of parotid and mixed saliva in the diagnosis of chronic pancreatitis, *Digestion*, 19, 180, 1979.

135. **Abelson, D. C., Mandel, I. D., and Karmiol, M.,** Salivary studies in alcoholic cirrhosis, *Oral Surg.*, 41, 188, 1976.

136. **Lundström, I. M. C., Anneroth, G. B., and Bergstedt, H. F.,** Salivary gland function and changes in patients with oral lichen planus, *Scand. J. Dent. Res.*, 90, 443, 1982.

137. **Gandara, B. K., Izutsu, K. T., Truelove, E. L., Ensign, W. Y., and Sommers, E. E.,** Age-related salivary flow rate changes in controls and patients with oral lichen planus, *J. Dent. Res.*, 64, 1149, 1985.

138. **Blomfield, J., Warton, K. L., and Brown, J. M.,** Flow rate and inorganic components of submandibular saliva in cystic fibrosis, *Arch. Dis. Child.*, 48, 267, 1973.

139. **Blomfield, J., Rush, A. R., Allars, H. M., and Brown, J. M.,** Parotid gland function in children with cystic fibrosis and child control subjects, *Pediat. Res.*, 6, 574, 1976.

140. **Worthington, J. J.,** Parotid enlargement bilaterally in a patient on thioridazine, *Am. J. Psychiatry*, 121, 813, 1965.

141. **Diamant, H., Ekstrand, I., and Wiberg, A.,** Prognosis of idiopathic Bell's palsy, *Arch. Otolaryngol.*, 95, 431, 1972.

142. **Davis, M. J.,** Parotid salivary secretion and composition in cerebral palsy, *J. Dent. Res.*, 58, 1808, 1979.

143. **Karmiol, M. and Walsh, R. F.,** Dental caries after radiotherapy of the oral regions, *J. Am. Dent. Assoc.*, 91, 838, 1975.

144. **Dreizen, S. and Brown, L. R.,** Xerostomia and dental caries, in *Proceedings Microbial Aspects of Dental Caries*, Stilles, Loesche, and O'Brien, Eds., Sp. Supp. Microbiology Abstracts, 1976, 263.

145. **Brown, L. R., Dreizen, S., Daly, T. E., Drane, J. B., Handler, S., Riggan, L. J., and Johnston, D. A.,** Interrelations of oral microorganisms, immunoglobulins, and dental caries following radiotherapy, *J. Dent. Res.*, 57, 882, 1978.

146. **Ben-Aryeh, H., Gutman, D., Szargel, R., and Laufer, D.,** Effects of irradiation on saliva in cancer patients, *Int. J. Oral Surg.*, 4, 205, 1975.

147. **Dreizen, S., Daley, T. E., Drane, J. B., and Brown, L. R.**, Oral complications of caries therapy, *Postgrad. Med.*, 61, 85, 1977.
148. **Shannon, I. L., Starcke, E. N., and Wescott, W. B.**, Effect of radiotherapy on whole saliva flow, *J. Dent. Res.*, 56, 693, 1977.
149. **Kashima, H. K., Kirkham, W. R., and Andrew, R. J.**, Postirradiation sialadenitis: a study of the clinical feature, histopathologic changes and serum enzyme variations following irradiation on human salivary glands, *Am. J. Roentgenol.*, 94, 271, 1965.
150. **Shannon, I. L., Trodahl, J. N., and Starcke, E. N.**, Radiosensitivity of the human parotid gland, *Proc. Soc. Exp. Biol. Med.*, 157, 50, 1978.
151. **Eneroth, C.-M., Henrikson, C. O., and Jakobsson, P. Å.**, The effect of irradiation in high doses on parotid glands, *Acta Oto-Laryngol.*, 71, 349, 1971.
152. **Mira, J. G., Wescott, W. B., Starcke, E. N., and Shannon, I. L.**, Some factors influencing salivary function when treating with radiotherapy, *Int. J. Radiat. Oncol. Biol.*, 7, 535, 1981.
153. **Enerth, C.-M., Henrikson, C. O., and Jakobsson, P. Å.**, Pre-irradiation qualities of a parotid gland predicting the grade of functional disturbance by radiotherapy, *Acta Oto-Laryngol.*, 74, 436, 1972.
154. **Wiesenfeld, D., Webster, G., Ferguson, M. M., MacFadyen, E. E., and MacFarlane, T. W.**, Salivary gland dysfunction following radioactive iodine therapy, *Oral Surg.*, 55, 138, 1983.
155. **Dawes, C.**, Rhythms in salivary flow rate and composition, *Int. J. Chronobiol.*, 2, 253, 1974.
156. **Shannon, I. L.**, Climatological effects on human parotid gland function, *Arch. Oral Biol.*, 11, 451, 1966.
157. **Dawes, C.**, Circadian rhythms in human salivary flow rate and composition, *J. Physiol. (London)*, 220, 529, 1972.
158. **Ferguson, D. B., Fort, A., Elliott, A. L., and Potts, A. J.**, Circadian rhythms in human parotid saliva flow rate and composition, *Arch. Oral Biol.*, 18, 1155, 1973.
159. **Dawes, C.**, Circadian rhythms in the flow rate and composition of unstimulated and stimulated human submandibular saliva, *J. Physiol. (London)*, 244, 535, 1975.
160. **Ferguson, D. B. and Botchway, C. A.**, Circadian variations in the flow rate and composition of whole saliva stimulated by mastication, *Arch. Oral Biol.*, 24, 877, 1980.
161. **Ericson, S.**, The importance of sialography for the determination of the parotid flow, *Acta Oto-Laryngol.*, 72, 437, 1971.
162. **Ericson, S., Hedin, M., and Wiberg, A.**, Variability of the submandibular flow rate in man with special reference to the size of the gland, *Odontol. Revy*, 23, 411, 1972.
163. **Dawes, C., Cross, H. G., Baker, C. G., and Chebib, F. S.**, The influence of gland size on the flow rate and composition of human parotid saliva, *Dent. J.*, 44, 21, 1978.
164. **Shannon, I. L.**, Body weight and parotid flow in the human, *J. Dent. Assoc. S. Afr.*, 23, 366, 1968.
165. **Mäkilä, E. and Vaaja, U.**, The relationship between the rate of flow, pH, buffer capacity and viscosity of the saliva and the number of extracted teeth, *Suom. Hammaslääk. Toim.*, 62, 195, 1966.
166. **Mäkilä, E.**, Properties of saliva in edentulous persons before and after wearing complete dentures. A longitudinal study, *Suom. Hammaslääk. Toim.*, 65, 115, 1969.
167. **Lantzman Gabay, E.**, Flow rate, sodium and potassium concentration in mixed saliva of complete denture-wearers, *J. Oral Rehabil.*, 7, 435, 1980.
168. **Parvinen, T.**, Stimulated salivary flow rate, pH and lactobacillus and yeast concentrations in persons with different types of dentition, *Scand. J. Dent. Res.*, 92, 412, 1984.
169. **Le Bell, Y., Söderling, E., Kirveskari, P., and Alanen, P.**, Flow rate, pH and buffer capacity of whole saliva before and after treatment of TMJ dysfunction, *Proc. Finn. Dent. Soc.*, 81, 226, 1985.
170. **Navazesh, M. and Ship, I. I.**, Xerostomia: diagnosis and treatment, *Am. J. Otolaryngol.*, 4, 283, 1983.
171. **Glass, J. B., Van Dis, M. L., Langlais, R. P., and Miles, D. A.**, Xerostomia: diagnosis and treatment planning considerations, *Oral Surg.*, 58, 248, 1984.
172. **Baum, B. J.**, Salivary gland function during aging, *Gerodontics*, 2, 61, 1986.
173. **Sonis, S. T., Sonis, A. L., and Lieberman, A.**, Oral complications in patients receiving treatment for malignancies other than of the head and neck, *J. Am. Dent. Assoc.*, 97, 468, 1978.
174. **Chen, M.-S., and Daly, T. E.**, Xerostomia and complete denture retention, *Tex. Dent. J.*, 97(9), 1979.
175. **Imfeld, T.**, Oligosialie und Xerostomie II: Diagnose, Prophylaxe und Behandlung, *Schweiz. Mschr. Zahnmed.*, 94, 1083, 1984.
176. **Shannon, I. L., McCrary, B. R., and Starcke, E. N.**, A saliva substitute for use by xerostomic patients undergoing radiotherapy to the head and neck, *Oral Surg.*, 44, 656, 1977.
177. **Nakamoto, R. Y.**, Use of a saliva substitute in postradiation xerostomia, *J. Prosthet. Dent.*, 42, 539, 1979.
178. **Shannon, I. L.**, A saliva substitute for dry mouth relief, in *Geriatric Dentistry*, Toga, C. J., Nandy, K., and Chaunsey, H. H., Eds., Lexington Books, Toronto, 1979, chap. 12.
179. **Klestov, A. C., Webb, J., Latt, D., Schiller, G., McNamara, K., Young, D. Y., Hobbes, J., and Fetherston, J.**, Treatment of xerostomia: a double-blind trial in 108 patients with Sjögren's syndrome, *Oral Surg.*, 51, 594, 1981.

180. s'Gravenmade, E. J. and Panders, A. K., Clinical applications of saliva substitutes, *Front. Oral Physiol.*, 3, 154, 1981.

181. Spielman, A., Ben-Aryeh, H., Gutman, D., Szargel, R., and Deutsch, E., Xerostomia — diagnosis and treatment, *Oral Surg.*, 51, 144, 1981.

182. Weisz, A. S., The use of a saliva substitute as treatment for xerostomia in Sjögren's syndrome — a case report, *Oral Surg.*, 51, 384, 1981.

183. Donatsky, O., Johnsen, T., Holmstrup, P., and Bertram, U., Effect of Saliment® on parotid salivary gland secretion and on xerostomia caused by Sjögren's syndrome, *Scand. J. Dent. Res.*, 90, 157, 1982.

184. Roberts, B. J., Help for the dry mouth patient, *J. Dent.*, 10, 226, 1982.

185. Epstein, J. B., Decoteau, W. E., and Wilkinson, A., Effect of Sialor in treatment of xerostomia in Sjögren's syndrome, *Oral Surg.*, 56, 495, 1983.

186. Vissink, A., s'Gravenmade, E. J., Panders, A. K., Vermey, A., Petersen, J. K., Visch, L. L., and Schaub, R. M. H., A clinical comparison between commercially available mucin- and CMC-containing saliva substitutes, *Int. J. Oral Surg.*, 12, 232, 1983.

187. Wiesenfeld, D., Stewart, A. M., and Mason, D. K., A critical assessment of oral lubricants in patients with xerostomia, *Br. Dent. J.*, 155, 155, 1983.

188. s'Gravenmade, E. J., Vissink, A., Panders, A. K., and Vermey, A., Artificial saliva in the management of patients suffering from xerostomia, *Gerodontology*, 3, 243, 1984.

189. Mandel, I. D., Relation of saliva and plaque to caries, *J. Dent. Res.*, 53, 246, 1974.

190. Shannon, I. L. and Terry, J. M., A higher parotid fluid flow rate in subjects with resistance to caries, *J. Dent. Med.*, 20, 128, 1965.

191. Kapsimalis, P., Rosenthal, S. L., Updegrave, W., Evans, R., Hurley, B., and Cobe, H. M., The relationship between caries activity, flow rate, total nitrogen and the mucin content of saliva, *J. Oral Med.*, 21, 107, 1966.

192. Rovelstad, G. H., Salivary components and their relationship to oral disease, in *Environmental Variables in Oral Disease*, Kreshover, S. J. and McClure, F. J., Eds., AAAS, Washington, D.C., 1966, 75.

193. Turtola, L. O., Salivary fluoride and calcium concentrations, and their relationship to the secretion of saliva and caries experience, *Scand. J. Dent. Res.*, 85, 535, 1977.

194. Lehtonen, O.-P., Gråhn, E. M., Ståhlberg, T. H., and Laitinen, L. A., Amount and avidity of salivary and serum antibodies against *Streptococcus mutans* in two groups of human subjects with different dental caries susceptibility, *Infect. Immun.*, 43, 308, 1984.

195. Ericsson, Y., Hellström, I., Jared, B., and Stjernström, L., Investigations into the relationship between saliva and dental caries, *Acta Odontol. Scand.*, 11, 179, 1954.

196. Gurley, W. B., Unilateral dental caries: report of a case, *J. Am. Dent. Assoc.*, 26, 163, 1939.

197. Hill, F. J., Rampant caries and the salivary glands. A case report, *Dent. Pract. Dent. Rec.*, 22, 454, 1972.

198. Crossner, C.-G. and Holm, A.-K., A descriptive and comparative study of oral health in 8-year-old Swedish children, *Acta Odontol. Scand.*, 33, 135, 1975.

199. Crossner, C.-G. and Holm, A.-K., Saliva tests in the prognosis of caries in children, *Acta Odontol. Scand.*, 35, 135, 1977.

200. van Dijken, J., von Knorring, A. L., von Knorring, L., Mörnstad, H., Rundegren, J., and Wahlin, Y.-B., Antidepressiva läkemedel kan ge tandskador hos barn och vuxna, *Läkartidningen*, 78, 4366, 1981.

201. Ericson, Th., Nordblom, A., and Ekedahl, C., Effect on caries susceptibility after surgical treatment of drooling in patients with neurological disorders, *Acta Oto-Laryngol.*, 75, 71, 1973.

202. Englander, H. R., Shklair, I. L., and Fosdick, T. S., The effects of saliva on the pH and lactate concentration in dental plaque, *J. Dent. Res.*, 38, 848, 1959.

203. Kleinberg, I. and Jenkins, G. N., The pH of dental plaques on the different areas of the mouth before and after meals and their relationship to the pH and rate of flow of resting saliva, *Arch. Oral Biol.*, 9, 493, 1964.

204. Abelson, D. C. and Mandel, I. D., The effect of saliva on plaque pH *in vivo*, *J. Dent. Res.*, 60, 1634, 1981.

205. Lagerlöf, F., Dawes, R., and Dawes, R., Salivary clearance of sugar and its effect on pH changes by *Strep. mitior* in an artificial mouth, *J. Dent. Res.*, 63, 1266, 1984.

206. Dawes, C., A mathematic model of salivary clearance of sugar from the oral cavity, *Caries Res.*, 17, 321, 1983.

207. Lagerlöf, F. and Dawes, C., The effect of swallowing frequency on oral sugar clearance and pH changes by *Strep. mitior in vitro* after sugar ingestion, *J. Dent. Res.*, 64, 1229, 1985.

208. Lilienthal, B., Buffering systems in the mouth, *Oral Surg.*, 8, 828, 1955.

209. Dreizen, S., Mann, A. W., Cline, J. K., and Spies, T. D., The buffer capacity of saliva as a measure of dental caries activity, *J. Dent. Res.*, 25, 213, 1946.

210. Leung, S. W., A demonstration of the importance of bicarbonate as a salivary buffer, *J. Dent. Res.*, 30, 403, 1951.

211. **Sellman, S.,** The buffer value of saliva and its relation to dental caries, *Acta Odontol. Scand.,* 8, 244, 1950.
212. **Lilienthal, B.,** An analysis of the buffer systems in saliva, *J. Dent. Res.,* 34, 516, 1955.
213. **Izutsu, K. T.,** Theory and measurement of the buffer value of bicarbonate in saliva, *J. Theor. Biol.,* 90, 397, 1981.
214. **Helm, J. F., Dodds, W. J., Hogan, W. J., Soergel, K. H., Egide, M. S., and Wood, C.,** Acid neutralizing capacity of human saliva, *Gastroenterology,* 83, 69, 1982.
215. **Leung, S. W.,** The apparent first dissociation constant ($pK_1$) of carbonic acid in saliva, *Arch. Oral Biol.,* 5, 236, 1961.
216. **Grøn, P. and Messer, A. C.,** An investigation of the state of carbon dioxide in human saliva, *Arch. Oral Biol.,* 10, 757, 1965.
217. **Izutsu, K. T. and Madden, P. R.,** Evidence for the presence of carbamino compounds in human saliva, *J. Dent. Res.,* 57, 319, 1978.
218. **Kreusser, W., Heidland, A., Hennemann, H., Wigand, M. E., and Knauf, H.,** Mono- and divalent electrolyte patterns, $pCO_2$ and pH in relation to flow rate in normal human parotid saliva, *Eur. J. Clin. Invest.,* 2, 398, 1972.
219. **Dreizen, S., Reed, A. I., Nidermeier, W., and Spies, T. D.,** Sodium and potassium as constituents of human salivary buffers, *J. Dent. Res.,* 32, 497, 1953.
220. **Thaysen, J. H., Thorn, N. A., and Schwartz, I. L.,** Excretion of sodium, potassium, chloride and carbon dioxide in human parotid saliva, *Am. J. Physiol.,* 178, 155, 1954.
221. **Dawes, C.,** The effects of flow rate and duration of stimulation on the concentrations of protein and the main electrolytes in human parotid saliva, *Arch. Oral Biol.,* 14, 277, 1969.
222. **Parvinen, T.,** Flow rate, pH, and lactobacillus and yeast counts of stimulated whole saliva in adults, *Proc. Finn. Dent. Soc.,* 80, (Suppl. 10), 1985.
223. **Sullivan, J. H. and Storvick, C. A.,** Correlation of saliva analyses with dental examinations of 574 freshmen at Oregon state college, *J. Dent. Res.,* 29, 165, 1950.
224. **Chauncey, H. H., Lisanti, V. F., and Winer, R. A.,** Human parotid gland secretion: flow rate and interrelationship of pH and inorganic components, *Proc. Soc. Exp. Biol. Med.,* 97, 539, 1958.
225. **Shannon, I. L. and Prigmore, J. R.,** Parotid fluid flow rate. Its relationship to pH and chemical composition, *Oral Surg.,* 13, 1488, 1960.
226. **Agus, H. M. and Schamschula, R. G.,** Lithium content, buffering capacity and flow rate of saliva and caries experience of Australian children, *Caries Res.,* 17, 139, 1983.
227. **Sand, H. G.,** Source of the bicarbonate of saliva, *J. Appl. Physiol.,* 4, 66, 1951.
228. **Burgen, A. S. V. and Emmelin, N.,** *Physiology of the Salivary Glands,* Arnold, London, 1961.
229. **Niedermeier, W., Stone, R. E., Dreizen, S., and Spies, T. D.,** Effect of a 2-acetyl-amino-1,3,4, thiadiazole-5-sulfonamide (Diamox) on sodium, potassium, bicarbonate, and buffer content of saliva, *Proc. Soc. Exp. Med.,* 88, 273, 1955.
230. **Chauncey, H. H. and Weiss, P. A.,** Composition of human saliva. Parotid gland secretion, flow rate, pH and inorganic composition after oral administration of a carbonic anhydrase inhibitor, *Arch. Intern. Pharmacodyn,* 113, 377, 1958.
231. **Van Goor, H.,** Carbonic anhydrase, its properties, distribution and significance for carbon dioxide transport, *Enzymologia,* 13, 73, 1948.
232. **Yoshimura, H., Iwasaki, H., Nishikawa, T., and Matsumoto, S.,** Role of carbonic anhydrase in the bicarbonate excretion from salivary glands and mechanisms of ionic excretion, *Jpn. J. Physiol.,* 9, 106, 1959.
233. **Maren, T. H.,** Carbonic anhydrase: chemistry, physiology and inhibition, *Physiol. Rev.,* 47, 595, 1967.
234. **Anderson, D. J.,** The relationship between hydrogen-ion concentration and rate of flow of saliva, *J. Dent. Res.,* 28, 583, 1949.
235. **Hildes, J. A.,** Glandular secretion of electrolytes, *Can. J. Biochem. Physiol.,* 33, 481, 1955.
236. **Hildes, J. A. and Ferguson, M. H.,** The concentration of electrolytes in normal human saliva, *Can. J. Biochem. Physiol.,* 33, 217, 1955.
237. **Ericsson, Y.,** Enamel-Apatite Solubility, thesis, Stockholm, 1949.
238. **Rae, J. J. and Clegg, C. T.,** The relation between buffering capacity, viscosity and lactobacillus count of saliva, *J. Dent. Res.,* 28, 589, 1949.
239. **Feldman, H.,** Salivary buffer capacity, pH and stress, *J. Am. Soc. Psychosom. Dent. Med.,* 21, 25, 1974.
240. **Mann, A. W., Dreizen, S., Spies, T. D., and Hunt, F. M.,** A comparison of dental caries activity in malnourished and well-nourished patients, *J. Am. Dent. Assoc.,* 34, 244, 1947.
241. **Bratthall, D. and Hager, B.,** Enkel metod för bedömning av salivens buffringskapacitet samt sekretionshastighet, *Tandlaekartidningen,* 69, 677, 1977.
242. **Frostell, G.,** A colourimetric screening test for evaluation of the buffer capacity of saliva, *Swed. Dent. J.,* 4, 81, 1980.

243. **Wikner, S. and Nedlich, U.**, A clinical evaluation of the ability of the Dentobuff® method to estimate buffer capacity of saliva, *Swed. Dent. J.*, 9, 45, 1985.
244. **Linder, L., Sund, M. L., and Branting, C.**, Ett salivtest för bestämning av kariesriskfaktorer, *Tandlaekartidningen*, 77, 283, 1985.
245. **Dewar, M. R.**, Laboratory methods for assessing susceptibility to dental caries, *J. Dent. Austr.*, 21, 509, 1949.
246. **Jenkins, G. N.**, *The Physiology and Biochemistry of the Mouth*, 4th ed., Blackwell Scientific, Oxford, 1978.
247. **Ericson, T.**, Secretion of salivary glycoproteins, in *Oral Physiology*, Emmelin, N. and Zotterman, Y., Eds., Pergamon Press, Oxford, 1972, 75.
248. **Mörnstad, H., Ryberg, M., and Sjöström, R.**, Flow rate, pH and buffer capacity of chewing stimulated saliva in an adult population, *J. Dent. Res.*, 63, 303, 1984.
249. **Krasse, B.**, *Caries Risk: A Practical Guide for Assessment and Control*, Quintessence, Chicago, 1985.
250. **Söderling, E., Le Bell, Y., Alanen, P., and Kirveskari, P.**, Salivary buffer systems and the Dentobuff® test, *Proc. Finn. Dent. Soc.*, 81, 284, 1985.
251. **Suddick, R. P., Hyde, R. J., and Feller, R. P.**, Salivary water and electrolytes and oral health, in *The Biologic Basis of Dental Caries*, Menaker, L., Ed., Harper & Row, New York, 1980.
252. **Forbes, J. C. and Gurley, W. B.**, Effect of diet on the acid-neutralizing power of saliva, *J. Dent. Res.*, 12, 637, 1932.
253. **Wills, J. H. and Forbes, J. C.**, Dietary effects upon the acid neutralising power of the saliva, *J. Dent. Res.*, 18, 409, 1939.
254. **Swenander Lanke, L.**, Salivens buffringsförmåga i relation till kariesaktivitet och olika kost, *Sven. Tandlaek. Tidskr.*, 45, 255, 1952.
255. **Swenander Lanke, L.**, Salivens pH vid olika kariesaktivitet, *Sven. Tandlaek. Tidskr.*, 45, 246, 1952.
256. **Shannon, I. L. and Chauncey, H. H.**, Hyperhydration and parotid flow in man, *J. Dent. Res.*, 46, 1028, 1967.
257. **Hunt, J. N. and Knox, M. T.**, Regulation of gastric emptying, in *Handbook of Physiology*, Vol. 4, Code, C. F., Ed., American Physiological Society, Washington, D.C., 1968, p. 1917.
258. **Cantarow, A. and Schepartz, B.**, *Biochemistry*, 4th ed., W. B. Saunders, Philadelphia, 1967, 840.
259. **Dodds, E. C.**, Variations in alveolar carbon dioxide pressure in relation to meals, *J. Physiol. (London)*, 54, 342, 1921.
260. **Kinirons, M. J.**, Increased salivary buffering in association with a low caries experience in children suffering from cystic fibrosis, *J. Dent. Res.*, 62, 815, 1983.
261. **Mandel, I. D., Eriv, A., Kutscher, A., Denning, C., Thompson, R. H., Kessler, W., and Zegarelli, E.**, Calcium and phosphorus levels in submaxillary saliva, *Clin. Pediatr. (Bologna)*, 8, 161, 1964.
262. **Mandel, I. D., Kutscher, A. H., Denning, C. R., Thompson, R. H., Jr., and Zegarelli, E. V.**, Salivary studies in cystic fibrosis, *Am. J. Dis. Child.*, 113, 431, 1967.
263. **Flodhammar, B.**, Tandhälsoförhållanden och kostvanor hos en grupp gravida, *Tandlaekartidningen*, 67, 1050, 1975.
264. **Orosz, M., Vasko, A., Gabris, K., and Banoczy, J.**, Changes in salivary pH and lactobacilli count in pregnant women, *Proc. Finn. Dent. Soc.*, 76, 204, 1980.
265. **Kreusser, W., Heidland, A., Hennemann, A., and Wigand, M. E.**, Die Speichelchemie beim primären Hyperaldosteronismus (Conn-Syndrom), *Arch. Klin. Exp. Ohren Nasen Kehlkopfheilkd.*, 202, 430, 1972.
266. **Heintze, U. and Dymling, J.-F.**, Buffer effect, secretion rate, pH and electrolytes of stimulated whole saliva in relation to the renin-aldosterone system, *Swed. Dent. J.*, 9, 249, 1985.
267. **Kakizaki, G., Soeno, T., Sasahara, M., Sanada, M., and Aikawa, T.**, Reevaluation of parotid saliva test in the diagnosis of pancreatic disorders, *Acta Med. Port.*, 4, 311, 1983.
268. **Lankisch, P. G., Chilla, R., Luerssen, K., Koop, H., Arglebe, C., and Creutzfeldt, W.**, Parotid saliva test in the diagnosis of chronic pancreatitis, *Digestion*, 19, 52, 1979.
269. **Costa, P. T., Chauncey, H. H., Rose, C. L., and Kapur, K. K.**, Relationship of parotid saliva flow rate and composition with personality traits in healthy men, *Oral Surg.*, 50, 416, 1980.
270. **Münzel, M.**, Die Biochemie der menschlichen Speicheldrüsensekrete, *Arch. Otorhinolaryngol.*, 213, 209, 1976.
271. **Trell, E.**, Community-based preventive medical department for individual risk factor assessment and intervention in an urban population, *Prev. Med.*, 12, 397, 1983.
272. **Janzon, L., Lindell, S.-E., and Trell, E.**, Smoking and disease. Attitudes and knowledge in middle-aged men, *Scand. J. Soc. Med.*, 9, 127, 1981.
273. **Bynum, T. E., Solomon, T. E., Johnson, L. R., and Jacobson, E. D.**, Inhibition of pancreatic secretion in man by cigarette smoking, *Gut*, 13, 361, 1972.
274. **Brown, P.**, The influence of smoking on pancreatic function in man, *Med. J. Aust.*, 2, 290, 1976.
275. **Feyerabend, C., Higenbottam, T., and Russell, M. A. H.**, Nicotine concentrations in urine and saliva of smokers and non-smokers, *Br. Med. J.*, 284, 1002, 1982.

276. **Dawes, C.,** Inorganic constituents of saliva in relation to caries, in *Cariology Today,* Guggenheim, B., Ed., S. Karger, Basel, 1984, 70.
277. **Frostell, G.,** The effect of chewing on the pH of dental plaques after carbohydrate consumption, *Acta Odontol. Scand.,* 32, 79, 1979.
278. **Lamberts, B. L., Pedersen, E. D., and Shklair, I. L.,** Salivary pH-rise activities in caries-free and caries-active naval recruits, *Arch. Oral Biol.,* 28, 605, 1983.
279. **Edgar, W. M.,** The role of saliva in the control of pH changes in human dental plaque, *Caries Res.,* 10, 241, 1976.
280. **McNamara, T. F., Friedman, B. K., and Kleinberg, I.,** The microbial composition of human incisor tooth plaque, *Arch. Oral Biol.,* 24, 91, 1979.
281. **Young, G., Resca, H. G., and Sullivan, M. T.,** The yeasts of the normal mouth and their relation to salivary acidity, *J. Dent. Res.,* 30, 426, 1951.
282. **Arendorf, T. M. and Walker, D. M.,** The prevalence and intra-oral distribution of *Candida albicans* in man, *Arch. Oral Biol.,* 25, 1, 1980.
283. **Mäkinen, K. K.,** Defence mechanisms in health and disease, *Proc. Finn. Dent. Soc.,* 76, 3, 1980.
284. **Marlay, E.,** The relationship between dental caries and salivary properties at adolescence, *Aust. Dent. J.,* 15, 412, 1970.
285. **Valentine, A. D., Anderson, R. J., and Bradnock, G.,** Salivary pH and dental caries, *Br. Dent. J.,* 144, 105, 1978.
286. **Afonsky, D.,** *Saliva and Its Relation to Oral Health,* University of Alabama Press, Tuscaloosa, 1961.
287. **Nyman, S., Bratthall, D., and Böhlin, E.,** The Swedish dental health programme for adults, *Int. Dent. J.,* 34, 130, 1984.
288. **Ravald, N., Hamp, S.-E., and Birkhed, D.,** Long-term evaluation of root surface caries in periodontally treated patients, *J. Clin. Periodontol.,* 13, 758, 1986.
289. **Rundegren, J. and Ericson, T.,** Actual caries development compared with expected caries activity, *Community Dent. Oral Epidemiol.,* 6, 97, 1978.
290. **Klock, B. and Krasse, B.,** A comparison between different methods for prediction of caries activity, *Scand. J. Dent. Res.,* 87, 129, 1979.
291. **Schröder, U. and Granath, L.,** Dietary habits and oral hygiene as predictors of caries in 3-year-old children, *Community Dent. Oral Epidemiol.,* 11, 308, 1983.
292. **Bergendal, B. and Hamp, S.-E.,** Dietary pattern and dental caries in 19-year-old adolescents subjected to preventive measures focused on oral hygiene and/or fluorides, *Swed. Dent. J.,* 8, 1, 1985.
293. **Imfeld, T. N.,** Identification of low caries risk dietary components, in *Monographs in Oral Science,* Vol. 11, Myers, H. M., Ed., Philadelphia, 1983.

Chapter 3

# SALIVARY ELECTROLYTES

## D. B. Ferguson

## TABLE OF CONTENTS

# I. INTRODUCTION

Salivary electrolytes have been extensively studied, and the normal concentrations of the principal electrolytes are well documented (Tables 1 to 5). Unfortunately, from a diagnostic viewpoint, there is wide variation in values observed both between and within subjects. Concentrations of electrolytes alter as salivary flow rate alters and may vary with time of day in any one individual, while age and possibly sex may be sources of variation between individuals. Diet affects plasma concentrations of some ions and may therefore indirectly affect salivary concentrations.

If saliva is to be used in diagnosis, samples have to be collected, and the method of collection is important. This problem has already been discussed in Chapters 1 and 2 of this volume. In general it is more convenient for untrained investigators and subjects to collect samples of oral fluid by expectoration, although for ease of analysis, samples of saliva from individual glands are usually preferable. There are slight differences in ionic composition between oral fluid and the separate salivary secretions, and the varying degree to which the different gland secretions contribute to the oral fluid under different conditions will vary the composition of oral fluid. In some instances collection of a particular gland secretion may be indicated because changes are seen only, or perhaps more readily, in this one secretion.

It is rare for either oral or systemic conditions to affect concentrations of any particular ion by itself: in most of the pathological conditions studied, attempts have been made to detect patterns of change across a spectrum of electrolytes. There are a few ions, however, whose assay gives direct information about the state of the subject. If sodium concentrations

## Table 1
## CONCENTRATIONS OF INORGANIC COMPONENTS OF WHOLE SALIVA IN mmol/l[1-19]

| Electrolyte | Unstimulated Mean ± s.d. | Unstimulated Range | Stimulated Mean ± s.d. | Stimulated Range | Effect of flow | Comments |
|---|---|---|---|---|---|---|
| Sodium | 7.7 ± 3.0 | 2 — 26 | 32 ± 20 | 13 — 80 | Increases | Higher in very young and old |
| Potassium | 21 ± 4 | 13 — 40 | 22 ± 12 | 13 — 38 | Unchanged | |
| Calcium | 1.35 ± 0.45 | 0.5 — 2.8 | 1.7 ± 1.0 | 0.2 — 4.7 | Decreases | |
| Magnesium | 0.31 ± 0.22 | 0.15 — 0.6 | 0.18 ± 0.15 | | | |
| Copper (μmol/l) | 0.4 | 0.2 — 0.8 | 0.4 | 0.2 — 0.8 | | Ref. 1 (Ref. 4 gives mean of 4.03) |
| Lead (μmol/l) | | | 0.55 | 0.14 — 1.11 | | |
| Cobalt (μmol/l) | | | 1.2 | 0 — 2.0 | | |
| Strontium (μmol/l) | 0.4 ± 0.01 | 0.1 — 33 | 1.0 ± 0.1 | 0.1 — 1.2 | | |
| Chloride | | | | 10 — 56 | | |
| Hydrogen carbonate | 24 ± 8 | | 25 ± 18 | | Increases | |
| | 2.9 ± 2.4 | | 20 ± 8 | | Increases | (0.16 ± 0.02 also given in resting) |
| Phosphate | | | | 1.5 — 25 | | |
| Iodide (μmol/l) | 5.5 ± 4.2 | 2 — 22 | 10 ± 7 | | Decreases | |
| Bromide | | | 14 ± 8 | 0.01 — 0.1 | Decreases | |
| Thiocyanate(mmol/l) | | | 1.2 ± 0.7 | | Decreases | |
| Hypothiocyanite (μmol/l) | 10 | 2 — 84 | 1.1 ± 0.5 | | Decreases | |
| Nitrate (μmol/l) | | | 178 ± 11 | 79 — 183 | | |
| Nitrite (μmol/l) | | | 68 ± 11 | | | |
| Fluoride (μmol/l) | 1.45 ± 0.6 | | 5.8 ± 0.25 | | | |
| Sulfate (μmol/l) | | | 72 ± 4 | | | |

*Note*:   The figures given for the principal electrolytes are pooled from several sources.

**Table 2**
## CONCENTRATIONS OF INORGANIC COMPONENTS IN PAROTID SALIVA[5,10,16,20-37]

| Electrolyte | Unstimulated | | Stimulated | | Effect of flow |
|---|---|---|---|---|---|
| | Mean ± s.d. | Range | Mean ± s.d. | Range | |
| Sodium | 1.3 ± 1.5 | 0.5 — 6 | 36 ± 12 | 8 — 80 | Increases |
| Potassium | 24 ± 6.5 | 30 — 80 | 21 ± 5 | 8 — 44 | Unchanged |
| Calcium | 1.05 ± 0.35 | 0.5 — 2.1 | 1.6 ± 0.8 | 0.2 — 2.7 | Increases |
| Magnesium | 0.16 ± 0.07 | 0.07 — 0.5 | 0.12 ± 0.15 | 0.01 — 0.4 | |
| Copper (μmol/l) | | | 0.04 | 0.02 — 0.08 | |
| Chloride | 22 ± 6 | 17 — 40 | 28 ± 15 | 4 — 56 | Increases |
| Hydrogen carbonate | 1.1 + 0.1 | 0.5 — 5.0 | 30 ± 9.6 | 5 — 60 | Increases |
| Phosphate | 9 ± 3.5 | 3.9 — 20 | 3.7 ± 1.0 | 2.3 — 9.3 | Decreases |
| Iodide (μmol/l) | | 0.5 — 2.3 | | 0.2 — 1.2 | Decreases |
| Fluoride (μmol/l) | 1.5 | | 1.0 ± 0.3 | 4.0 — 13 | |

*Note:* Figures for the principal electrolytes are pooled from several sources and based on several thousand observations.

**Table 3**
## CONCENTRATIONS OF INORGANIC COMPONENTS IN SUBMANDIBULAR SALIVA[5,10,20,38-40]

| Electrolyte | Unstimulated | | Stimulated | | Effect of flow |
|---|---|---|---|---|---|
| | Mean ± s.d | Range | Mean ± s.d. | Range | |
| Sodium | 3.3 ± 3.9 | | 45 ± 23 | 10 — 60 | Increases |
| Potassium | 14.4 ± 2.2 | 10 — 22 | 17 ± 4 | 10 — 22 | Unchanged |
| Calcium | 1.56 ± 0.45 | 0.5 — 5.0 | 2.4 ± 0.6 | 0.7 — 3.7 | Decreases |
| Magnesium | 0.07 ± 0.03 | | 0.04 ± 0.01 | − 0.5 | |
| Chloride | 12 ± 4.6 | 3 — 24 | 25 ± 11 | 10 — 42 | Increases |
| Hydrogen carbonate | 4 | | 18 | 3 — 36 | Increases |
| Phosphate | 5.6 ± 1.9 | 3 — 12 | 5.5 ± 4.0 | 0.2 — 7.3 | Decreases |
| Iodide (μmol/l) | 1.0 | | 0.5 | | Decreases |

*Note:* Figures for the main electrolytes are pooled from several sources.

**Table 4**
## CONCENTRATIONS OF INORGANIC COMPONENTS IN SUBLINGUAL SALIVA[5,20]

| Electrolyte | Unstimulated | | Stimulated | | Effect of flow |
|---|---|---|---|---|---|
| | Mean ± s.d.[a] | Range | Mean ± s.d. | Range | |
| Sodium | | | 32.7 ± 10.4 | 21.6 — 55 | Increases |
| Potassium | | | 13.2 ± 2 | 9.8 — 17.3 | Unchanged |
| Calcium | | | 2.1 ± 0.4 | 1.7 — 2.95 | Increases |
| Chloride | | | 26.2 ± 9.6 | 11.6 — 37.6 | Increases |
| Hydrogen carbonate | | | 10.9 ± 3.6 | 4.5 — 16.5 | Increases |
| Phosphate | | | 4.1 ± 0.8 | 2.5 — 5.0 | Decreases |

[a]  Data not available.

**Table 5**
**CONCENTRATIONS OF INORGANIC COMPONENTS IN SALIVA FROM ACCESSORY GLANDS[5,41,42]**

| Electrolyte | Unstimulated | | Stimulated | | Effect of flow |
|---|---|---|---|---|---|
| | Mean ± s.d. | Range | Mean ± s.d. | Range | |
| Sodium | 13.9 ± 12.0 | 2.6 — 37.5 | 37.3 ± 22.7 | 11 — 97.7 | Increases |
| Potassium | 19.3 ± 4.9 | 10 — 29 | 17.3 ± 3.9 | 11 — 25 | Unchanged |
| Calcium | 2.29 ± 0.47 | 1.6 — 3.2 | 2.03 ± 0.38 | 1.64 — 2.48 | Decreases |
| Magnesium | 0.65 ± 0.25 | 0.41 — 1.22 | 0.54 ± 0.14 | 0.38 — 0.8 | |
| Chloride | 31.4 ± 14.0 | 16 — 54 | 56.5 ± 29.7 | 19 — 109 | Increases |
| Phosphate | 0.62 ± 0.23 | 0.25 — 1.07 | 0.45 ± 0.11 | 0.2 — 0.6 | Decreases |

at low salivary flow rates are high, it suggests that there is damage to the cells of the striated ducts of the salivary glands. The same is true of chloride concentrations. Thiocyanate concentrations are high in subjects who are heavy tobacco smokers, and the concentrations of nitrate and of some of the toxic metal ions may reflect the total intake of these ions into the body.

In this chapter, I will consider first the variations in salivary electrolyte concentrations due to physiological factors, then describe the observations which have been made in pathological conditions, and, finally, deal in turn with each component and its significance.

## II. SOURCES OF NORMAL VARIATION

### A. Variation in Electrolyte Composition in Oral Fluid (Whole or Mixed Saliva) Due to Variation in the Relative Contribution of Saliva from Different Sources

With the exception of calcium, the mean concentrations of ions in parotid saliva are higher than those in submandibular, sublingual, or accessory gland salivas (Tables 2 to 5). There is, however, considerable overlap in the ranges. Mean calcium concentrations in parotid saliva are only two thirds of those in the secretions of the other glands, and although the ranges overlap, they are clearly different. Thus, if samples of oral fluid are collected, the calcium content will be greater in resting conditions or when the level of stimulation is low, because of the lesser contribution from the parotid glands under these conditions (see Reference 5 for a discussion of the relative contributions of different glands to oral fluid). While this is true of total calcium concentrations, it is probably less so of ionic calcium concentrations. There are very few data on ionic calcium concentrations in saliva from the different glands, but the glycoproteins of nonparotid saliva bind calcium more strongly, and a greater proportion of nonparotid saliva calcium is in a bound form.

At slow flow rates a nonsalivary source of variation in oral fluid composition may become important. Gingival crevicular fluid[43] normally contributes a small volume of plasma-like composition to the oral fluid. This contribution is increased when any form of mechanical stimulation to salivary flow is used (e.g., chewing of inert material). The sodium concentration in plasma is at least one and a half times that in saliva, and so small amounts of gingival fluid may increase salivary sodium concentrations if salivary flow rates are low. The lower potassium concentrations in gingival crevicular fluid probably do not affect oral fluid concentrations.

### B. Variations in Composition Due to Variations in Salivary Flow Rate (Figure 1)[22,26,27,30,31,38]

The concentration of an ion in saliva is governed to a major extent by the mechanisms which cause that ion to appear in saliva. The concentration of the ion in plasma or in the

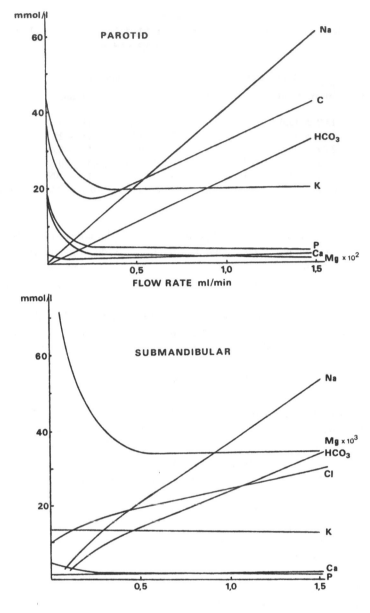

FIGURE 1.   The changes in concentrations of electrolytes as the salivary flow rate increases. Data from Dawes.[21,22,38]

interstitial fluid of the gland usually has little influence because of the separate nature of the mechanism for providing the water, and hence the volume flow. Thus, any substance which is lipid soluble or small enough to cross the epithelial cell membranes will diffuse across the glandular epithelium at a rate which depends upon the concentration gradient. This rate is affected by flow rate only in that flow will maintain the gradient of concentration. Such substances, therefore, usually decrease in concentration in the final saliva as flow rate increases.

When an ion is actively pumped into saliva, particularly if that pumping takes place in the ducts, and the ion is not actively reabsorbed in subsequent parts of the duct, increasing flow rate will again lead to a decrease in concentration in the final saliva. Examples of this are calcium, iodide, thiocyanate, and nitrate.[27] If an ion is actively reabsorbed in the ductal system, there will be less time for this to occur as flow rate increases, and the concentration in the final saliva will increase with increasing flow rate. Examples of this phenomenon are provided by sodium and chloride. A special case is that of hydrogen carbonate (bicarbonate),[33] since the source of this ion is not the interstitial fluid or the plasma but the metabolism of the cells themselves. The production of hydrogen carbonate increases as the cells become more active, and its concentration in the final saliva, therefore, is directly related to flow rate. Chloride and hydrogen carbonate concentrations are balanced somewhat in the striated ducts because both are negatively charged and can accompany the positively charged sodium ions which are reabsorbed in this part of the ductal system.

### C. Effects of Diet and Plasma Composition upon the Electrolyte Concentrations in Saliva

In general, diet has little effect upon salivary composition because the concentrations of most plasma components are fairly closely controlled in the body.[44] Diet can, however, at least transiently, alter plasma concentrations of phosphate, fluoride, iodide, and nitrate,[17] and all these changes are, to a lesser extent, shown in saliva also.

### D. Effects of Different Foods upon Salivary Composition

The local effects of food in the mouth on salivary composition are indirect results of the different degrees of stimulation to salivary flow provided by the foodstuffs. Flow rate is the determining factor in any variations in composition.[45,46]

Ben-Aryeh et al.[47] found that there were no significant differences in composition between saliva of infants fed with breast milk, bottle milk feeds, or solid food, up to 1 year of age.

### E. Effects of Time of Day on the Concentration of Electrolytes in Saliva (Figure 2)

Circadian variation has been demonstrated in the flow rates of saliva from all the glands and in the concentrations of all electrolytes that have been studied.[6,23,24,39,40,48,49] The variations may be indirectly caused by the variation in flow rate, but there are also variations in activity of the active pumping processes which add ions to, or remove them from, saliva. The peaks of ion concentration are usually in either early morning (6:00 a.m. to 8:00 a.m.) or early evening (4:00 p.m. to 8:00 p.m.) (Table 6). Although the variation due to circadian rhythms can be quite substantial, it is less important than that due to differences in salivary flow rate.[50]

### F. Variation in Salivary Electrolytes over Periods Greater than 24 h

Week-by-week variation in salivary electrolytes was studied by Shannon and Segreto[29] who did not analyze their data for any sign of regular variation, and by Dawes and Chebib,[50] who found no consistent variations.

Seasonal variation was reported by Shannon,[51] but this was primarily an effect on flow rate.

### G. Effects of Duration of Stimulation on Concentrations of Salivary Electrolytes (Figure 3)

The concentrations of ions in the first few drops of saliva secreted by the glands are different from those found if stimulation of salivary secretion continues. It is recommended, therefore, that the saliva collected during the first minute of stimulation should be discarded as being nonrepresentative. The variations were investigated by Dawes.[22,38,50] He found that concentrations of sodium, chloride, and hydrogen carbonate rose sharply during the first 2 min of stimulation, while those of potassium, calcium, magnesium, and phosphate fell. These effects may be related simply to the change in flow rate — the initial samples containing saliva that has remained in the gland (acini and ducts) for some time or been slowly secreted,

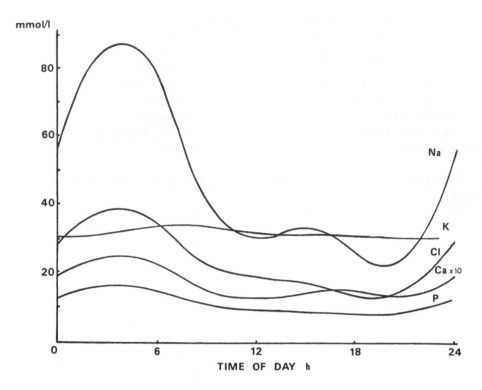

FIGURE 2.   Variations in concentrations of electrolytes in whole saliva samples collected from one subject at each hour of the day — smoothed curves. The usual midafternoon peaks for potassium and phosphate are not seen in this subject.

### Table 6
### TIMES OF MAXIMUM CONCENTRATIONS OF SALIVARY ELECTROLYTES AND THE RANGE OF VARIATION IN CONCENTRATION (EXPRESSED AS PERCENTAGE OF MEAN CONCENTRATION)

|  | Whole | | Parotid | | Submandibular | |
|---|---|---|---|---|---|---|
|  | Time (h) | Range (%) | Time (h) | Range (%) | Time (h) | Range (%) |
| Sodium | 3:00 a.m. - 5:00 a.m. | 76 | 3:00 a.m. - 6:00 a.m. | 52 | 2:00 a.m. - 4:00 a.m. | 46 |
| Potassium | 5:00 p.m. - 9:00 p.m. | 25 | 3:00 p.m. - 5:00 p.m. | 22 | 2:00 p.m. - 5:00 p.m. | 36 |
| Calcium | 4:00 a.m. - 7:00 a.m. | 61 | 5:00 a.m. or 1:00 p.m. | 46 | 5:00 a.m. or 7:00 p.m. | 53 |
| Chloride | 4:00 a.m. - 5:00 a.m. | 69 | 3:00 a.m. - 6:00 a.m. | 37 | 3:00 a.m. - 6:00 a.m. | 46 |
| Phosphate | 2:00 a.m. - 5:00 a.m. | 48 | 6:00 a.m. or 5:00 p.m. | 24 | 7:00 p.m. - 10:00 p.m. | 51 |

and the later samples being more homogeneous. Drop-by-drop analysis of saliva[50] shows that even with a constant stimulus saliva composition is variable, but these variations are smoothed if samples are collected over at least 2 min.

Even after the first 2 min of collection, with the flow rate held constant, some electrolytes vary in concentration. Hydrogen carbonate concentrations rise steadily, increasing by 50% over 10 min, while both calcium and phosphate concentrations rise to a lesser extent. One way to avoid these difficulties is to standardize a collection time of, say, 10 min, which is sufficiently long to compensate for the initial variation and provide a steady state for most ions.

Continued stimulation of the salivary glands leads eventually to a general decrease in

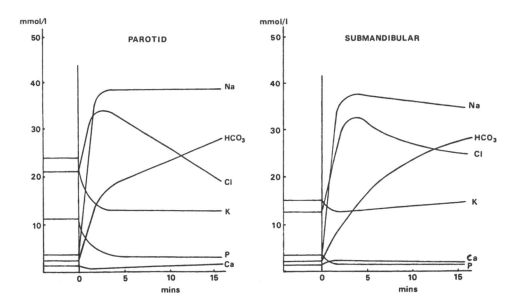

FIGURE 3.   The effect of duration on stimulation on the concentrations of electrolytes in saliva. Smoothed data from Dawes[22,38] for changes observed at a constant secretion rate of 1 ml/min/gland. Resting concentrations are shown on the left.

concentration of inorganic components as well as organic. The decrease in concentrations, however, is not usually noticeable in less than about 3 h.

The changes in salivary composition resulting from continued secretion do persist over some time, and Dawes[51] concluded that at least 1 and preferably 2 h should be allowed to elapse after a meal or other stimulation of salivary flow before samples were collected for estimation of "normal" concentrations.

## H. Effects of Sex Hormones on the Concentration of Electrolytes in Saliva

The only comparison of salivary composition in prepubertal subjects appears to be that of Ben-Aryeh et al.,[47] in which male and female infants were compared up to the age of 1 year. No significant differences were observed.

There have been a few reports that the pattern of ion concentrations in saliva varies at different points in the menstrual cycle. Puskulian[53] found a decrease in calcium concentration, a decrease in the sodium to potassium ratio, and a decrease in flow rate of submandibular saliva at mid-cycle in 8 women. Ben-Aryeh et al.[54] found that phosphate concentrations were higher at mid-cycle in unstimulated whole saliva in 14 women. Tenovuo et al.[55] measured potassium, calcium, and thiocyanate concentrations in wax-stimulated whole saliva from 12 women and found no significant variations during the menstrual cycle and no reliable indicator of ovulation. I was unable to find any consistent variation in acid-stimulated parotid saliva electrolytes through the menstrual cycle in 10 women, and the variations appeared more cyclic over 28 d in a group of 10 men then they did in the women.[56]

## I. Effects of Exercise on Salivary Electrolytes

Salminen and Konttinen[57] reported that sodium concentrations in whole saliva doubled after exercise, although potassium concentrations were unchanged. Shannon,[58] however, found no change in sodium, potassium, and chloride concentrations in acid-stimulated parotid saliva when collected after exercise. Dawes[59] studied changes in salivary composition after jogging for 3 to 8 mi. Although there were changes in protein concentrations, the effects on ionic composition were small and not significant.

## J. Changes in Salivary Composition at Different Ages

The ionic composition of unstimulated whole saliva in infants was studied by Ben-Aryeh et al.[47] Their subjects were 41 infants aged 3 to 30 d, 40 infants aged 2 to 3 months, 41 infants aged 4 to 6 months, and 46 infants aged 7 to 12 months. They observed that calcium, magnesium, and chloride concentrations were higher in infants than in adults, calcium and magnesium concentrations remaining high throughout the first year of life while chloride concentrations fell toward adult levels. The concentrations of sodium and potassium were high in the youngest group of subjects and fell steadily during the first year but were not significantly different from adult values. Phosphate concentrations were significantly lower in the youngest subjects than in adults and rose over the first year of life. In another study,[60] salivary composition was compared in a group of children, young adults, and older subjects. Sodium concentrations were slightly lower in the young adults than in the other groups.

Salivary secretion in older subjects has been studied by a number of investigators, but most of these have examined flow rates only.[61-67] These effects are discussed elsewhere in this book. Changes in composition were described by Chauncey et al.[68] in parotid saliva. They reported that sodium, calcium, and chloride concentrations were lower in acid-stimulated parotid saliva from older subjects in the Boston VA Normative Aging Study. Baum et al.[69] confirmed their observations for sodium concentrations in parotid saliva. In the Boston study the results were corrected for differences in flow rate by using regression analysis, and in the other study no significant difference in the salivary flow rates was recorded in older and younger subjects. The decrease in sodium concentrations cannot be attributed, therefore, to a reduction in flow rates. Variations in salivary composition due to age and sex have been further described recently in Portuguese subjects.[70]

## III. PATTERNS OF CHANGES IN ELECTROLYTE COMPOSITION OF SALIVA OBSERVED IN DIFFERENT DISEASE STATES AND AFTER THERAPEUTIC DRUGS

Most of the studies of changes in electrolyte composition have been attempts to find typical salivary electrolyte patterns in diseases of the mouth or salivary glands. These latter include diseases which may be systemic but are known to affect salivary glands, such as Sjögren's syndrome and cystic fibrosis (Table 7).

It has also been realized that salivary composition can be altered by drugs used systemically to treat nonsalivary disorders.

## A. Salivary Changes in Oral Disease

### 1. Dental Caries

No consistent variations in salivary electrolyte concentrations have been observed in subjects who are caries free or caries susceptible or have active carious lesions. Some investigators found lower concentrations of calcium in caries-resistant subjects, but this is not sufficiently significant to act as a predictor of future freedom from dental caries; others found no relation between calcium concentrations and caries susceptibility. Mandel[71] reexamined previous reports and carried out further studies but concluded that there were no significant differences in the calcium and phosphate concentrations in stimulated parotid and submandibular saliva from caries-resistant and caries susceptible subjects. Dulce and Hardel[72] found the concentrations of ionised calcium in resting parotid, but not whole, saliva to be directly related to caries experience. Shannon[73] found the phosphate levels in unstimulated parotid saliva to be related to caries experience, but the spread of results was such that the observation had no diagnostic value. In a rather unusual approach to this question Shaw et al.[74] have studied the composition of the mixed secretions of the submandibular and sublingual glands by isolating the parotid glands and collecting fluid from the floor of the mouth

**Table 7**
## EFFECTS OF DISEASE ON SALIVARY ELECTROLYTE CONCENTRATIONS

| Disease | Na | K | Ca | Mg | Cl | HCO$_3^-$ | P | Suggested derived indices |
|---|---|---|---|---|---|---|---|---|
| Dental caries | | | | | | | ML ↓ | Ca/P |
| Periodontal disease | | | | | | | | |
| Sialadenitis | WP ↑ | P ↓ | WP ↑ | | | | P ↓ | |
| Radiation damage | W ↑ | | W ↑ | W ↑ | W ↑ | | | |
| Sjögren's syndrome | P ↑ | | | | P ↑ | | P ↓ | |
| Cystic fibrosis | A ↑ | | Sm ↑ | | | | Sm ↑ | Ca + P |
| Aldosteronism | WPSm ↓ | Sm ↑ | | | | | | Na/K |
| Hypertension | WPSm ↓ | | | | | | | |
| Alcoholic cirrhosis | | P ↑ | | | | | | |
| Hyperparathyroidism | | | W ↑ | | | | W ↑ | |
| Diabetes | | | PSm ↑ | | | | | |
| Chronic pancreatitis | | | | | | WP ↓ | | |
| Psychiatric illness | ?P ↑ | | | | | | | |
| Digitalis toxicity | | W ↑ | W ↑ | | | | | Ca × K |

*Note:*   See text for individual references. Letter refers to types of saliva: W (whole), P (parotid), Sm (submandibular), A (accessory gland), and ML (sublingual and submandibular).

From Ferguson, D. B., *J. Dent. Res.*, 66, 420, 1988. With permission.

with an aspirator. They report that phosphate concentrations were significantly higher, and calcium concentrations slightly higher, in caries-free subjects.

### 2. Periodontal Disease

Again there is no consistent correlation of salivary electrolyte pattern with periodontal disease.[75] Subjects with high concentrations of pyrophosphate in their saliva have been reported to form less calculus[37] although Sawinski and Cole[28] stated, without giving data, that both phosphate and pyrophosphate concentrations were higher in stimulated parotid saliva from subjects who formed calculus readily. In Vogel and Amdur's study[37] the ranges of values for the subject groups were overlapping.

## B. Diseases of the Salivary Glands

### 1. Inflammatory Diseases

Rausch[77] reported that salivary sodium concentrations were raised in sialadenitis while potassium levels were unaffected. This was confirmed in a series of studies by Mandel and Baurmash,[78,79] who reported that sodium and chloride concentrations in parotid saliva from affected glands were almost as high as the levels in plasma. Potassium concentrations and phosphate concentrations were low, but calcium concentrations were normal. These observations apply to saliva collected during the acute phases of chronic recurrent sialadenitis; during the quiescent phases, sodium and chloride levels fall but remain above normal levels, while potassium levels become normal and phosphate levels remain low. These changes can be used to differentiate sialadenitis from sialadenosis, or noninflammatory enlargement of salivary glands.

### 2. Immunological Changes

Changes in allergic parotitis have not been studied.
Changes in glands affected by Sjögren's syndrome are discussed later.

### 3. Neoplastic Changes

Salivary neoplasms occur relatively infrequently, and there do not appear to be any data on changes in salivary electrolytes which might result from neoplastic conditions.

### 4. Effects of Radiation

Neoplasms of the head and neck are, however, sufficiently common and radiosensitive for there to be a substantial body of information on the effects of radiation-induced damage to salivary glands. Most of this refers to flow rates, but changes in salivary electrolyte composition have been reported by Ben-Aryeh et al.[80] and Dreizen et al.[81] Ben-Aryeh et al. examined unstimulated whole saliva in a group of 15 patients. The salivary flow rates were reduced, and concentrations of sodium increased. Dreizen et al. studied stimulated whole saliva in 30 patients and found that concentrations of sodium, chloride, calcium, and magnesium rose markedly, concentrations of bicarbonate decreased significantly, and concentrations of potassium and phosphate were unchanged. I have unpublished data on stimulated parotid saliva from 2 patients: both these exhibited very high sodium and chloride concentrations. These results would be consistent with acinar damage affecting processes involved in water movement but sparing, to a greater or lesser extent, secretion of protein and ions not involved in water movement (calcium and magnesium), and ductal damage abolishing or reducing reabsorption of sodium and chloride. A reduction in bicarbonate concentration might result from the reduced metabolic activity in secretion. The lack of change in potassium and phosphate concentrations is difficult to explain. Potassium ions are probably secreted into saliva throughout the acinar and ductal regions, and therefore, the concentrations may be less affected if radiation damage is selective, but the only evidence on phosphate movement comes from studies on sheep parotid glands, where it has been suggested that there is active phosphate secretion in the acinar region and that ductal changes are limited to those due to equilibration.[82] It may be that there is a maximum gradient which can be maintained for these ions across the ductal epithelium.

Although these changes in electrolytes may be diagnostic of radiation damage to the salivary glands, this condition is always characterized by a marked reduction in flow rate, and this is a much simpler test. Since the only treatment possible is to ameliorate the effect of the xerostomia, analysis of the electrolyte changes offers no particular advantage.

## C. Changes in Salivary Function Due to Systemic Diseases

### 1. Sjögren's Syndrome

Sjögren's syndrome is a connective-tissue disease which also affects a number of epithelial structures. In its classical form it consists of three manifestations — xerostomia, keratoconjunctivitis sicca (due to impaired secretion from the lacrimal glands), and rheumatoid arthritis. In 30 to 50% of cases rheumatoid arthritis is not present. In some of these its place is taken by another connective-tissue disease such as systemic lupus erythematosis, polymyositis, or polyarteritis nodosa, but in others the gland symptoms only are seen. When this is so, the name "sicca syndrome" is given.

Associated with the xerostomia are characteristic changes in the electrolyte content of the saliva.[83-85] Sodium and chloride concentrations in acid-stimulated parotid saliva are markedly increased, and phosphate concentrations are lower than usual.[84] These effects are the reverse of what would be expected from the reduced rate of flow and are consonant with the damage to the glands being particularly noticeable in the ducts.[86] Potassium and calcium concentrations in acid-stimulated parotid saliva are not significantly different from those in normal subjects. These changes in ionic concentrations in parotid saliva are similar to those in sialadenitis; it is unlikely that measurement of these ions will provide any diagnostic advantage.

## 2. Systemic Immunological Reactions

Although effects of systemic immunological reactions on individual organs or tissues may be poorly defined and variable in intensity and location, some changes in salivary gland function have been reported. Thus, the generalized reaction seen in patients after rejection of bone marrow transplants is easily detected in the minor salivary glands of the lip and results in very high sodium concentrations in the saliva from these glands.[87] Changes in parotid saliva and lacrimal secretion have been observed in psoriasis.[88]

## 3. Cystic Fibrosis

Cystic fibrosis is a congenital disease affecting exocrine glands generally, probably arising from some metabolic defect. The gland which is clinically important is the pancreas, but salivary secretions are affected and have been studied in attempts to discover the underlying mechanisms of the disease. Of the salivary glands, the parotid is little affected, the submandibular and sublingual secretions show changes in chemical composition, and the minor salivary glands also show a decreased flow rate.[89]

Sodium concentrations are slightly raised in whole saliva, variable in parotid and submandibular saliva,[90,91] and high in minor gland saliva.[92] Calcium concentrations are slightly raised in parotid saliva but more markedly raised in submandibular saliva.[42,91-98] Phosphate concentrations are said by some observers to be raised in submandibular saliva.[90,95,97]

## 4. Endocrine Disturbances
### a. Aldosterone

The activity of the sodium-pumping mechanisms in the ducts of the salivary glands is responsive to aldosterone in the same manner as those in the distal convoluted tubules of the kidney. The reabsorption of sodium is increased by the hormone, and so concentrations in saliva fall, even in stimulated saliva. Sodium-to-potassium ratios also fall, although potassium concentrations are not necessarily increased.[99-101] Frawley and Thorn[102] measured the sodium-to-potassium ratio in whole wax-stimulated saliva from normal patients, patients with Cushing's syndrome, and both treated and untreated patients with Addison's disease. In Cushing's syndrome excess aldosterone is secreted by the adrenal glands, and in Addison's disease secretion of the hormone falls to very low levels. The ratios were 1.3:1, 0.5:1, 1.8:1, and 5:1, respectively. Similar results were obtained by Conn,[103] Morris,[105] Lauler et al.,[104] and others. Wotman et al.[106] examined sodium to potassium ratios in wax-stimulated whole saliva, acid-stimulated parotid saliva, and acid-stimulated submandibular saliva before and after surgical treatment of primary aldosteronism in seven patients. The sodium to potassium ratios increased in all the saliva types after surgery in the five cases treated successfully but not in the unsuccessful cases. In another group of subjects Wotman et al.[107] found the most significant response to aldosterone to be an increase in potassium concentrations in submandibular saliva. Salivary estimations were unable to differentiate between primary and pseudo-primary aldosteronism.[107]

Changes in sodium and potassium concentrations and in the sodium to potassium ratio have also been observed in systemic diseases in which circulating aldosterone levels are known, or suspected, to be raised. These include hypertension, where sodium concentrations and sodium to potassium ratios are low in parotid and submandibular saliva[108] and in whole saliva,[109,110] and possibly alcoholic cirrhosis, where sodium and potassium concentrations are increased in parotid saliva, but the increase in sodium concentration is less than would be expected at the high flow rates observed.[111] In cirrhosis there is also an increase in calcium concentrations.

### b. Parathormone

In seven patients with hyperparathyroidism the whole saliva concentrations of calcium and phosphate were both raised.[112] Infusion of parathormone in six young adults resulted in an increase in calcium and phosphate concentrations in unstimulated and acid-stimulated parotid saliva.[113] Sodium concentrations were also raised in the stimulated saliva.

### c. Insulin

In diabetic patients Francois and Guest[114] reported that sodium concentrations were increased in the parotid saliva of ten children, while Marder et al.[115] were unable to confirm this in adults but did find that calcium concentrations were raised in parotid saliva from ten men, and in both parotid and submandibular saliva in ten men and ten women.

The similarities between the salivary glands, particularly the parotid, and the pancreas would suggest that diseases affecting the pancreas might also affect the salivary glands. In patients with chronic pancreatitis Kakizaki et al.[116] reported that pilocarpine-stimulated parotid saliva was low in bicarbonate. Descos et al.[117] made a similar observation in unstimulated and hormone-stimulated whole saliva, but found no difference in wax-stimulated whole saliva. In both sets of observations the low bicarbonate might be due to the low flow rates. Dobrilla et al.[118] found no significant differences in pilocarpine-stimulated parotid and whole saliva from 29 patients not suffering from chronic pancreatitis and 19 with the condition.

### d. Thyroid Hormones

Salivary concentrations of iodine are very similar in hypothyroid, euthyroid, and hyperthyroid patients.[119]

### e. Psychiatric Illness

In general, patients with either chronic depression or manic depression have low salivary flow rates; schizophrenics may have high flow rates. Glen et al.[120] reported that parotid saliva from 18 subjects suffering from depression had higher concentrations of sodium than that from 31 nondepressed patients when flow rate was taken into consideration. Bolwig and Rafaelsen,[121] however, found no consistent differences in electrolyte composition in whole saliva from depressed patients. Costa et al.[122] also found that subjects with a number of personality traits, usually exhibiting some degree of anxiety, had increased salivary flow rates with consequent changes in salivary electrolyte composition. Similar results are reported by Ben-Aryeh et al.[123]

### 5. Effects of Various Pharmacological Agents

Any drugs which stimulate or inhibit either sympathetic or parasympathetic activity will have effects on the secretion of saliva. A number of writers have compiled lists of such drugs, the most recent list being that given by Mandel.[11] The effects of these drugs on salivary composition are principally determined by their effects on flow rate and are usually nonspecific. Drugs which affect transport mechanisms, though, may affect both flow rate and composition.

The example which has been most thoroughly studied is digitalis, used in the treatment of congestive heart failure. With the cardiac glycosides, the correct dosage is critical, since overdoses are toxic and the symptoms of overdosage are similar to the symptoms being treated. The observation that calcium and potassium concentrations in whole saliva were raised as digitalis dosage was increased and were very high in digitalis toxicity led to a number of groups exploiting the measurement of these ions in saliva as a test of digitalis poisoning.[124-130] Gould et al.[131] were unable to detect increased levels of calcium and potassium in saliva in digitalis intoxication. Sodium concentrations are unchanged.[126]

Diuretic drugs which produce their effects by altering the transport of ions in the kidney will alter the same transport processes in other parts of the body. If they affect sodium or chloride reabsorption in the kidney, then they are likely to affect either the flow rate of saliva or the reabsorption of sodium and chloride in the striated ducts of the salivary glands. An example is furosemide, a diuretic used widely in the U.K. This drug inhibits sodium and chloride reabsorption in the kidney but does not affect the quabain-sensitive sodium-potassium pumps. In the parotid glands, therefore, it reduces secretion (a process involving several different ion pumps) but not sodium reabsorption in the striated ducts (via the quabain-sensitive sodium pump). Concentrations of sodium and chloride are therefore lower but appropriate to the reduced rate of flow. Potassium concentrations are unchanged, but calcium concentrations rise slightly.[132]

## IV. THE ANALYSIS OF INDIVIDUAL ION SPECIES AND THEIR SIGNIFICANCE

### A. Sodium and Chloride

Since sodium and chloride concentrations are usually linked except at high flow rates, they may be considered together.

These two ions reach saliva in the acinus, and their concentrations in acinar fluid are similar to those in interstitial fluid and plasma. The current view is that there are at least two transport processes involved — a $Na^+/K^+$-ATP-ase, which is quabain sensitive, and a sodium/potassium/chloride co-transport system, which is furosemide sensitive.[133] From experiments in the rabbit, Case et al.[134] also suggest that there is a $Na^+/H^+$ pump, which is hydrogen carbonate dependent (being inhibited by carbonic anhydrase inhibitors) and may be linked to the $Cl^-/HCO_3^-$ pump. As a result of the transport of these ions across the basolateral walls of the acinar cells, an osmotic gradient is created between the cells, and water follows the ionic movement. The final concentrations of sodium and chloride in saliva, however, depend upon the extent of reabsorption of these two ions which occurs in the striated ducts. The mechanism of reabsorption is a $Na^+/K^+$-ATP-ase system situated in the walls of the ductal cells distant from the lumen. The extent of reabsorption is directly related to the time the secretion takes to traverse the ducts and is therefore inversely related to flow rate. Thus sodium concentrations are low in the final saliva at slow flow rates, and high at fast flow rates. Damage to the acinar cells, therefore, reduces flow rate but does not affect sodium and chloride concentrations in the primary secretion; damage to the ductal cells may affect reabsorption of sodium and chloride and therefore results in inappropriately high concentrations of these ions relative to flow rate.

Sodium concentrations may be measured by flame photometry. Most flame photometers are designed for routine measurement of plasma sodium and potassium concentrations and will give reasonable estimations of these ions in stimulated saliva. Samples of unstimulated or slow-flowing saliva, however, with sodium concentrations down to 1% of plasma concentrations, should be diluted less than plasma samples during the measurement of sodium concentration. An alternative to flame photometry is the use of atomic absorption spectrophotometry. Chloride concentrations are measured by the standard potentiometric method for plasma chloride concentrations, but the sample size may need to be increased at least tenfold for samples collected at low flow rates.

The major physiological influence on concentrations of sodium and chloride is the flow rate. Duration of stimulation is important in considering chloride concentrations, which fall over a period of time as bicarbonate concentrations rise. The highest concentrations of sodium and chloride are observed in early morning samples, and the lowest in samples collected in the evening. The circadian rhythms of these two ions are almost pure sine curves. However, time of day does not introduce a major variation into the relationship between flow and concentration[5] and observations on very large numbers of subjects and at various times of day can be pooled to give a highly significant correlation between the two variables. Prader et al.[100] calculated regression equations for both sodium and potassium concentrations in whole saliva; only the one for sodium concentrations was significant.

$$[Na^+] = 8.3 + 7.9F$$

The 4 value was 0.74. The correlation for Na/K with flow rate was also significant with a similar value for r. My own data yields the following equations for sodium and potassium concentrations in stimulated parotid saliva

$$[Na^+] = 18 + 24.5F \ (r = 0.68)$$

$$[Cl^-] = 14 + 18.1F \ (r = 0.69)$$

These equations are derived from over 1000 observations on some 44 subjects, male and female. No significant differences were observed between male and female parotid salivas. The correlations between sodium concentrations and flow rate in submandibular saliva are much weaker.[40] In whole saliva the correlations become stronger at faster flow rates, as parotid saliva provides an increasing proportion of the mixed secretion.[135] Some data for whole saliva suggest that at low flow rates sodium concentrations fall slightly as flow rate increases whilst other observations show no relationship with flow rate. Similar statements can be made about chloride concentrations, with the additional complication that chloride concentrations may level off or even fall as hydrogen carbonate concentrations increase at high flow rates.

In very young subjects sodium and chloride concentrations tend to be high,[47] while in older subjects sodium concentrations are lower at equivalent flow rates than in young adults.[69]

In general, sodium and chloride concentrations give diagnostic information relating to the efficiency of ductal transport systems. Variations from normal values are readily detectable in parotid saliva, but concentrations in submandibular and whole saliva are much less predictable. Such measurements, however, are of value in linear studies of individuals, when changes over a period of time can be studied. Examples are in the assessment of recurrent parotitis, in the response to radiation, and in following the progress of transplant acceptance or rejection. The value of salivary sodium estimations in adrenocortical disorders has been questioned, and although Na/K ratios differ in different groups of patients, individual variation reduces the value of this in diagnosis. Again, the measure may be of more value in assessing the response to treatment or the progress of the diseases in individual patients.

## B. Potassium

Potassium concentrations in saliva are five to ten times as high as in plasma, but the mechanisms by which potassium reaches saliva have not been so extensively studied as those for sodium transport. The review by Schneyer et al.,[136] although old, probably summarizes present views fairly accurately: potassium reaches saliva by active processes in both the acini and the ducts, and sodium-potassium exchange in the ducts accounts for only a part of the secretory processes in that situation. Thus, potassium concentrations are relatively flow rate independent. Similarly, the effect of mineralocorticoids on the reabsorption of sodium in the striated duct is accompanied by very little change in potassium concentrations, as noted in the original reports (e.g., Reference 99). The use of sodium-to-potassium ratios gives some weighting to this small change.

Potassium concentrations in older subjects are similar to those in young adults.

In clinical situations where potassium concentrations are changed, it is usually in association with other ions. Thus in chronic sialadenitis, potassium and phosphate concentrations usually fall. In digitalis intoxication both potassium and calcium concentrations rise, and so the diagnostic values of the test is improved by taking the product of these two concentrations.

## C. Calcium

Calcium reaches the primary saliva in the acinus by active transport and by movement in association with protein during exocytosis.[137] Although concentrations increase with flow rate, they tend to plateau at higher rates of flow. This would be consistent with the increase in protein concentration as flow rate increases, and with any active movement of calcium being limited to the acini. Concentrations are said to relate to blood concentrations[138] and are affected by parathyroid hormone. In whole saliva, concentrations fall as flow rate increases because of the diminishing proportion of the secretion contributed by the submandibular gland, whose saliva contains more calcium.

The significance of calcium concentrations in saliva is difficult to evaluate, since calcium is normally measured by atomic absorption spectrophotometry, which gives a value for total calcium, that is, both bound and free. In the oral cavity it is the free calcium that is probably most important. Other methods of analysis, such as complexometric titration or spectrophotometric assay of color changes when complexing agents bind with calcium, suffer from problems associated with differential binding capacities. Indeed, attempts have been made to separate different fractions of bound calcium by these methods. Dreisbach[139] used ultrafiltration to separate calcium fractions. The selective calcium ion electrode has been used to measure ionic calcium by Maier et al.[26] and by Lagerlof and Lindqvist.[25] The latter succeeded in separating three complexed fractions of total calcium by a gel filtration method. They found that about 10% was protein bound, about 40% was bound to phosphate, citrates, and lactate, about 5% was complexed with hydrogen carbonate, and about 45% was in free ionic form. This is a little lower than the estimate of 54% by Maier et al.[26]

All the measurements of calcium concentration which have been obtained in clinical situations have been of total calcium. Of these, the most significant are the increase in calcium concentrations in digoxin-intoxicated patients (taken in conjunction with raised potassium levels) and the increase in concentration in submandibular saliva in cystic fibrosis. These observations distinguish control groups from groups of children with asthma and from groups of children with cystic fibrosis, but there is overlap between the groups, and the estimation of calcium concentration is not sufficient by itself to characterize a patient as having cystic fibrosis.

## D. Magnesium

Little is known of how magnesium reaches saliva or of how far concentrations are related to blood levels. Concentrations fall as flow rate increases.[21,30] As with calcium, magnesium concentrations in submandibular and whole saliva are higher than in parotid saliva; both magnesium and calcium concentrations in submandibular saliva may exceed blood concentrations. The method of choice for analysis would be atomic absorption spectrophotometry. Although a number of investigators have measured magnesium concentrations in parotid and whole saliva in different disease states,[42,75,81,95,110,123] no diagnostic role has been suggested.

## E. Mercury

Salivary mercury levels reflect blood levels and can be used to evaluate exposure to mercury poisioning.[9,140] Mercury is easily measured by atomic absorption spectrophotometry. There are no data on how mercury concentrations may vary with flow rate, but it is likely that mercury reaches saliva by diffusion and, therefore, its concentration decreases as flow rate increases.

## F. Lead

Although lead also reaches saliva, the correlation of lead concentrations in wax-stimulated whole saliva with those in plasma is poor.[8] Atomic absorption spectrophotometry would be the method of choice for analysis. In view of the poor correlation with blood levels, salivary estimations would not be suitable for monitoring exposure to lead as an atmospheric pollutant, although it is possible that there might be a better correlation if parotid saliva or even unstimulated whole saliva were used.

### G. Copper

Copper levels in saliva were reported to be around 25 times as high as in plasma.[4,14] There is a more recent report from Czechoslovakia on copper levels in saliva.[141] The use of atomic absorption spectrophotometry would be appropriate for further work on copper.

### H. Cadmium

Cadmium is another metal ion found in biological tissues as a result of environmental pollution.[142]

### I. Cobalt

This was one of the metal ions investigated by Dreizen et al.[4] in saliva. I do not know of any further work on it, although it is possible that its presence is related to environmental pollution. In the study referred to, only 10 of the 37 subjects had detectable levels in saliva.

### J. Lithium

Although lithium is not normally present in detectable amounts in parotid or submandibular salivas, in patients receiving lithium medicinally the concentrations in resting whole saliva, unstimulated parotid and submandibular saliva, and acid-stimulated parotid saliva are some 2.25 times the level in plasma.[13] Concentrations are higher in unstimulated saliva.[35]

### K. Hydrogen Carbonate (Bicarbonate)

Hydrogen carbonate is produced in the cells of the salivary gland as a result of metabolic production of carbon dioxide and its hydration in the presence of the enzyme carbonic anhydrase. It reaches the secretion by active transport, probably mainly in the ducts, although there are species differences and there are no data for human glands. Its concentration increases almost linearly with the rate of flow. Changes with age have not been investigated. The estimation of the ion concentration is not easy, partly because it is in equilibrium with carbon dioxide, and so precautions must be taken against the loss of dissolved gas — such as collected under paraffin oil — and partly because direct estimations usually measure carbon dioxide as well.[143] Thus, the Natelson apparatus measures the carbon dioxide evolved by adding acid manometrically, while the Corning apparatus measures it by thermal conductivity. Many investigators have avoided the difficulties by taking the hydrogen carbonate concentration to be the difference between the sum of the main cations (sodium, potassium, calcium) and the sum of the other anions (chloride and phosphate). When hydrogen carbonate has been measured, it has been taken as an indication of buffering capacity or as an indication of the activity of the glands. In this latter context, the hydrogen carbonate concentration in whole saliva stimulated by chewing was low after irradiation of the glands.[81]

### L. Phosphate

Phosphate concentrations in saliva, although related to plasma levels, are much higher than in blood. Most of the phosphate is inorganic; a small amount is present as pyrophosphate.[37,38] It is actively tranported into saliva, probably mainly in the acini, but possibly also in the ducts. Concentrations decrease as flow rate increases in all the secretions. There do not appear to be any differences in concentration in stimulated parotid saliva in different age groups.[68]

Phosphate concentrations are measured by a number of methods, all based on that of Kuttner and Cohen,[144] in which the phosphate reacts with molybdic acid to form phosphomolybdate, which in turn forms "molybdenum blue" with a reducing agent. In the original method this was stannous chloride, but others such as Chen et al.[145] use different reagents.

The lack of relationship between salivary phosphate levels and dental calculus formation has already been mentioned. The more recent evidence,[74] however, suggests that high salivary phosphate levels may be associated with lower caries rates. Phosphate concentrations are increased in cystic fibrosis and hyperparathyroidism, and decreased in chronic parotitis and Sjögren's syndrome. In all these diseases the phosphate concentration by itself would not be sufficient for diagnostic purposes.

### M. Iodide[18,27,36,148]

Iodide is concentrated by the salivary glands, being actively transported in the proximal parts of the ducts. Concentration decreases with increasing flow rate. No data exist on variation with age. The salivary glands will take up radioiodine and other ions transported by the same mechanism in a manner similar to that of the thyroid glands.[146,147,149] Salivary iodide levels, however, are not related to levels of thyroid activity (see earlier). Since iodide and thiocyanate share the same transport system, cigarette smokers, who secrete more thiocyanate in their saliva, have lower concentrations of iodide.[18,148]

### N. Bromide

Although bromide concentrations in saliva have been measured,[1] and it would be predicted that it would be transported by a route similar to that for iodide, no detailed studies have been carried out.

### O. Thiocyanate and Hypothiocyanite

Thiocyanate is concentrated in saliva by the same transport system that secretes iodide. Its concentration falls as flow rates increase, and it exhibits a circadian rhythm.[19] Variations due to age have not been studied. It is of interest for two reasons — it is a component in an antibacterial system in saliva, and its concentration is higher in the saliva of cigarette smokers. In whole saliva it is converted by bacterial generation of peroxide and by peroxidase enzymes into hypothiocyanite, the actual antibacterial agent.

Thiocyanate is assayed by spectrophotometric measurement of the ferrous salt.[150] Hypothiocyanite is assayed by measuring the oxidation of 5-thio-2-nitrobenzoic acid.[151]

The relationship between salivary thiocyanate and cigarette smoking has been used to identify adolescents who are heavy smokers.[152] This would seem to be a useful diagnostic role. The method, though, will not detect small differences in cigarette consumption and may be affected by exposure of subjects to other people's smoking.[153] Nicotine-containing chewing gum does not affect salivary thiocyanate levels.[154] It would be interesting to see whether thiocyanate as an indicator of smoking would be more sensitive if it were combined with iodide estimation and the thiocyanate-to-iodide ratio was used.

### P. Nitrate and Nitrite

There has been growing interest in salivary nitrate concentrations over recent years since it was discovered that the nitrate content of saliva reflected the nitrate intake of the body.[7,17] Nitrate is transported into saliva by the iodide transport system but is converted in the mouth by bacteria into nitrite. In individual secretions nitrate concentrations fall as flow rate increases. In whole saliva both nitrate and nitrite can be detected and estimated by the method of Phazackerley and Al Dallagh.[155] Nitrites are thought to be converted in the gut to nitrosamines which are carcinogenic. Nitrate estimation in saliva, then, not only provides a means of monitoring nitrate uptake, but also may be a pointer to the future development of carcinoma, particularly in the gastric region. Thiocyanate may be another nitrosamine precursor.

## Q. Fluoride

Ionized fluoride levels in gland saliva, as measured with the fluoride-specific ion electrode, follow plasma fluoride levels.[156] Whole saliva levels have been studied during ingestion of fluoride-containing foods, drinks, and tablets to determine the concentrations of fluoride around the teeth and the duration of effectiveness of fluoride administered in these forms. Shannon,[32] reviewing previous work and reporting new data, concluded that fluoride reached saliva by passive diffusion in the acini and that some concentration might occur if water were reabsorbed in the ductal system. This results in slightly higher fluoride levels in unstimulated saliva but virtually no change with rate of flow once stimulation has begun. Peak concentrations of fluoride in gland saliva are observed some 30 to 60 min after ingestion of a fluoride dose. No data are available as to whether fluoride levels differ in different age groups.

## V. CONCLUDING REMARKS

The diagnostic areas in which analysis of salivary electrolytes would seem to be useful with our present state of knowledge, therefore, are those in which sodium transport is affected — aldosteronism, damage to salivary ductal tissue, diseases such as Bartther's syndrome, drug-induced conditions such as digitalis toxicity, and situations in which toxic or potentially toxic ions are taken into the body and their intake is reflected in saliva concentrations. It is the medical profession rather than the dental profession who are likely to make use of these tests, and it is increasingly likely that new tests involving the use of saliva will be sought by our medical colleagues.

## REFERENCES

1. **Arwill, T., Myrberg, N., and Soremark, R.,** The concentrations of Cl, Na, Br, Cu, Sr, and Mn in human mixed saliva, *Odontol. Revy,* 18, 1, 1967.
2. **Cole, D. E. and Landry, D. A.,** Determination of inorganic sulphate in human saliva and sweat by controlled flow anion chromatography. Normal values in adult humans, *J. Chromatog.,* 337, 267, 1985.
3. **Curzon, M. E. J.,** Strontium concentrations in whole human saliva, *Arch. Oral Biol.* 29, 211, 1984.
4. **Dreizen, S., Spies, H. A., and Spies, T. D.,** The copper and cobalt levels of human saliva and dental caries activity, *J. Dent. Res.,* 31, 137, 1952.
5. **Ferguson, D. B.,** Salivary glands and saliva, in *The Applied Physiology of the Mouth,* Lavelle, Ed., John Wright, Bristol, 1975.
6. **Ferguson, D. B. and Botchway, C. A.,** Circadian variations in flow rate and composition of whole saliva stimulated by mastication, *Arch. Oral Biol.,* 24, 877, 1979.
7. **Forman, D., Al-Dabbagh, S., and Doll, R.,** Geographic and social class variation within the UK in levels of salivary nitrates and nitrites, a preliminary report, *IARC Sci. Publ.,* 57, 901, 1984.
8. **Fung, H. L., Yaffee, S. J., Mattar, M. E., and Lanighan, M. C.,** Blood and salivary lead levels in children, *Clin. Chim. Acta,* 61, 423, 1975.
9. **Joselow, M. M., Ruiz, R., and Goldwater, L. J.,** Adsorption and excretion of mercury in man. XIV. Salivary excretion of mercury and its relationship to blood and urine mercury, *Arch. Environ. Health,* 17, 35, 1968.
10. **Mandel, I. D. and Wotman, S.,** The salivary secretions in health and disease, *Oral Sci. Rev.,* 8, 25, 1976.
11. **Mandel, I. D.,** Sialochemistry in diseases and clinical situations affecting salivary glands, *Crit. Rev. Clin. Lab. Sci.,* 12, 321, 1980.
12. **McClure, F. J.,** Domestic water and dental caries. III. Fluorine in human saliva, *Am. J. Dis. Child.,* 72, 512, 1941.
13. **Neu, C., DiMascio, A., and Williamds, D.,** Saliva lithium levels: clinical implications, *Am. J. Psychiatry,* 132, 66, 1975.
14. **Nilner, K. and Glantz, P. O.,** The prevalence of copper, silver, tin, mercury and zinc ions in human saliva, *Swed. Dent. J.,* 6, 71, 1982.

15. **P'an, A. Y.,** Lead levels in saliva and blood, *J. Toxicol. Environ. Health,* 7, 273, 1981.
16. **Shannon, I. L., Suddick, R. P., and Down, F. J.,** *Saliva Composition and Secretion,* S. Karger, Basel, 1974.
17. **Srianujata, S., Tangbanleukal, L., Bunyaratvej, S., and Valyasevi, A.,** Nitrate and nitrate in saliva and urine of inhabitants of areas of low and high incidence of cholangiocarcinoma in Thailand, *IARC Sci. Publ.,* 57, 921, 1984.
18. **Tenovuo, J. and Mäkinen, K. K.,** Concentration of thiocyanate and ionisable iodine in saliva of smokers and non-smokers, *J. Dent. Res.,* 55, 661, 1976.
19. **Tenovuo, J., Pruitt, K. M., and Thomas, E. L.,** Peroxidase antimicrobial system of human saliva: hypothiocyanite levels in resting and stimulated saliva, *J. Dent. Res.,* 61, 982, 1982.
20. **Chauncey, H. H., Feller, R. P. and Henriques, B. L.,** Comparative electrolyte composition of parotid, submandibular and sublingual secretions, *J. Dent. Res.,* 45, 1230, 1966.
21. **Dawes, C.,** The secretion of magnesium and calcium in human parotid saliva, *Caries Res.,* 1, 333, 1967.
22. **Dawes, C.,** The effect of flow rate and duration of stimulation on the concentrations of protein and the main electrolytes in human parotid saliva, *Arch. Oral Biol.,* 14, 277, 1969.
23. **Ferguson, D. B., Elliott, A. L., Fort, A., and Potts, A. J.,** Circadian rhythms in human stimulated parotid saliva flow rate and composition, *Arch. Oral Biol.* 18, 1155, 1973.
24. **Ferguson, D. B. and Fort, A.,** Circadian variations in calcium and phosphate secretion from human parotid and submandibular salivary glands, *Caries Res.,* 7, 19, 1973.
25. **Lagerlof, F. and Lindqvist, L.,** A method for determining concentrations of calcium complexes in human parotid saliva by gel filtration, *Arch. Oral Biol.* 27, 735, 1982.
26. **Maier, H., Coroneo, M. T., Antonczyk, G., and Heidland, A.,** The flow-rate-dependent excretion of ionized calcium in human parotid saliva, *Arch. Oral Biol.,* 24, 225, 1979.
27. **Mason, D. K., Harden, R., McG., and Alexander, W. D.,** The influence of flow rate on the salivary iodide concentration in man, *Arch. Oral Biol.,* 11, 235, 1966.
28. **Sawinski, V. J. and Cole, D. F.,** Phosphate concentrations of sterile human parotid saliva and its relationship to dental disorders, *J. Dent. Res.,* 44, 827, 1965.
29. **Shannon, I. L. and Segreto, V. A.,** Periodic Variations in Flow Rate and Chemical Constituents of Human Parotid Fluid, Publication SAM-TR-68-7, USAF School of Aerospace Medicine, Brooks Air Force Base, Texas, 1968.
30. **Shannon, I. L.,** Effect of rate of gland function on pH, viscosity, total solids, calcium, and magnesium in unstimulated parotid fluid, *Proc. Soc. Exp. Biol. Med.,* 130, 874, 1969.
31. **Shannon, I. L.,** Reference table for human parotid saliva collected at varying levels of exogenous stimulation, *J. Dent. Res.,* 52, 1157, 1973.
32. **Shannon, I. L.,** Biochemistry of fluoride in saliva, *Caries Res.,* 11 (Suppl. 1), 206, 1977.
33. **Shannon, I. L.,** Effect of rate of gland function on human parotid fluid bicarbonate concentration, *IRCS Med. Sci.,* 9, 62, 1981.
34. **Shannon, I. L.,** Physiologic baselines for human parotid saliva, *IRCS Med. Sci.,* 9, 90, 1981.
35. **Spring, K. R. and Spirtes, M. A.,** Salivary excretion of lithium in human parotid and submaxillary secretions, *J. Dent. Res.,* 48, 546, 1969.
36. **Stephen, K. W., Harden, R., McG., and Mason, D. K.,** Effect of stimulus on iodide concentration in human parotid saliva, *Arch. Oral Biol.,* 16, 581, 1971.
37. **Vogel, J. J. and Amdur, B. H.,** Inorganic pyrophosphate in parotid saliva and its relation to calculus formation, *Arch. Oral Biol.,* 12, 159, 1967.
38. **Dawes, C.,** The effects of flow rate and duration of stimulation on the concentrations of protein and the main electrolytes in human submandibular saliva, *Arch. Oral Biol.,* 19, 887, 1974.
39. **Ferguson, D. B. and Fort, A.,** Circadian variations in human resting submandibular saliva flow rate and composition, *Arch. Oral Biol.,* 19, 47, 1974.
40. **Ferguson, D. B. and Botchway, C. A.,** Circadian variations in flow rate and composition of human stimulated submandibular saliva, *Arch. Oral Biol.,* 24, 433, 1979.
41. **Dawes, C. and Wood, C. M.,** The composition of lip mucous gland secretion, *Arch. Oral Biol.,* 18, 343, 1973.
42. **Weissman, U. N., Boat, T. F., and DiSant'Agnese, P. A.,** Flow rates and electrolytes in minor salivary gland saliva in normal subjects and patients with cystic fibrosis, *Lancet,* 2, 510, 1972.
43. **Cimasoni, G.,** Crevicular fluid updated, *Monographs in Oral Science,* No 12, S. Karger, Basel, 1983.
44. **Dawes, C.,** Effects of diet on salivary secretion and composition, *J. Dent. Res.,* 49, 1263, 1970.
45. **Dawes, C.,** Stimulus effects on protein and electrolyte concentrations in parotid saliva, *J. Physiol. (London),* 346, 579, 1984.
46. **Dawes, C. and Jenkins, G. N.,** The effect of the type of stimulus on the composition of saliva, *J. Physiol. (London),* 170, 86, 1964.
47. **Ben-Aryeh, H., Lapid, S., Szargel, R., Benderly, A., and Gutman, D.,** Composition of whole unstimulated saliva in infants, *Arch. Oral Biol.,* 29, 357, 1984.

48. **Dawes, C.,** Circadian rhythms in human salivary flow rate and composition, *J. Physiol. (London),* 220, 525, 1972.

49. **Ferguson, D. B. and Botchway, C. A.,** A comparison of circadian variation in the flow rate and composition of stimulated human parotid, submandibular and whole salivas from the same individuals, *Arch. Oral Biol.,* 25, 559, 1980.

50. **Dawes, C. and Chebib,** The influence of previous stimulation and the day of the week on the concentrations of protein and the main electrolytes in human parotid saliva, *Arch. Oral Biol.,* 17, 1289, 1972.

51. **Shannon, I. L.,** Climatological effects on human parotid gland function, *Arch. Oral Biol.,* 11, 451, 1966.

52. **Ferguson, D. B.,** Physiological, pathological, and pharmacological variations in salivary composition, in *The Environment of the Teeth,* D. B. Ferguson, Ed., S. Karger, Basel, 1981, 138.

53. **Puskulian, L.,** Salivary electrolyte changes during normal menstrual cycle, *J. Dent. Res.,* 51, 1212, 1972.

54. **Ben-Aryeh, H., Filman, S., Gutman, D., Szargel, R., and Paldi, E.,** Salivary phosphate as an indicator of ovulation, *Am. J. Obstet, Gynecol.,* 125, 871, 1976.

55. **Tenovuo, J., Laine, M., Söderling, E., and Irjala, K.,** Evaluation of salivary markers during the menstrual cycle: peroxidase, protein, and electrolytes, *Biochem. Med.,* 25, 337, 1981.

56. **Ferguson, D. B.,** Protein and phosphate concentrations in saliva from young adults, *J. Dent. Res.,* 62, 493, Abstr., 1982.

57. **Salminen, S. and Konttinen, A.,** Effect of exercise on Na and K concentration in human saliva and serum, *J. Appl. Physiol.,* 812, 1963.

58. **Shannon, I. L.,** Effect of exercise on parotid fluid corticosteroids and electrolytes, *J. Dent. Res.,* 46, 608, 1966.

59. **Dawes, C.,** The effects of exercise on protein and electrolyte secretion in parotid saliva, *J. Physiol. (London),* 320, 139, 1981.

60. **Gutman, D. and Ben-Aryeh, H.,** The influence of age on salivary content and rate of flow, *Int. J. Oral Surg.,* 3, 314, 1974.

61. **Baum, B. J.,** Evaluation of stimulated parotid saliva flow rate in different age groups, *J. Dent. Res.,* 60, 1292, 1981.

62. **Becks, H. and Wainwright, W. W.,** Human saliva. XIII. Rate of flow of resting saliva of healthy individuals, *J. Dent. Res.,* 22, 391, 1943.

63. **Bertram, U.,** Xerostomia, *Acta Odontol. Scand.,* 25 (Suppl. 25), 1967.

64. **Chisholm, D. M. and Mason, D. K.,** Salivary gland function in Sjögren's syndrome, a review, *Br. Dent. J.,* 135, 393, 1973.

65. **Mäkila, E.,** Oral health among the inmates of an old people's homes. II. Salivary secretion, *Proc. Finn. Dent. Soc.,* 75, 64, 1977.

66. **Heft, M. W. and Baum, B. J.,** Unstimulated and stimulated parotid salivary flow rate in individuals of different ages, *J. Dent. Res.,* 63, 1182, 1984.

67. **Pederson, W., Schubert, M., Izutsu, K., Mersai, T., and Truelove, E.,** Age-dependent decreases in human submandibular gland flow rates as measured under resting and post-stimulation conditions, *J. Dent. Res.,* 64, 822, 1985.

68. **Chauncey, H. H., Borkan, G. A., Wayler, A. H., Feller, R. P., and Kapur, K. K.,** Parotid fluid composition in healthy aging males, *Adv. Physiol. Sci.,* 28, 323, 1981.

69. **Baum, B. J., Costa, P. T., Jr., and Izutsu, K. T.,** Alteration in sodium handling by human parotid glands during aging: failure to support a simple two stage secretion model, *Am. J. Physiol.,* 246, R35, 1984.

70. **Kalipatnapu, P., Kelly, R. H., Rao, K. N., and van Thiel, D. H.,** Salivary composition: effects of age and sex, *Acta Med. Port.,* 4, 327, 1983.

71. **Mandel, I. D.,** Relation of saliva and plaque to caries, *J. Dent. Res.,* 53, 246, 1974.

72. **Dulce, H. J. and Hardel, M.,** Calciumionen-Aktivität im Löslichkeits-gleichgewicht Zwischen dem Apatit des Zahnschmelzes und dem Speichel, *Naturwissenschaften,* 55, 137, 1968.

73. **Shannon, I. L.,** Parotid fluid flow rate, parotid fluid and serum inorganic phosphate concentrations as related to dental caries status in man, *J. Dent. Res.,* 43, 1029, 1964.

74. **Shaw, L. Murray, J. J., Burchell, C. K., and Best, J. S.,** Calcium and phosphorus content of plaque and saliva in relation to dental caries, *Caries Res.,* 17, 543, 1983.

75. **Mandel, I. D.,** Biochemical aspects of calculus formation. II. Comparative studies of saliva in heavy and light calculus formers, *J. Periodontal Res.,* 9, 211, 1974.

76. **Wotman, S., Mercadente, J., Mandel, I. D., Goldman, R. S., and Denning, C.,** The occurrence of calculus in normal children, children with cystic fibrosis, and children with asthma, *J. Periodontol.,* 44, 278, 1973.

77. **Rausch, S.,** Diseases of the salivary glands, in *Thoma's Oral Pathology,* Vol. 2, 6th ed., Gorlin, R., Ed., C. V. Mosby, St. Louis, 1974, chap. 22.

78. **Mandel, I. D. and Baurmash, H.,** Biochemical profile in salivary gland disease, *J. Dent. Res.,* 52, 226, Abstr., 1973.

79. **Mandel, I. D. and Baurmash, H.,** Sialochemistry in chronic recurrent parotitis: electrolytes and glucose, *J. Oral Pathol.,* 9, 92, 1980.

80. **Ben-Aryeh, H., Gutman, D., Szargel, R., and Laufer, D.,** Effects of irradiation on saliva in cancer patients, *Int. J. Oral Surg.,* 4, 205, 1975.

81. **Dreizen, S., Brown, L. R., Handler, S. and Levy, B. M.,** Radiation-induced xerostomia in cancer patients: effect on salivary and serum electrolytes, *Cancer (Philadelphia),* 38, 273, 1976.

82. **Compton, J. S., Nelson, J. F., Wright, R. D., and Young, J. A.,** A micropuncture investigation of electrolyte transport in the parotid glands of sodium-replete and sodium-depleted sheep, *J. Physiol. (London),* 309, 429, 1980.

83. **Ben-Aryeh, H., Spielman, A., Szargel, R., Gutman, D., Scharf, J., Nahir, M., and Scharf, Y.,** Sialochemistry for diagnosis of Sjögren's syndrome in xerostomic patients, *Oral Surg., Oral Med. Oral Pathol.,* 52, 487, 1981.

84. **Mandel, I. D. and Baurmash, H.,** Sialochemistry in Sögren's syndrome, *Oral Surg., Oral Med. Oral Pathol.,* 41, 182, 1976.

85. **Spielman, A., Ben-Aryeh, H., Lichtig, C., Szargel, R., Gutman, D., Scharf, J., Nahir, M., and Scharf, Y.,** Correlation between sialochemistry and lip biopsy in Sjögren's syndrome patients, *Int. J. Oral Surg.,* 11, 326, 1982.

86. **Bertram, U. and Theilade, J.,** Ultrastructural changes in the striated ducts of salivary glands of mice with autoimmune chronic sialoadenitis, *J. Dent. Res.,* 56, A87, Abstr., 1977.

87. **Izutsu, K. T., Schubert, M. M., Truelove, E. L., Shulman, H. M., Sale, G. E., Morton, T. H., Ensign, W. Y., Mersai, T., Sullivan, K. M., Oberg, S., and Thomas, E. D.,** The predictive value of elevated labial saliva sodium concentration: its relation to labial gland pathology in bone marrow transplant recipients, *Human Pathol.,* 14, 29, 1983.

88. **Syrjänen, S. M.,** Chemical analysis of parotid saliva and lacrimal fluid in psoriatics, *Arch. Dermatol. Res.,* 275, 152, 1983.

89. **Kutscher, A. H., Denning, C. R., Zegarelli, E. V., Kessler, W., Eriv, A., Phelan, J., and Ellgood, K.,** Capillary tube tests for minor salivary gland secretion in cystic fibrosis, *N.Y. State J. Med.,* 68, 2812, 1968.

90. **Mandel, I. D., Kutscher, A. H., Denning, C. R., Thompson, R. H., Jr., and Zegarelli, E. V.,** Salivary studies in cystic fibrosis, *Am. J. Dis. Child.,* 113, 431, 1967.

91. **Mandel, I. D., Thompson, R. H., Wotman, S., Taubman, M., Kutscher, A. H., Zegarelli, E. V., Denning, C. R., Botwick, J. T., and Fahn, B. S.,** Parotid saliva in cystic fibrosis. II. Electrolytes and protein-bound carbohydrates, *Am. J. Dis. Child.,* 110, 646, 1965.

92. **Tannenbaum, P., Posner, A. S., and Mandel, I. D.,** Formation of calcium phosphates in saliva and dental plaque, *J. Dent. Res.,* 55, 997, 1976.

93. **Blomfield, J., Allars, H. M., Rush, A. R., VanLenner, E. W., and Brown, J. M.,** Parotid serous hypersecretion in cystic fibrosis, *Aust. Paediatr. J.,* 10, 75, 1974.

94. **Blomfield, J., Rush, A. R., Allars, H., and Brown, J. M.,** Parotid gland function in children with cystic fibrosis and child control subjects, *Pediatr. Res.,* 10, 574, 1976.

95. **Blomfield, J., Warton K. L., and Brown, J. M.,** Flow rate and inorganic components of submandibular saliva in cystic fibrosis, *Arch. Dis. Child.,* 48, 267, 1977.

96. **Chernick, W. S., Barbero, G. J., and Parkins, F. M.,** Studies on submaxillary saliva in cystic fibrosis, *J. Pediatr.,* 59, 890, 1968.

97. **Mandel, I. D., Eriv, A., Kutscher, A., Denning, C., Thompson, R. H., Kessler, W., and Zegarelli, E.,** Calcium and phosphorus levels in submaxillary saliva. Changes in cystic fibrosis and in asthma, *Clin. Pediatr. (Philadelphia),* 8, 161, 1964.

98. **Wotman, S., Mandel, I. D., Mercadente, J., and Denning, C. R.,** Parotid and submaxillary calcium in human cystic fibrosis, *Arch. Oral Biol.,* 16, 663, 1971.

99. **Grad, B.,** Influence of ACTH on the sodium and potassium concentration of human mixed saliva, *J. Clin. Endocrinol.,* 12, 708, 1952.

100. **Prader, A., Gautier, E., Gautier, R., Naf, D., Semer, J. M. and Rothschild, E. J.,** The Na and K concentration in mixed saliva: influence of secretion rate, stimulation, method of collection, age, sex, time of day and adrenocortical activity, in *Ciba Foundation Colloquia on Endocrinology,* Vol. 8, Wolstenholme, G. E. W. and Cameron, M. P., Eds., J. & A. Churchill, London, 1955.

101. **Warming-Larsen, A., Hamburger, C., and Sprechler, M.,** The influence of ACTH on the sodium and potassium concentrations of human saliva, *Acta Endocrinol.,* 11, 400, 1952.

102. **Frawley, T. F. and Thorn, G. W.,** The relation of the sodium:potassium ratio to adrenal cortical activity, in *Proceedings 2nd Annual ACTH Conf.,* Mote, J. R., Ed., Churchill Livingstone, Edinburgh, 1951, 115.

103. **Conn, J. W.,** Primary aldosteronism, a new clinical syndrome, *J. Lab. Clin. Med.,* 45, 6, 1955.

104. **Lauler, D. E., Hickler, R. B., and Thorn, G. W.,** The salivary sodium:potassium ratio: a useful "screening test" for aldosteronism in hypertensive subjects, *N. Engl. J. Med.,* 267, 1136, 1962.

105. **Morris, G. C. R.,** Factors Determining Sodium and Potassium Concentrations of Saliva with Special Reference to Aldosterone, Thesis, University of Oxford, 1963.
106. **Wotman, S., Goodwin, F. J., Mandel, I. D., and Laragh, J. H.,** Changes in salivary electrolytes following treatment of primary aldosteronism, *Arch. Intern. Med.,* 124, 477, 1969.
107. **Wotman, S. Baer, L., and Mandel, I. D.,** Submaxillary potassium concentration in true and pseudo-primary aldosteronism, *Arch. Intern. Med.,* 126, 248, 1970.
108. **Wotman, S., Mandel, I. D., Thompson, R. H., Jr., and Laragh, J. H.,** Salivary electrolytes, urea nitrogen, uric acid, and salt taste thresholds in hypertension, *J. Oral Ther. Pharmacol.,* 3, 239, 1967.
109. **Niedermeier, W., Dreizen, S., Stone, R. E., and Spies, T. D.,** Sodium and potassium concentrations in the saliva of normotensive and hypertensive subjects, *Oral Surg. Oral Med. Oral Pathol.,* 9, 426, 1956.
110. **Ben-Aryeh, H., Schiller, M., Shasha, S., Szargel, R., and Gutman, D.,** Salivary composition in patients with essential hypertension and the effect of Pindolol, *J. Oral Med.,* 36, 76, 1981.
111. **Abelson, D., Mandel, I. D., and Karmiol, M.,** Salivary studies in alcoholic cirrhosis, *Oral Surg. Oral Med. Oral Pathol.,* 41, 188, 1976.
112. **Weinberger, A., Sperling, O., and DeVries, A.,** Calcium and phosphate in saliva of patients with primary hyperparathyroidism, *Clin. Chim. Acta,* 50, 5, 1974.
113. **Schneider, P., Paunier, L., Sizonero, P. C., and Wyss, M.,** Effects of parathyroid hormone on total protein, calcium, magnesium, phosphorus, sodium and potassium concentration of normal human parotid saliva, *Eur. J. Clin. Invest.,* 7, 121, 1977.
114. **Francois, R. and Guest, G.,** Etude clinique et experimentale de quelque electrolytes et de quelque constituants organiques de la salive. Etude comparee chez le chien et chez l'enfant, *C. R. Soc. Biol.,* 147, 700, 1953.
115. **Marder, M., Abelson, D. C., and Mandel, I. D.,** Salivary alterations in diabetes mellitus, *J. Periodontol.,* 46, 567, 1975.
116. **Kakizaki, G., Noto, N., Saito, T., Fujiwara, Y., Ohizumi, T., Soeno, T., and Ishidate, T.,** Laboratory diagnosis test for pancreatic disorders by examination of parotid saliva, *Tohuko J. Exp. Med.,* 109, 121, 1973.
117. **Descos, L., Lambert, R., and Minaire, Y.,** Comparison of human salivary secretion in health and chronic pancreatitis, *Digestion,* 9, 76, 1973.
118. **Dobrilla, G., Valentine, M., Fillipeni, M., Bonoldi, M. C., Felder, M., and Moroder, E.,** The study of parotid and mixed saliva in the diagnosis of chronic pancreatitis, *Ir. J. Med., Sci.,* 146 (Suppl. 1), 13, Abstr., 1977.
119. **Harden, R. McG. and Mason, D. K.,** Quantitative studies of iodide excretion in saliva in euthyroid, hypothyroid and thyrotoxic patients, *J. Clin. Endocrinol.,* 25, 957, 1965.
120. **Glen, A. I. M., Ongley, G. C., and Robinson, K.,** Diminished membrane transport in manic depressive psychosis and recurrent depression, *Lancet,* 2, 241, 1968.
121. **Bolwig, T. G. and Rafaelson, O. J.,** Salivation in affective disorders, *Psychol. Med.,* 2, 232, 1972.
122. **Costa P. T. Jr., Chauncey, H. H., Rose, C. L., and Kapur, K. K.,** Relation of parotid saliva flow rate and composition with personality traits in healthy men, *Oral Surg. Oral Med. Oral Pathol.,* 50, 416, 1980.
123. **Ben-Aryeh, H., Laor, R., Szargel, R., Gutman, D., Naon, H., Pascal, M., and Hefetz, A.,** Saliva for monitoring of patients with primary affective disorders, *Isr. J. Med. Sci.,* 20, 197, 1984.
124. **Avissar, R., Menache, R., and Mandel, E.,** Increased salivary calcium levels as an indication of digitalis intoxication, *Arch. Intern. Med.,* 135, 1029, 1975.
125. **Ben-Aryeh, H. Bergman, S., Gutman, D., Barzilai, B., Hammerman, H., and Szargel, R.,** Salivary levels of calcium and potassium as indicators of digitalis toxicity, *Chest,* 72, 131, 1977.
126. **Ben-Aryeh, H., Gutman, D., and Szargel, R.,** Salivary sodium concentration in digitalised patients, *J. Oral Med.,* 33, 90, 1978.
127. **Kahn, N., Bartelstone, H. J., and Mandel, I. D.,** Salivary potassium concentration as an indicator of digitalis toxicity, *J. Dent. Res.,* 48, 169, Abstr., 1969.
128. **Lankisch, P. G., Buckesfeld, R. P., Bolte, H. D., and Larbir, D.,** Salivary electrolytes and digitalis intoxication, *N. Engl. J. Med.,* 288, 326, 1973.
129. **Swanson, M., Cacace, L., Chun, G., and Itano, M.,** Salivary calcium and potassium concentrations in the detection of digitalis toxicity, *Circulation,* 47, 736, 1977.
130. **Wotman, S., Bigger, T. J., Mandel, I. D., and Bartelstone, H. J.,** Salivary electrolytes in the detection of digitalis toxicity, *N. Engl. J. Med.,* 285, 871, 1971.
131. **Gould, L., Reddy, R., and Gomprecht, R. F.,** Evaluation of digitalis toxicity by salivary electrolytes, *N. Engl. J. Med.,* 286, 47, 1972.
132. **Crook, M., Ferguson, D. B., and Vites, N.,** Effects of furosemide on the flow rate and composition of human saliva, *J. Physiol. (London),* 257, 60P, 1976.

133. **Poulsen, J. H., Laugesen, L. P., and Nielsen, J. O. D.,** Evidence supporting that basolaterally located $Na^+$-$K^+$-ATP-ase and a co-transport system for sodium and chloride are key elements in the secretion of primary saliva, in *Electrolyte and Water Transport Across Gastrointestinal Epithelia,* Case, R. M., Garner, A., Turnberg, L. A., and Young, J. A., Eds., Raven Press, New York, 1982, 157.

134. **Case, R. M., Hunter, M., Novak, I., and Young, J. A.,** The anionic basis of fluid secretion by the rabbit mandibular salivary gland, *J. Physiol. (London),* 349, 619, 1984.

135. **White, A. G., Entmacher, P. S., Rudin, G., and Leiter, L.,** Physiological and pharmacological regulation of human salivary electrolyte concentrations, *J. Clin. Invest.,* 34, 246, 1955.

136. **Schneyer, L. H., Young, J. A., and Schneyer, C. A.,** Salivary secretion of electrolytes, *Physiol. Rev.,* 53, 720, 1972.

137. **Wallach, D. and Schramm, M.,** Calcium and the exportable protein in rat parotid gland. Parallel subcellular distribution and concomitant secretion, *Eur. J. Biochem.,* 21, 433, 1971.

138. **Freeman, R. M. and Welt, L. G.,** Parotid fluid calcium and phosphate levels in patients with hypercalcaemia, *Proc. Soc. Exper. Biol., Med.,* 120, 627, 1965.

139. **Dreisbach, R. H.,** Calcium binding by normal human saliva, *J. Dent. Res.,* 39, 1133, 1960.

140. **Nixon, G. S. and Smith, H.,** Hazard of mercury poisoning in the dental surgery, *J. Oral Ther.,* 1, 512, 1965.

141. **Richter, J., Kral, V., Zukov, I., Subrt, P., and Rahm, J.,** Circadian changes of the SIgA, lysozyme, albumin and copper content of saliva, *Czech. Med.,* 3, 249, 1980.

142. **Gervais, L., Lacasse, Y., Brodeur, J., and P'an, A.,** Presence of cadmium in the saliva of adult male workers, *Toxicol. Lett.,* 8, 63, 1981.

143. **Izutsu, K. T.,** Theory and measurement of the buffer value of bicarbonate in saliva, *J. Theoret. Biol.,* 90, 397, 1981.

144. **Kuttner, T. and Cohen, H. B.,** Microcolorimetric studies. I. A molybdic acid, stannous chloride reagent. The microestimation of phosphate and calcium in pus, plasma, and spinal fluid, *J. Biol. Chem.,* 75, 517, 1927.

145. **Chen, P. S., Toribaba, T. Y., and Warner, H.,** Microdetermination of phosphorus, *Anal. Chem.,* 28, 1756, 1956.

146. **Mason, D. K., Harden, R. McG., and Alexander, W. D.,** The salivary and thyroid glands, *Br. Dent. J.,* 122, 485, 1963.

147. **Myant, N. B.,** Iodine metabolism of salivary glands, *Ann. N. Y. Acad. Sci.,* 85, 208, 1960.

148. **Tenovuo, J., Söderling, S., and Anttonen, T.,** Distribution and forms of iodine in the human oral cavity, *Scand. J. Dent. Res.,* 88, 430.

149. **Talner, L. B., Coel, M. N., and Lang, J. H.,** Salivary secretion of iodine after urography, *Radiology,* 106, 263, 1973.

150. **Powell, W. N.,** Photoelectric determination of blood thiocyanates without precipitation of proteins, *J. Lab. Clin. Med.,* 30, 107, 1945.

151. **Thomas, E. L., Bates, K. P., and Jefferson, M. M.,** Hypothiocyanite ion: detection of the antimicrobial agent in human saliva, *J. Dent. Res.,* 59, 1466, 1980.

152. **Luepker, R. V., Pechacek, T. F., Murray, D. M., Johnson, C. A., Hund, F., and Jacobs, D. R.,** Saliva thiocyanate: a chemical indicator of cigarette smoking in adolescents, *Am. J. Public Health,* 71, 1320, 1981.

153. **Gillies, P. A., Wilcox, B., Coates, C., Kristmundsdottir, F., and Reid, D. J.,** Use of objective measurement in the validation of self-reported smoking in children aged 10 and 11 years: saliva thiocyanate, *J. Epidemiol. Commun. Health,* 36, 205, 208, 1982.

154. **Olson, B. L., McDonald, J. L., Jr., Gleason, M. R., Stookey, G. K., Schemehorn, B. R., Drook, B. B., Beiswanger, B. B., and Christen, A. G.,** Comparisons of various salivary parameters in smokers before and after the use of a nicotine-containing chewing gum, *J. Dent. Res.,* 64, 826, 1985.

155. **Phazackerley, P. J. R., and Al Dallagh, S. A.,** Estimation of nitrate and nitrite in saliva and urine, *Anal. Biochem.,* 131, 242, 1983.

156. **Ericsson, Y.,** Fluoride excretion in human saliva and milk, *Caries. Res.,* 3, 159, 1969.

Chapter 4

## SALIVARY GLYCOPROTEINS

**Robert E. Cohen and Michael J. Levine**

### TABLE OF CONTENTS

# I. INTRODUCTION

Saliva is a complex fluid composed of a wide variety of organic and inorganic constituents which collectively act to modulate the oral environment. The protective qualities of saliva become clinically evident when salivary flow is absent or markedly decreased. Such situations, clinically termed "xerostomia" or "dry mouth", may result from numerous factors, including removal of salivary glands following neck dissection for cancer therapy, specific disease, irradiation, and/or pharmacological agents. Nonspecific causes of xerostomia can include mouth breathing, nasal obstruction, and psychiatric distress.[1-5] Chronic xerostomia can lead to dry, red, sticky, and rough mucosal surfaces which bleed more easily and are increasingly susceptible to infection. The tongue becomes smooth, slimy, hypersensitive to irritation and loses taste acuity.[6-8] The accumulation of bacterial plaque and debris can lead to an increased incidence of dental caries and periodontal disease.[3,9] In addition, facility of speech and management of the edentulous patient become more difficult. Studies over the past two decades have suggested that many of the protective effects of saliva can be attributed to particular salivary glycoproteins, such as mucins, proline-rich glycoproteins, α-amylases, lactoferrin, salivary peroxidase, and secretory IgA. We are just beginning, however, to elucidate the precise structure, function, and salivary concentrations of these molecules. This information will be required in order for the dental scientist to develop sialochemical tests and artificial salivas which can be used by the clinician to monitor, regulate, and/or augment the healthy or diseased oral environment. This chapter summarizes current information on various aspects of the major salivary glycoproteins, including structure, synthetic pathways involved in construction and processing, function, their structural modulation, and future studies and clinical applications.

# II. CLASSIFICATION OF SALIVARY GLYCOPROTEINS

Salivary secretions can be classified according to a number of separate schemes, based on glandular origin, biological function, and/or biochemical features. Classification is usually complicated, however, by the diversity of salivary constituents with regard to many of these features. In addition, the limitations associated with the cellular and bacterial contamination inherent in whole saliva necessitate that salivary components be characterized from secretions obtained directly from the ductal orifices of the individual glands. Since the human salivary glands (with the notable exception of the parotid gland) contain a mixture of serous and mucous cells, classification based upon glandular origin may not be particularly useful. Classification of salivary molecules based on their cell origin, however, provides a workable framework for describing their structural and biosynthetic properties.[10-12] In Table 1, for example, human salivary glycoproteins are classified according to cell origin and then subclassified based upon biochemical properties associated with serous or mucous products. In general, one can group human salivary glycoproteins synthesized by acinar cells into families whose members share common structural features. For example, the salivary mucin glycoproteins constitute a family of at least two members: a multisubunit higher molecular weight species, designated MG1, and a lower molecular weight single subunit species, MG2.[10,11,13,14] Salivary proline-rich proteins and amylases also occur in multiple forms as glycosylated or nonglycosylated species.[15-20]

Although family members are structurally related, they may also exhibit structural and functional differences. The differences observed among the family members may be due to transcriptional and/or translational modifications. For example, genetic studies have revealed striking similarities in the amino acid sequence of a number of proline-rich proteins.[16,17,21] These studies have indicated that not only acidic but also some basic proline-rich proteins have a similar overall polypeptide structure, supporting the possibility that mRNAs for these

**Table 1**
## CLASSIFICATION OF SALIVARY GLYCOPROTEINS BASED UPON CELLULAR ORIGIN AND MOLECULAR FAMILIES

1. Salivary glycoproteins occuring as members of families (acinar cell origin)
   A. Mucous glycoproteins
      Mostly O-linked oligosaccharides (Ser/Thr-GalNAc)
      Higher molecular weight
      Greater than 40% carbohydrate
      Small amounts of mannose may be present

   Examples:  mucin glycoprotein 1 (MG1)
              mucin glycoprotein 2 (MG2)

   B. Serous glycoproteins
      N-linked oligosaccharides (Asn-GlcNAc)
      Lower molecular weight
      Less than 50% carbohydrate
      Significant amounts of mannose

   Examples:  proline-rich glycoproteins (PRG)
              α-amylases
              salivary peroxidase
              carbonic anhydrase

2. Salivary glycoproteins occurring as single species (ductal or stromal cell origin)

   Examples:  secretory IgA
              lactoferrin
              kallikrein
              fibronectin

different family members may have originated from a single gene by differential mRNA splicing. Recently, the molecular cloning of sequences encoding human submandibular gland statherin and a basic histidine-rich peptide have been described.[22] Sequence analyses revealed strong homology between their mRNAs, suggesting their evolution from a common ancestral sequence.[22] The presence of multiple amylase isoenzymes may be due to a variety of factors, including multiple alleles and posttranslational modifications. Indeed, each of the salivary amylase genes can occur in a number of alleles, giving rise to 12 distinct phenotypes.[23]

Posttranslational modifications may also account for structural differences among family members. These differences can be attributed to the degree of phosphorylation, acylation, deamidation, sulfation, and glycosylation. In addition, family members may be subject to a variety of proteolytic or glycosidic structural modifications which may be intrinsic (e.g., directly affecting biosynthetic pathways) or extrinsic (e.g., resulting from bacterial degradation).

A number of salivary glycoproteins do not occur as component members of structurally related families. These "individuals" include, among others, lactoferrin, kallikrein, and fibronectin. In general, these molecules are synthesized by ductal or stromal cells and have only been described as single species.[10-12] Secretory IgA provides an exception, since it exists as two subclasses (A1 and A2). Each of these glycoproteins may also undergo posttranslational modifications.

## III. BIOCHEMICAL PROPERTIES OF SALIVARY GLYCOPROTEINS

### A. Salivary Mucins
Human salivary mucins comprise a family of molecules which share general biochemical and biophysical properties but also possess distinct structural and functional differences.

Current evidence suggests that two mucins exist within submandibular-sublingual saliva — namely, a higher molecular weight species, mucin glycoprotein 1 (MG1), and a lower molecular weight species, mucin glycoprotein 2 (MG2).[11,13,14] Recent immunocytochemical studies using monoclonal antibody probes have localized each of the salivary mucins to mucous acini within human submandibular gland tissues.[24,25] These studies also demonstrate the existence of distinct cell subpopulations of MG1- and MG2-secreting acini within these glands, thereby suggesting that the two mucins are authentic cell products and not the result of posttranslational processing.

Selected structural features of each of these salivary mucins are summarized in Table 2. MG1 has been examined by a number of investigators and shown to consist of multiple disulfide-linked subunits composing a molecule of more than 1000 kDa.[13,26-31] The protein core of MG1 is responsible for less than 15% of the total weight. Within the protein core, approximately 43% of the total amino acid residues are composed of threonine, serine, proline, and alanine. Glycine constitutes 8.6% of the total amino acids. Covalently linked fatty acids are also associated with this salivary mucin. Initial characterization of the oligosaccharide units of MG1 has been performed following their release by mild alkaline/borohydride treatment.[13] These studies reveal that the glycopeptide linkage of MG1 involves O-glycosidic bonds between *N*-acetylgalactosamine and/or threonine and serine. The major oligosaccharides of MG1 range in size from 4 to 16 sugar residues. These are responsible for 78% of the total weight of this molecule, with sulfate contributing an additional 7%. However, the precise sequences of the MG1 oligosaccharide units have only been partly determined.[13] A representative oligosaccharide unit of MG1 is illustrated in Figure 1.[32]

Biophysical studies utilizing fluorescent hydrophobic probes have demonstrated the existence of hydrophobic pockets associated with MG1.[13] On the one hand, treatment of MG1 with dithiothreitol increases binding to these probes, implying that cleavage of disulfide bridges exposes additional hydrophobic domains. On the other hand, treatment of MG1 with Pronase results in diminished probe binding, implying destruction of hydrophobic domains associated with naked peptide regions.[13] Experiments designed to examine binding under conditions of varying pH also suggest that the hydrophobic pockets of MG1 contain negatively charge amino acids. In addition, preliminary circular dichroism data have revealed that the carbohydrate units of MG1 may be arranged in a biased (as opposed to random) configuration about the core peptide.[13]

The other human salivary mucin member, MG2, is a molecule of approximately 200 to 250 kDa. It is composed of a single peptide chain which accounts for about 30% of the total chemical composition.[13,14] Approximately 75% of the total amino acid residues are accounted for by threonine, serine, proline, and alanine, while glycine contributes only 1.4%. The carbohydrate content of MG2 is about 68% and consists of a high density of carbohydrate units attached via O-glycosidic linkages to the peptide core. These units are 2 to 7 residues in length. The structures of the major neutral and acidic oligosaccharides from MG2 have been determined and are also presented in Figure 1.[207] Based upon an estimated molecular weight of 250 kDa, approximately 170 such oligosaccharide chains are distributed over the single polypeptide backbone of MG2. This finding, coupled with the high content of proline, suggests that MG2 may have a "bottle-brush" conformation. Recent studies using well-characterized immunoaffinity purified MG2 have revealed small quantities of mannose within the MG2 molecule.[24,33] Subsequent structural studies using affinity purifed mucins have resulted in the isolation of MG2 glycopeptides enriched in mannose, providing preliminary evidence of 3 N-glycosidically linked oligosaccharides in this molecule.[33] MG2 does not bind fluorescent hydrophobic probes, implying the absence of hydrophobic regions.[13] Preliminary circular dichroism spectroscopy of MG2 has further suggested that this mucin exists primarily as a random coil, displaying little organized secondary structure.

## Table 2
## SELECTED BIOCHEMICAL PROPERTIES OF SALIVARY GLYCOPROTEINS

| Properties | MG1[a] | MG2[b] | PRG[c] | Amy[d] | SP[e] | CA[f] |
|---|---|---|---|---|---|---|
| Protein content | 14.9% | 30.4% | 60% | 93—94%[g] | 87.3% | 85.7% |
| Carbohydrate content | 78.1% | 69.0% | 40% | 6—7% | 12.7% | 14.3% |
| Sulfate content | 7% | 1.6% | 0% | 0% | ? | ? |
| Size (kDa) | >1000[h] | 200—250 | 38.9[i] | 55—60 | 72—78 | 42 |
| Subunits | Yes[j] | No | No | No | No | No |
| Size of oligosaccharides | 4—16 residues | 2—7 residues | 14 residues | 11—12 | ? | ? |
| No. of oligosaccharides | 292[k] | 170[k] | 6 | 4 | ? | 2 |
| No. of sialic-acid-containing units | 118 | 67 | 3 | 1 | Present | ? |
| Glycopeptide linkage | GalNAc-Thr/Ser | GalNAc-Thr/Ser & GlcNAc-Asn | GlcNAc-Asn | GlcNAc-Asn | GlcNAc-Asn | GlcNAc-Asn |
| Covalently bound fatty acids[l] | 5—10 | Negligible | 0 | 0 | 0 | ? |
| Quantity[m] | ? | 14—203 μg/ml[267] (HSMSL) | ? | 650—800 μg/ml[46] (HPS) | 5—6 μg/ml[268] (HPS) | ? |

a  High molecular weight salivary mucin.
b  Low molecular weight salivary mucin.
c  Proline-rich glycoprotein.
d  α-Amylase.
e  Salivary peroxidase.
f  Carbonic anhydrase.
g  Both glycosylated and nonglycosylated isoenzymes exist. Data are given for the glycosylated form.
h  Estimated by its elution at the void volume of Sepharose CL-2B columns.
i  Calculated from the carbohydrate structure[35] and the deduced amino acid sequence.[21]
j  Disulfide-linked.
k  Includes sialic-acid-containing, sulfate-containing, and neutral chains.
l  Moles fatty acids per mole glycoprotein. Contains C16:0, C18:0, and C18: derivatives.
m  HSMSL: human submandibular-sublingual saliva; HPS: human parotid saliva.

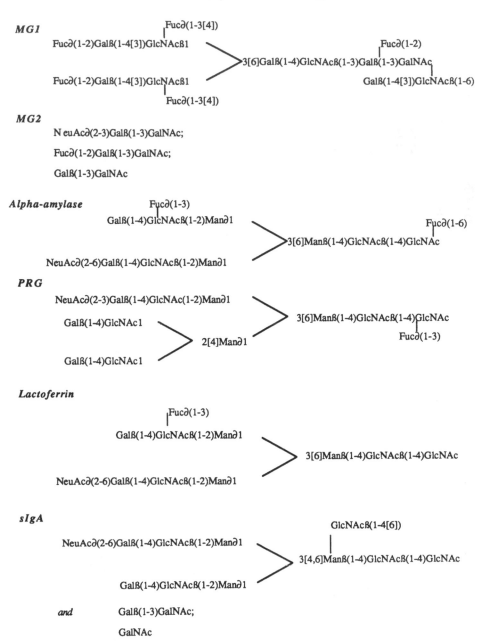

FIGURE 1.    Representative oligosaccharide structures of salivary glycoproteins. The structures presented illustrate typical or predominant oligosaccharide units of the named molecules. See text for references.

## B. Proline-Rich Glycoproteins

Human parotid and submandibular saliva contain proline-rich glycoproteins, of which several are phosphorylated.[15] The major human salivary proline-rich glycoprotein (PRG) is a nonphosphorylated molecule of 38.9 kDa consisting of 60% protein and 40% carbohydrate (Table 2). The peptide sequence of PRG has been deduced from the nucleotide sequence and has revealed that PRG exists as a single peptide chain containing 231 amino acids.[21] Amino acid analysis of PRG isolated from human parotid saliva[34] is identical to that derived from the nucleotide sequence data, suggesting that PRG's peptide moiety is not posttranslationally processed before entering the oral cavity. Studies performed on the carbohydrate moieties of PRG have demonstrated the presence of 6 triantennary oligosaccharide units which are attached to the protein core through N-glycosidic bonds to asparagine residues (Figure 1 and Table 2).[35] The carbohydrate units are evenly distributed along the peptide; three units contain a sialic acid residue, while three units are neutral.

The conformation of PRG is determined, in part, by a series of β-turns within a larger secondary structure dominated by random coils.[34] Recent studies utilizing nuclear magnetic resonance (NMR) spectroscopy have localized the site of the β-turns to a heptapeptide sequence containing the N-glycosylation sites of PRG.[36] Additional studies employing computer modeling, NMR spectroscopy, and known structural characteristics of PRG have suggested that potential hydrogen-binding interactions are of relatively minor significance and that the polypeptide backbone exhibits considerable flexibility.[34] Collectively, these data suggest that the oligosaccharide domains of PRG may be free to assume a variety of orientations which are dependent upon the local conformation of the peptide core at different tissue-environmental interfaces.

## C. α-Amylases

Alpha-amylase is a calcium-requiring metalloenzyme which is responsible for the enzymatic hydrolysis of internal α(1-4) glycosidic linkages in starch, glycogen, and glucose polymers.[37-40] Immunofluorescence and immunocytochemical methodologies have been utilized to detect amylase within serous acinar cells of the major salivary glands.[41-43] Amylase is the most abundant and best characterized enzyme found in saliva and occurs as a single polypeptide with a molecular weight of 55 to 62 kDa.[44,45] The concentration of α-amylase in human parotid saliva has recently been determined by immunochemical techniques, with average values ranging from 650 to 800 μg/ml.[46] The biochemistry of human α-amylases has been extensively reviewed,[39,40] and the biochemical properties of these molecules are summarized in Table 2. Briefly, the family of salivary amylases can be divided into glycosylated and nonglycosylated members.[47-49] Glycosylated salivary α-amylase contains four biantennary N-glycosidically linked oligosaccharide units, one of which possesses a terminal sialic acid residue (Figure 1.)[50] From nucleotide sequencing studies, the primary amino acid sequence of salivary α-amylase has been shown to contain 511 residues.[51,52] While human salivary and pancreatic α-amylases are produced by the expression of different genes,[51,52] immunological studies have demonstrated antigenic similarities between these molecules.[53-55]

## D. Salivary Peroxidase

The salivary peroxidase system consists of the peroxidase enzyme, the thiocyanate ion (SCN⁻), and hydrogen peroxide. A number of studies utilizing antiperoxidase antibodies have localized these molecules to acinar cells within bovine parotid, submandibular, and sublingual glands.[56-57] The biochemical properties of salivary peroxidase are summarized in Table 2. Analysis by SDS-polyacrylamide gel electrophoresis revealed the presence of a closely spaced doublet at approximately 77 kDa, as well as a higher molecular weight band of about 280 kDa. Reducing conditions result in an apparent increase in molecular weight by 16 kDa on SDS-PAGE, supporting the existence of intrachain disulfide linkages within the peroxidase polypeptide core. Such reduction also results in the inactivation of the enzyme. Salivary peroxidase contains approximately 12.7% carbohydrate,[58] and the majority of the oligosaccharide units appear to be of the high-mannose type which are N-glycosidically linked via asparagine to the protein core. The identification of both *N*-acetylglucosamine and *N*-acetylgalactosamine, however, suggests that both N- and O-glycosidically linked carbohydrate units may be present within the molecule. Predominant amino acid residues appear to be aspartic acid, glutamic acid, and leucine, which together compose 37% of the total residues; serine, proline, glycine, and alanine compose an additional 33%.

## E. Carbonic Anhydrase

Carbonic anhydrase is a zinc metalloenzyme comprising a family of at least six distinct isoenzymes. This enzyme is responsible for the reversible hydration of carbon dioxide and occurs in a variety of species, including birds, reptiles, and mammals.[59,60] Two nonglycosylated soluble isoenzymes, carbonic anhydrase I and carbonic anhydrase II, appear to be the major nonhemoglobin protein constituents of the erythrocyte, while a similar species (carbonic anhydrase III) predominates in red skeletal muscle.[61,62] Other membrane-associated glycosylated isoenzymes have been identified in liver, lung, and kidney (isoenzyme IV) and in mitochondria (as nonglycosylated isoenzyme V).[59, 63-71] In addition, immunocytochemical analysis of murine parotid tissue, utilizing enzyme histochemistry and immunofluorescence techniques, has demonstrated carbonic anhydrase within the acinar cells and lumina of the excretory duct system, but not within the ductal cells themselves.[72]

Carbonic anhydrase from human whole saliva has recently been isolated and subjected to initial structural and immunochemical characterization.[73] This enzyme, designated carbonic anhydrase VI, is a glycoprotein of 42 kDa and consists of a single peptide chain. Each molecule of the salivary enzyme contains two N-linked oligosaccharide chains of approximately 3 kDa each, which are of the complex type. Although significant charge heterogeneity was encountered,[73] the isoelectric point was determined to be approximately 6.8. Rabbit antiserum raised against the human salivary isoenzyme demonstrated cross-reactivity with isoenzyme II, but not with isoenzymes I or III. In addition, the sensitivity of the salivary carbonic anhydrase to inhibitors such as iodide, sulfanilamide, and bromopyruvic acid was similar to isoenzyme II, but the sensitivity to other inhibitors, such as acetazolamide and methazolamide, was diminished. In studies with patients deficient in carbonic anhydrase II, the amount of salivary isoenzyme was similarly deficient.[73] As a result, salivary carbonic anhydrase is most likely immunologically and genetically related, but not identical to, carbonic anhydrase II.

## F. Fucose-Rich Glycoprotein

A fucose-rich glycoprotein (FRG) was initially described as a calcium-dependent salivary agglutinin capable of binding serotype *c* strains of *Streptococcus mutans*.[74,75] FRG has been obtained from human parotid saliva by affinity adsorption of the presumptive microbial agglutinin to bacterial cells, and then desorption from the bacteria using dilute phosphate buffer. Purification was accomplished by use of preparative ultrafiltration and gel filtration methodologies, ultimately yielding a preparation of apparent electrophoretic homogeneity. Subsequent chemical analyses of the isolated agglutinin revealed a multisubunit glycoprotein occurring in a complex of at least 5,000 to 10,000 kDa, with subunits of approximately 440 kDa. The biochemical properties of FRG are summarized in Table 3. This molecule contains 45% carbohydrate, but the nature of the glycosidic linkages to the protein core has not been determined. Analysis of the carbohydrate content of FRG reveals that 12.5% of the total molecular weight is contributed by fucose, with hexosamines (10.5%), neutral hexoses (16.2%), and sialic acid (5.7%) accounting for the remaining residues. Aspartic acid, serine, threonine, and glycine compose 41.5% of the total number of amino acid residues. The contribution of proline is relatively small, representing just 4.3% of the total amino acids.

## G. Secretory IgA (sIgA)

Secretory IgA is the predominant immunoglobulin within human mucosal secretions, including saliva. As the IgA system is described in more detail in Volume II, Chapter 8, only a brief overview of its structural features and functional properties will be presented here. Salivary sIgA is produced by plasma cells within the major and minor human salivary glands. Immunofluorescence studies[41,43,76] have localized IgA-containing plasma cells in the connective tissue around intercalated or intralobular ducts, as well as around a lesser number

Table 3
## SELECTED BIOCHEMICAL PROPERTIES OF SALIVARY GLYCOPROTEINS

| Properties | FRG[a] | sIgA[b] | Lf[c] | Klk[d] | Fn[e] |
|---|---|---|---|---|---|
| Protein content | 55% | 89—93% | 92.8% | 88—90% | 88—95% |
| Carbohydrate content | 45% | 7—11% | 7.2% | 10—12% | 5—12% |
| Sulfate content | ? | 0% | 0% | ? | ? |
| Size (kDa) | 440[f] | 385[g] | 76.5 | 2.7—4.0 | 450 |
| Subunits | Yes[h] | Yes[i] | No | No | Yes[j] |
| Size of oligosaccharides | ? | 1—12 | 11—12 | 5—18 | 9—13 |
| No. of oligosaccharides | ? | 4—9 | 2 | ? | 3—6 |
| No. of sialic-acid-containing units | Present | 4 | Present | Present | Present |
| Glycopeptide linkage | ? | GalN-Ser/Thr & GlcN-Asn | GlcN-Asn | GlcN-Asn | GalN-Ser/Thr & GlcN-Asn |
| Covalently bound fatty acids | 0 | 0 | 0 | 0 | 0 |
| Quantity[k] | ? | 96—102 μg/ml[46] (HPS) | 1—2 μg/ml[102] (HPS/HSMSL) | ? | 0.2—2 μg/ml;[114] 2—6 μg/ml[117] (HWS/HSMSL);[114] (HPS)[117] |

a   Fucose-rich glycoprotein.
b   Secretory IgA.
c   Lactoferrin.
d   Kallikrein.
e   Fibronectin.
f   Monomeric molecular weight.
g   Dimeric molecular weight.
h   >10 noncovalently linked subunits which dissociate in the presence of sodium dodecyl sulfate.
i   Secretory IgA exists primarily as dimers; higher multimers may also occur. J-chain and secretory component are also covalently linked to the IgA molecule via disulfide bonds.
j   Two disulfide-linked subunits.
k   HPS: human parotid saliva; HSMSL: human submandibular-sublingual saliva; HWS: human whole saliva.

of acini. Striated duct cells are also capable of demonstrating IgA in some cases. J-chain is usually found within IgA-secreting plasma cells as well.[76] Secretory component has been localized within epithelial cells of the intercalated and intralobular ducts.[41,76]

As are other immunoglobulin classes, IgA is made up of two identical light polypeptide chains and two identical heavy polypeptide chains linked together by disulfide bonds (Table 3). The class and subclass of immunoglobulins are determined by their distinct heavy-chain type where, in the case of IgA (as well as IgM), an additional C-terminal extension onto the heavy-chain permits monomer cross-linking and IgA dimer formation via interchain disulfide bonds. The N-terminal region of this molecule contains the two antibody combining sites. Within serum, IgA exists primarily as monomers, while within secretions, secretory IgA (sIgA) is composed of a 385-kDa complex consisting of a 300-kDa IgA dimer, a 70-kDa secretory component, and a 15-kDa J-chain. All of these components, with the exception of the immunoglobulin light chain, contain N-linked oligosaccharide units, as noted in Table 3 and Figure 1.[77-78]

Two subclasses of IgA heavy chains are known to exist, IgA1 and IgA2. These subclasses differ primarily with regard to their amino acid sequence in the hinge region of the immunoglobulin. IgA1 includes a duplicated eight amino acid, proline-rich sequence, which also contains five O-linked oligosaccharides.[78,79] The disulfide linkage between the immunoglobulin light and heavy chain also occurs in this region. In contrast, IgA2 contains a short sequence of consecutive proline residues in the hinge region and does not contain O-linked oligosaccharide units.[80] Further, two allotypes of the IgA2 subclass exist. Light chains of the IgA2m(2) allotype form disulfide linkages with each other and are not covalently linked to the heavy chains. The IgA2m(1) allotype is apparently a recombinant between IgA2m(2) and IgA1.[77] In serum, approximately 90% of the IgA occurs as the IgA1 subclass, while in secretions there appears to be approximately equal quantities of each type.[81,82]

The primary structure of the polypeptide and carbohydrate moieties of the sIgA molecule has been elucidated.[78,80,83] The free secretory component is a monomeric glycoprotein, consisting of 558 amino acids, with 7 N-glycosidically linked carbohydrate chains representing 23.4% of the total weight of this species.[84,85] The protein contains 20 cysteine residues which form 10 internal disulfide bonds, but no methionine residues. The polypeptide chain also appears to be divided into 5 regions of internal homology, of 104 to 114 amino acids in length. J-chain is also a glycoprotein containing a single N-linked oligosaccharide.[86] As mentioned previously, the carbohydrate content of IgA is variable and depends on the heavy chain subclass; both O- and N-glycosidically linked oligosaccharide units may be present, representing 7 to 11% of the total weight of the IgA molecule (Table 3).[78,80,81]

## H. Kallikrein

Kallikreins are a group of serine proteases which possess specific proteolytic activities. Kallikrein has been localized by immunocytochemistry to the granular tubules, striated ducts, and occasionally to the main duct cells of the rat submandibular gland.[87] Nonacinar localization has also been confirmed in mice submandibular gland tissues by *in situ* hybridization techniques using cDNA probes.[88] Kallikrein has also been identified, in somewhat lower quantities, within parotid and sublingual glands of these animals[89] and in man.[90]

Kallikreins are glycoproteins containing a single polypeptide chain with a molecular weight of 27 to 40 kDa. Glandular kallikreins are biochemically distinct from plasma kallikrein, the latter having a higher molecular weight (100 to 163 kDa),[91] different enzymatic activity, and a function in the intrinsic circulatory system coagulation pathway.[92] Since detailed biochemical analyses have not been performed on human salivary kallikrein, most of the chemical properties of glandular kallikreins have utilized enzymes either derived from human nonsalivary sources or obtained from animals. Analyses of partial amino acid sequences from a number of these sources have revealed considerable homology.[93-95] Structural similarities among human urinary, pancreatic, and salivary kallikreins have also been suggested by immunological cross-reactivity of antikallikrein antisera produced in rabbits.[96] Recently, the isolation of both active and inactive forms of human urinary kallikrein has been accomplished.[97] These studies reveal that the inactive prokallikrein contains an additional seven amino acids at the amino terminus of the kallikrein, which is capable of being cleaved by trypsin to yield the active form. The carbohydrate content of glandular kallikreins is usually within a range of 10 to 12%.[89] Urinary kallikrein has been used to investigate the carbohydrate domains of this molecule.[96] These studies have revealed the presence of asparagine-linked oligosaccharide units containing bi-, tri-, and tetraantennary structures of the complex type. However, the precise structure and number of oligosaccharide chains have not been elucidated.

## I. Lactoferrin

Lactoferrin is an iron-binding glycoprotein synthesized by glandular epithelial cells, as well as by neutrophils, and has been detected within most of the secretions which bathe human mucosal surfaces.[98-102] Immunocytochemical studies using fluorescence techniques have localized lactoferrin primarily within intercalated duct cells of the major human salivary glands, although it has also been found to a lesser extent within serous acinar cells.[41]

Lactoferrin exists as a single polypeptide chain of 76.5 kDa, with two asparagine-linked biantennary oligosaccharide units per molecule (Table 3). The structure of the lactoferrin oligosaccharides is illustrated in Figure 1. Lactoferrin displays considerable homology with the circulating iron-transport protein transferrin.[103-106] Despite similarities in the primary polypeptide sequence, lactoferrin and transferrin differ in a number of ways. First, there is relatively little immunological cross-reactivity unless the molecules are denatured.[107] Second, the affinity of lactoferrin for iron at various pH ranges is markedly different from that observed with transferrin.[107] Finally, lactoferrin differs significantly from its transferrin homologue in possessing two fucose residues per molecule, whereas the biantennary asparagine-linked oligosaccharide chains of transferrin do not contain fucose.[103] Studies performed on the primary structure of the lactoferrin glycans revealed that these carbohydrate domains exhibited considerable heterogeneity, since as many as five distinct structures could be isolated.[108]

Lactoferrin possesses two domains which can be separated by mild proteolysis, and each is capable of reversibly binding one molecule of $Fe^{3+}$. Repeating sequences within the amino acid sequence of lactoferrin[109-111] have also supported the concept of a bilobular lactoferrin structure, with one N-linked oligosaccharide present within each lobe. The concept of a bipolar structural conformation has been substantiated by X-ray crystallographic data.[112] Recently, investigators have begun to isolate structural domains from lactoferrin by hydrolysis with combinations of trypsin, chymotrypsin, and pepsin, and employed for functional characterization.[109] These techniques were used to isolate the N- and C-terminal domains, as well as a smaller 18.5 kDa subdomain derived from further hydrolysis of the N-terminal domain, each of which was able to retain iron-binding activity.[104]

## J. Fibronectin

Fibronectins are large molecular weight glycoproteins which occur at cell surfaces, within basement membranes, in the extracellular matrix, the connective tissues, and the circulatory system, and within a wide variety of body fluids.[113] Immunocytochemical techniques have been used to localize fibronectin within ductal cells of human minor salivary glands. Fibronectin has been detected within the gingival crevicular fluid, in small amounts in human whole saliva, and possibly in the major and minor salivary gland secretions.[114-117]

In general, human fibronectins have monomeric molecular weights between 210 to 260 kDa and contain 5 to 12% carbohydrate.[118] The salient biochemical features of fibronectin are summarized in Table 3. Human plasma fibronectin occurs as a disulfide-linked dimer joined near the carboxyterminus of both chains, with one polypeptide chain being slightly larger than the other. Cellular fibronectin, while structurally similar but not identical to plasma fibronectin,[119] occurs as monomers, dimers, or as higher multimers.[120-121] The polypeptide chains of fibronectin appear to be composed of discrete globular functional domains arranged over the linear structure of the molecule,[120-123] each responsible for one of the binding functions of fibronectin to other molecules or to cells.

Primary sequence information obtained from cDNA clones revealed that different subunits, which differ in parts of their primary sequence, all arise from a single large gene composed of multiple small exons that are identical over much of their sequence.[124,125] Fibronectin consists of a series of homologous repeats, containing disulfide-bonded loops of 45 to 50 and 90 amino acids long, which make up about 90% of the entire sequence of this molecule.[126,127] Biophysical studies indicate that fibronectins are composed of highly structured globular domains separated by flexible, relative unstructured regions.[128,129] Under physiological conditions, fibronectin is a relatively compact, asymmetric molecule, which becomes more extended and flexible at extreme salt concentrations of pH.[122,128-130] After binding collagen, or following reduction and carboxymethylation of intrachain disulfide bonds, fibronectin becomes more extended, suggesting a partial loss of structure.[131,132]

Fibronectin experiences a substantial amount of posttranslational modification. Transglutaminase reactive sites have been localized within some of the homologous repeat sequences, and the positions of some of the oligosaccharide side chains have been located within the collagen-binding domains.[124] Evidence also exists for the variable phosphorylation of serine residues throughout the fibronectin molecule.[124] However, the functional significance of these various posttranslational modifications remains obscure.

## IV. OVERVIEW OF BIOSYNTHETIC PATHWAYS

### A. Protein Core

Glycoproteins are conjugated proteins which contain oligosaccharide covalently attached to the peptide backbone through selected amino acid residues. Synthesis of both the peptide core and carbohydrate portions of glycoproteins occurs by distinctly different mechanisms; the peptide portions of both proteins and glycoproteins, however, are synthesized in the same manner.[133-135] The entire process of protein synthesis involves over 100 molecules, including messenger RNA, transfer RNAs (tRNA), activating enzymes, protein factors, and ribosomes, whose interactions occur within a number of cell organelles. Protein synthesis is initiated by the activation of individual amino acids by specific aminoacyl-tRNA synthetases. These enzymes couple the carboxyl group of an amino acid to the 2' or 3'-hydroxyl group of an adenosine unit located at the 3'-end of each tRNA. These are single RNA chains containing approximately 80 nucleotides which have been shown to possess an L-shaped conformation by X-ray crystallography studies.

Initiation of protein synthesis (translation) occurs following replication and transcription of genomic DNA to mRNA. A 30 to 40S ribosomal subunit, formylmethionyl-tRNA, and mRNA condense to form an initiation complex. The initiation sequence coded within the mRNA is recognized by formylmethionyl-tRNA. Addition of a larger, 50 to 60S ribosomal subunit then forms a 70 to 80S initiation complex. Elongation consists of codon recognition by aminoacyl-tRNA, peptide bond formation between amino acid residues delivered by tRNAs, and translocation from the amino- to the carboxyterminus of the growing peptide. Protein synthesis is terminated by release factors which recognize specific termination codons in mRNA.

Nascent polypeptides destined to be secreted from the cell are generally considered to carry a "signal" peptide sequence which serves to fix the ribosomes through their large subunits to the endoplasmic reticulum (ER) membrane.[136-138] Ribosomal fixation is also accomplished with the aid of numerous ER membrane proteins (ribophorins) which specifically bind to surface components of the ribosome.[139-140] During translation, the peptide is directed into the cisternal space of the rough ER through a "tunnel" created in the membrane. The cleavage of the signal peptide is also thought to occur in most cases during polypeptide synthesis, although there are some examples of posttranslational cleavage.[141,142] The primary structure of the signal sequence is not highly conserved, as was initially thought. A number of studies, however, have suggested that this sequence is primarily α-helical, enriched in hydrophobic amino acids, and possesses a β- turn near the carboxyl end of the signal.[143-145]

## B. N-Linked Glycoproteins

Addition of carbohydrate units to the peptide portion of a glycoprotein is a posttranslational event which depends of the availability of glycosyltransferases and varies according to the nature of the glycosidic linkage of the carbohydrate to the peptide. Asparagine-linked oligosaccharides contain a pentasaccharide core structure of Manα(1-3)[Manα(1-6)]Manβ(1-4) GlcNAcβ(1-4)GlcNAc-Asn. Complex-type oligosaccharides contain peripheral branches, typically composed of sialic acid, galactose, N-acetylglucosamine, and fucose, added onto the core structure. High mannose-type oligosaccharides have two to six additional mannose residues extending from the core. Finally, hybrid-type structures contain elements of both the high-mannose and complex-type oligosaccharides. Considerable variation in both complex- and hybrid-type carbohydrate structures are commonly observed.

The synthesis of the Asn-GlcNAc linkage is a complex process which involves the preassembly of a large oligosaccharide on a lipid carrier within the ER, with subsequent transfer of the oligosaccharide from the carrier to the peptide backbone within the rough ER.[146-149] The intermediate (Dollichol) is a phosphorylated, polyisoprenoid alcohol containing from 17 to 21 isoprene units. Each sugar is added to the intermediate in a stepwise fashion, in the presence of specific glycosyltransferases, with the first seven sugars (two GlcNAc and five Man residues) derived from nucleotide sugars. The resulting structure is thus Manα(1-2)Manα(1-2)Manα(1-3)[Manα(3-6)]Manβ(1-4)GlcNAcβ(1-4)GlcNAc-P-P-Dol, where P represents a phosphate group. Subsequent addition of 4 Man and 3 Glc residues to this structure are derived from the lipid intermediates Dol-P-Man and Dol-P-Glc.[133-135] This final major product is then transferred *en bloc* to asparagine residues in the peptide core, having the sequence Asn-X-Ser/Thr, where X can be almost any amino acid residue except proline, or possibly aspartic acid.[135] The complete oligosaccharide of the lipid intermediate undergoes extensive modifications after transfer to polypeptide. Initial processing of the oligosaccharide moieties is accomplished by removal of the glucose residues, which is thought to facilitate the movement of the nascent glycoprotein from the ER to the Golgi apparatus.[150-151] Subsequent processing reactions include the rapid removal of four mannose residues by α-mannosidase. These steps result in the formation of the heptasaccharide pentamannosyl-di-N-acetylglucosamine [Man$_5$(GlcNAc)$_2$] linked to protein. Conversion of the heptasaccharide into the common core pentasaccharide, as well as additional processing and elongation of some oligosaccharide units, are also accomplished by specific N-acetylglucosaminyltransferases during the progression of the oligosaccharide through the Golgi apparatus.[135] Finally, the newly synthesized glycoproteins leave the Golgi to become packaged into secretory vesicles for their release by secretory cells.

## C. O-Linked Glycoproteins

Biosynthesis of O-glycosidically linked oligosaccharide units occurs by the direct and sequential addition of one monosaccharide at a time to the core polypeptide. Synthesis of O-linked carbohydrates thus occurs via transfer of nucleotide sugar derivatives to glycoproteins without the participation of any lipid-linked intermediate and appears to involve transferases which are associated with the Golgi apparatus membrane.[152] The initial step in the formation of these units involves the establishment of the linkage to serine or threonine residues using UDP N-acetylgalactosamine in the presence of the appropriate specific transferases. Additional residues are added to the growing oligosaccharide in similar manner (i.e., transfer of UDP galactose, UDP N-acetylgalactosamine, CMP neuraminic acid, and GDP fucose). In general, the relative proportion of available sialyltransferases, galactosyltransferases, etc., and the specificity of these transferases for the elongating substrate significantly influences the eventual structure of the final O-linked oligosaccharide unit. That is, a predominance of a particular transferase will favor the addition of its specific carbohydrate residue. Addition of a particular carbohydrate, however, may also be inhibitory to the action of another transferase.[153]

The precise biosynthetic pathways involved in the synthesis of salivary glycoproteins have not been specifically determined for each of the individual components. It is reasonable to assume, however, that the assembly of N- and O-linked oligosaccharide units of these glycoproteins occurs in accordance with the general scheme discussed previously. The existence of such multiple pathways has important implications for the study of these molecules. For example, assembly of the polypeptide portion of glycoproteins is representative of a primary gene product and thus displays little (if any) variation in its primary sequence. Biosynthesis of N- and O-linked oligosaccharides produce secondary gene products, where genetic control is exerted on the primary gene product, the glycosyltransferases. As a result, the microheterogeneity observed in these molecules, especially the mucin glycoproteins, may be due, in part, to lack of direct genetic control of glycoprotein structure. Although the basis of such structural diversity has not been established, it has been suggested that it might be deliberate or contrived, rather than random, and such modulation may be necessary for the expression of biological function or to facilitate the transfer of biological information.[154-155]

## V. FUNCTIONS OF SALIVARY GLYCOPROTEINS

It has been proposed that salivary glycoproteins consist of discrete structural domains, each of which may be responsible for a particular biological function (Table 4).[10-12,14,155] Indeed, many of the protective functions of saliva can be attributed to the physical, structural, and rheological characteristics of salivary glycoproteins.[10,11,18,20] The concept of the structural domain as a fundamental unit of protein structure first arose from studies on the primary sequence of immunoglobulins, where it was found that the heavy and light chains of these molecules were composed of functional units which could be isolated as stable fragments following limited proteolysis.[156,157] Identification and characterization of domain structure have subsequently been extended to a number of molecules, including fibronectin,[113,118,124,158-161] collagens,[162-163] and to a variety of enzymes.[164-166] Classically, domains have been identified within globular proteins on the basis of spatial separation, composition from a single linear peptide region, the recognition of similar structures on the same or a different molecule, and their association with a particular catalytic or binding function.[167-169] In nonglobular proteins and glycoproteins, the concept of structural domains may also be extended to include recognition of discrete carbohydrate, peptide, or subunit domains. In the case of the human salivary glycoproteins, the detailed identification, distribution, and orientation of structural domains have only begun to be elucidated.

### A. Tissue Coating and Formation of Intraoral Pellicles

A salivary covering on the hard and soft oral structures protects them from desiccation and exogenous insult.[155] For example, salivary glycoproteins are thought to play important

**Table 4**
**PROPOSED FUNCTIONS OF SALIVARY GLYCOPROTEINS**

| Function | MG1[a] | MG2[b] | PRG[c] | Amy[d] | SP[e] | FRP[f] | CA[g] | sIgA[h] | Lf[i] | Klk[j] | Fn[k] |
|---|---|---|---|---|---|---|---|---|---|---|---|
| Tissue coating and formation of intraoral pellicles | + | + | + | + | | | | + | + | | + |
| Lubricating film at hard and soft tissue interfaces | + | + | + | | | | | ? | | | |
| Selective clearance and adherence of microbial flora | + | + | + | + | | + | | + | + | | + |
| Antimicrobial activity | | | | + | + | | | | + | | |
| Utilization as a microbial metabolic substrate | + | + | + | | | | | | | | + |
| Posttranslational processing | | | | | | | | | | + | |
| Digestion | + | + | | + | | | | | | | |
| Buffering capacity | | | | | + | | + | | | | |
| Heterotypic complexing | + | + | | + | | + | | + | | | + |

[a]  High molecular weight salivary mucin.
[b]  Low molecular weight salivary mucin.
[c]  Proline-rich glycoprotein.
[d]  α-amylase.
[e]  Salivary peroxidase.
[f]  Fucose-rich glycoprotein.
[g]  Carbonic anhydrase.
[h]  Secretory IgA.
[i]  Lactoferrin.
[j]  Kallikrein.
[k]  Fibronectin.

roles in the formation of the acquired enamel pellicle. Among the glycoproteins identified within 2-h *in vivo* enamel pellicle are salivary mucins, proline-rich glycoprotein, lactoferrin, sIgA, and α-amylase.[170-177] In addition, cysteine-containing phosphoproteins (cystatins), lysozyme, albumin, and acidic proline-rich proteins are also important contributors to enamel pellicle.[172-175,177] Recent *in vitro* studies have indicated that MG1 has a higher affinity for hydroxyapatite than does MG2, supporting the concept of selective binding of salivary glycoproteins to enamel surfaces.[171,177] Factors which may be potential mediators of (glyco)protein binding to surfaces include surface charge, pH, ionic strength, protein-protein interactions, and primary and/or secondary conformation of the adsorbate.[178]

The tissue coating function of MG1 at both hard and soft tissue interfaces may be due, in part, to the viscoelastic properties of this molecule.[11] Indeed, the viscoelastic properties of mucins may be regulated by hydration kinetics which involve water, inorganic ions, pH microenvironments, and noncovalent heterotypic complexing with other salivary components. Covalent interactions which occur between MG1 and fatty acids or noncovalent interactions between mucins and lipids have also been demonstrated.[31] Disulfide cross-linking between mucin subunits may also contribute to the viscoelastic properties usually associated with large mucin glycoproteins.

Immunoglobulins also protect mucosal surfaces from the local establishment of pathogens, and participate in the local oral immune response. For example, sIgA exhibits direct antiviral activity with the poliovirus system[179,180] and is known to inhibit the attachment of *Streptococcus mutans*.[181] Secretory IgA may also enhance the function of other salivary molecules, such as salivary peroxidase, by direct interaction with these molecules.[182]

Fibronectin has been identified along the interface between the tooth and the gingival connective tissue, as well as between the junctional epithelium-cementum interface.[183] Recently, it was found that *Pseudomonas aeruginosa* adherence to buccal epithelial cells was associated with this organism's ability to degrade fibronectin present on the cell surface.[184-186] Similar results were obtained by incubation of buccal epithelial cells with salivary proteinases.[184] It has also been found that treatment of buccal epithelial cells with saliva leads to the dose-dependent adherence of type 1 fimbriated strains of *Escherichia coli* adherence to these cells.[187] This adherence was blocked by exogenous fibronectin, since both *E. coli* and fibronectin bind to salivary component(s) having the same electrophoretic mobility as $\alpha$-amylase.[187]

## B. Lubrication

During and after mastication, saliva provides protection by lubricating and mechanically cleansing the oral tissues and flushing away debris. The role of salivary glycoproteins in lubrication has recently been demonstrated.[188-191] Lubrication is a property of oral pellicles which may protect surfaces against mechanical disruption or abrasion. These properties appear to be dependent on the presence of glycoproteins capable of forming boundary interfaces at tissue surfaces moving relative to each other and not directly related to the viscosity of the fluid.[192-193] Recently, we have reported on the use of a modified friction testing device (lubometer) to measure the lubricating properties of the higher molecular weight salivary mucin (MG1), the lower molecular weight salivary mucin (MG2), and the proline-rich glycoprotein (PRG).[194] On a molar basis, their relative lubricating ability was found to be MG1 > MG2 > PRG. Other salivary glycoproteins, including lactoferrin, amylase, and secretory IgA also possessed lubricating abilities which were found to be significantly higher than either human serum albumin or a simulated salivary buffer control. The lubricating properties of a number of salivary glycoproteins may be derived, to a significant extent, from the carbohydrate domains of these molecules.[188] Deglycosylation of the PRG using trimethylphenylsufonyl fluoride resulted in a marked decrease in the lubricating ability relative to the intact molecule.[188]

## C. Clearance/Adherence of Microflora

Studies from several laboratories have implicated salivary glycoproteins as playing an important role in modulating bacterial colonization of oral surfaces.[29,177,194-204] These interactions may involve both fluid-phase (in saliva) and solid-phase (on tissue surfaces) interactions and may involve both specific and nonspecific interactions, heterotypic and homotypic complexing, and extrinsic modifications of salivary glycoproteins.

Using both a glass adherence assay[198] and bacterial agglutination,[205] it has been demonstrated that MG2 interacts with several strains of *S. sanguis* and *S. mutans* and that removal of the sialic acid residues of MG2 diminishes interaction with *S. sanguis* but not *S. mutans*. Studies by Murray et al.[206] using a hemagglutination inhibition assay, whereby the red blood cell (RBC) surface serves as a mucin analogue, revealed that a NeuAc$\alpha$2,3Gal$\beta$1,3GalNAc sequence is a potent inhibitor of RBC-*S. sanguis* interactions. This sialic-acid-containing trisaccharide corresponds to the major acidic oligosaccharide of MG2.[207] Murray et al.[208] have utilized the homobifunctional cross-linking reagent disuccinimidyl suberate to identify an adhesion on *S. mitis* which binds the NeuAc$\alpha$2,3Gal$\beta$1,3GalNAc sequence. We have recently described a system in which monoclonal antibodies specific for salivary mucins were linked to agarose supports and used for the selective depletion of MG1 or MG2 from submandibular-sublingual saliva.[12,209] These studies demonstrated that saliva depleted of MG2, but not MG1, lost its ability to agglutinate selected strains of *S. sanguis* and *S. mitis*.

We have also examined the ability of PRG to interact with strains of oral streptococci. Studies using a bacterial agglutination assay revealed that MG2, but not PRG, agglutinated the test strains.[205] These results suggest that the density and/or distribution of oligosaccharides along the peptide backbone of PRG may not be sufficient to agglutinate organisms. Studies by Nagata et al.[196] and Shibata et al.[197] have used tritiated PRG to demonstrate binding with *S. mitis* and reported the presence of a galactose-binding adhesin on this bacterium. Recently, we have utilized a photoreactive heterobifunctional cross-linking agent (e.g., *N*-hydroxy-succinimidyl-4-azidosalicylic acid [ASA] to examine in a quantitiative fashion the nature of specific interactions between salivary glycoproteins and oral streptococci.[195] Specific binding between PRG and *S. sanguis* strain G9B was saturable, reversible, and inhibited by structural glycoprotein analogues. This study also indicated that PRG binding was mediated by a bacterial adhesin which recognizes either separately or together complex oligosaccharide structures consisting of sialic acid, galactose, and *N*-acetylgalactosamine. These observations were consistent with previous findings[206,208] which demonstrated the presence of a *S. sanguis* lectin having specificity for a NeuAc$\alpha$2,3Gal$\beta$1,3GalNAc sequence. We have also compared MG2 and PRG interactions with *S. sanguis* and *S. mutans* in a glass adherence assay.[11] The higher number of carbohydrate units in MG2 provides an explanation why this molecule binds more bacteria than PRG. Since MG2 has many more sialic-acid-containing units than PRG, neuraminidase treatment of each had the more profound effect on MG2.

The secretory immune system performs a range of biological functions which are well suited to mucosal defense. In general, secretory immunoglobulins are thought to participate in the local regulation of environmental antigens (i.e., soluble antigens) by providing a "first line of defense" via immunological means in the oral cavity.[210] The ability of sIgA to bind to antigens is by itself a beneficial process, whereby local aggregation of microorganisms would retard their movement and impair their subsurface invasion into deeper host tissues.[211] Williams and Gibbons[212] have demonstrated the ability of sIgA derived from parotid saliva to inhibit specifically the adherence of certain strains of streptococci to human buccal epithelial cells. Other investigators have suggested that sIgA may inhibit the adherence of these organisms to hard tissue surfaces within the oral cavity.[213-216] The presence of local antibody has also been shown to play a role in viral neutralization and in the attenuation of viral growth and replication on these surfaces.[179,217]

Fibronectin has also been shown to possess bacterial binding ability. Previous studies have demonstrated the binding of a number of Gram-positive bacteria to fibronectin, and that fibronectin was capable of mediating the binding of these microorganisms to epithelial cells.[218,219] In contrast, fibronectin appears to have a barrier effect against the adhesion of Gram-negative bacteria, whereupon this molecule possessed little or no affinity for a large variety of Gram-negative bacterial strains.

Little information is available regarding the role of other salivary glycoproteins in microbial interactions. The selective binding of $\alpha$-amylase to *S. sanguis* and *Neisseria gonorrheae* has recently been demonstrated,[220-222] as has the interaction of the fucose-rich glycoprotein with *S. mutans*.[74] The mechanisms of these interactions, however, have not been determined.

## D. Antimicrobial Activity

Salivary glycoproteins such as peroxidase and lactoferrin have been shown to have antimicrobial activities. The salivary peroxidase system catalyzes the oxidation of SCN$^-$ by H$_2$O$_2$, generating highly reactive oxidized forms of thiocyanate such as OSCN$^-$.[223] These products have demonstrated direct toxicity for a variety of microorganisms, including *S. mutans*, *S. fecalis*, *S. albus*, *E. coli*, and *B. megatherium*.[224-228] To date, all strains of *S. mutans* tested are inhibited by the peroxidase system.[227,229,230] Salivary peroxidase can also function by neutralizing the deleterious effects of hydrogen peroxide produced by a number of oral microorganisms.[229-232] In addition, the peroxidase system is effective in reducing acid production by glucose-stimulated homologous plaque[182] and can inhibit glucose uptake by *S. mutans*.[229]

Retardation of microbial growth may also be accomplished through direct effects of lactoferrin.[101,233-236] This effect is reversible upon addition of iron in excess of the lactoferrin binding capacity, suggesting that the glycoprotein's antimicrobial activity may be due in part to its ability to sequester iron. In addition, lactoferrin may also possess a direct, iron-independent, bacteriocidal effect on various strains of streptococci and vibrio.[101,139,236,237] While the mechanisms involved in the direct bacteriocidal effect of lactoferrin have not been completely elucidated, recent work by Arnold et al.[101,139,238] and by Lassiter et al.[236] using a *S. mutans* model system has supported the concept of an anionic target site for lactoferrin on the surface of these microorganisms.

Evidence also exists for direct microbiocidal effects of sIgA on microorganisms. Several studies have demonstrated receptors specific for the Fc region of IgA on macrophages, lymphocytes, and neutrophils and have been shown to promote antibody-dependent cell-mediated cytotoxicity of IgA-sensitized target cells *in vitro*.[239-241] Also, the limited ability of sIgA to activate complement by the alternative pathway could represent an additional mechanism of bacterial killing on mucosal surfaces.[242,243]

Salivary amylases have been shown to be specific inhibitors of *N. gonorrheae* by possibly acting on the gonococcal outer cell wall.[222] The precise mechanism of the antimicrobial activity, however, has not been determined.

### E. Utilization as a Microbial Substrate

It has recently been proposed that specific binding of salivary glycoproteins by oral bacteria constitutes a mechanism to collect nutrients in the vicinity of the cell.[244] It has been demonstrated that various strains of *S. sanguis* are capable of growth while using saliva as their sole source of nutrients. Concurrent degradation of salivary glycoproteins has been observed and likely represent the effects of liberated enzymes on these molecules. Accordingly, the lectin-like receptors present on the surface of many strains of *S. sanguis* may also be important in the binding of salivary glycoproteins, which then can be used as a microbial substrate. Indeed, neuraminidase-containing strains are able to exhibit a selective advantage over strains deficient in this enzyme when grown in enrichment cultures.[244] The metabolic specificity of these microorganisms, however, has not yet been determined.

### F. Posttranslational Processing

Kallikreins, which are present in lymph, plasma, and interstitial fluids in mammals, are responsible for the release of kinin from kininogen.[89] Glandular or tissue kallikrein is a regulatory protease which possesses a variety of direct biological activities separate from the indirect effects mediated by the liberation of kinin. While the precise function of salivary kallikrein is not well understood, its function has been postulated to include the processing of a number of hormones, including epidermal growth factor and nerve growth factor.[245] A recent study has suggested that kallikrein is capable of cleaving an arginine-glycine bond within human salivary proline-rich protein C, thus giving rise to proline-rich protein A.[246] Histochemical evidence indicated that the postsynthetic cleavage of protein C by kallikrein would have to take place during the passage of saliva through the secretory ducts, since in secreted saliva, cleavage of salivary protein C can only be observed after 72 h of incubation.[246]

### G. Digestion

Saliva's contribution to the digestive process, in relation to its diverse protective and homeostatic functions, is relatively minimal. Saliva facilitates formation of the food bolus to allow for efficient mastication and swallowing and aids in the maintenance of an appropriate fluid environment for the optimal functioning of taste bud receptors.[1,2] In this regard, the salivary amylases and, to a lesser extent, lipases[247] most likely contribute to the initial stages of digestion. Salivary amylases function in the initial steps of food breakdown by initiating the breakdown of susceptible foods via hydrolysis of $\alpha(1-4)$ glycosidic linkages within carbohydrates in starch, glycogen, and glucose polymers.[37,38,40] Due to the comparatively short time that food actually remains within the oral cavity, it is likely that the digestive role of salivary amylase is minor at best.[1,2,20] In addition, salivary glycoproteins (e.g., mucins) may also assist in preparation of the food bolus by imparting their lubricatory and viscosity properties to the food.[1,2,20,155,188]

## H. Buffering Capacity

Several components within saliva help to maintain a relatively neutral pH in the oral cavity, in bacterial plaque, and in the esophagus.[20,248] This effect is due largely to the presence of bicarbonate, although histidine-rich peptides and phosphates may also contribute.[1] The tissue-coating properties of the larger molecular weight salivary mucins are also ideally suited to act as permeability and diffusion barriers and thereby maintain local pH gradients. Indeed, human intestinal mucins can provide an unstirred surface layer upon mucosal surfaces which act to localize and concentrate bicarbonate ions and form a barrier for excluding hydrogen ions.[249,250]

## I. Heterotypic Complexing

Several salivary glycoproteins are known to interact noncovalently with other salivary molecules. These interactions, which are termed "heterotypic complexing", can be mediated by ionic, hydrophobic, and/or hydrogen bonding forces. One function of heterotypic complexing is for one molecule to act as a "carrier" to target other molecules to oral surfaces. The complexes themselves could also serve as functional units by possessing properties different from those of the individual constituents. Salivary mucins display complexing with sIgA, lysozyme, cysteine-containing phosphoproteins (cystatins), and lipids.[10,11,31,251-253] In this regard, the mucins may act as "carrier molecules", which bind to and concentrate protective molecules at various oral tissue-environmental interfaces. Heterotypic complexing between the PRG and human serum albumin has been shown to enhance the *in vitro* lubricatory ability of PRG between an enamel-glass interface. Ionic interactions can occur *in vitro* between α-amylase and neutral salivary cystatins.[195] Even though both of these molecules are found in 2 h *in vivo* enamel pellicle,[172] the biological consequence, if any, of their interaction at the tooth surface remains to be determined. Recently, fibronectin has been shown to interact with a salivary glycoprotein with characteristics similar to α-amylase.[187] This interaction results in the inhibition of adherence of type 1 fimbriated stains of *E. coli* to buccal epithelial cells.

## VI. STRUCTURAL MODULATION OF GLYCOPROTEIN FUNCTION

The structural domains of salivary glycoproteins are subject to a wide variety of extracellular or extrinsic modifications in order to meet dynamically changing biological needs within the oral cavity.[10,11] This concept is referred to as structural modulation. The structural modulation of salivary glycoproteins is primarily mediated by bacterial proteases whose effects can regulate microbial colonization in several ways.

Enzymatic modification of salivary mucins could alter their conformation, which in turn could affect their adsorption to teeth.[199,204,254] Subsequent enzymatic modification of glycoproteins already adsorbed to the tooth could expose new binding sites for bacterial attachment and thereby affect the microbial succession characteristic of dental plaque formation.[177,255,256]

The existence of bacterial IgA proteases is well established. These proteases, which are elaborated by microorganisms such as *S. sanguis* and *Haemophilus influenzae,* can cause specific cleavage of sIgA in its hinge region and thereby modulate this immunoglobulin's role in microbial adherence to oral surfaces.[257-259] In general, the IgA2 subclass appears to be more resistant to these enzymes, due to the lack of susceptible Pro-Ser and Pro-Thr bonds in the hinge region.[210,258]

Evidence also exists for the presence within saliva of an enzyme which can convert the glycosylated forms of amylase into nonglycosylated forms.[260] Amylase may also undergo chemical and enzymatic deamidation, where an amide group is lost from glutamine and/or asparagine to generate negatively charged glutamic acid or aspartic acid residues. The deamidation of amylase can occur in the presence of proteases or protease inhibitors, and this effect may be pH and temperature dependent.[261-263] The functional significance of the deamidation of amylase remains largely unknown but may correspond to the half-life of amylase in the oral cavity.

The structure of other salivary glycoproteins can also be modified by the action of bacterial proteases. Modification of fibronectin by bacterial proteases, including those from *B. gingivalis,* may facilitate attachment of bacterial species on buccal epithelial cells.[114,118,124,160,264] The integrity of sialic-acid-containing glycoproteins may be maintained by salivary peroxidases which prevent the decarboxylation of sialic acid residues by hydrogen peroxide.[265]

## VII. FUTURE STUDIES AND CLINICAL APPLICATIONS

The increasing body of knowledge dealing with salivary glycoprotein structure is shedding more light upon the precise mechanisms by which these molecules perform their biological functions. Such studies are greatly enhanced through the utilization of specific probes of glycoprotein domains. Current work in our laboratory is directed to the development of such probes, in particular, the use of monoclonal antibodies and genetic reagents. For example, we have employed monospecific antimucin antibodies directed to epitopes on MG1 or MG2 for the localization of these molecules *in situ* within salivary gland tissues, and for their immunoquantitation within saliva.[10,12,24,209,266,267] Identification and quantitation of defined structural domains within pellicle and plaque would provide useful information regarding the presence or accessibility of such domains on selected mucosal or hard tissue surfaces. The use of well-defined immunological reagents for the epitope mapping would enable us to determine the spatial orientation, conformation, and distribution of structural domains within salivary glycoproteins. Finally, immunological and genetic probes for structural domains would be useful adjuncts in the differential diagnosis of oral diseases and dysfunctions, such as Sjögren's syndrome, xerostomia, or salivary gland neoplasia, where alterations in the antigenic profile of salivary molecules may be manifested.

Knowledge of the precise structure and function of selected salivary glycoproteins will enable the purposeful design of custom-engineered salivary molecules. Such "super salivary substances" might be constructed which would combine desired properties of salivary molecules from a library of defined structural domains. As a result, it has been proposed that an ideal saliva substitute or additive could be custom synthesized to include structural domains concomitant with an individual's needs. For example, an artificial saliva incorporating the oligosaccharides of the PRG may facilitate masticatory lubrication and thereby diminish possible abrasion associated with xerostomia. Similarly, an adhesive domain, perhaps obtained from a salivary mucin or fibronectin, might be coupled to bacteriocidal domains derived from another molecule, such as lactoferrin or peroxidase. A mouth rinse composed of an adhesive domain, a cell proliferative/cell attachment domain, and/or bacteriocidal domains may provide an adjunct for treatment of plaque-mediated diseases. Such directions in the development and synthesis of artificial salivas require a knowledge of the structure-function relationships of salivary molecules. Consequently, further elucidation of these relationships, as well as the initial *in vitro* testing of these "chimeric" salivary molecules, are now under way in our laboratory.

## ACKNOWLEDGMENTS

This endeavor was supported in part by USPHS grants DE08448, DE08240, DE07585, and DE07034.

## REFERENCES

1. **Mandel, I. D. and Wotman, S.,** The salivary secretions in health and disease, *Oral Sci. Rev.,* 8, 25, 1976.
2. **Mandel, I.D.,** Sialochemistry in diseases and clinical situations affecting salivary glands, *Crit. Rev. Clin. Lab. Sci.,* 12, 321, 1980.
3. **Fox, P. C., van der Ven, P., Sonies, B. C., Weiffenbach, J. M., and Baum, B. J.,** Xerostomia: evaluation of a symptom with increasing significance, *J. Am. Dent. Assoc.,* 110, 519, 1985.
4. **Fox, P. C.,** Systemic therapy of salivary gland hypofunction, *J. Dent. Res.,* 66, (Sp. Issue), 689, 1987.
5. **Shubert, M. M. and Izutsu, K. T.,** Iatrogenic causes of salivary gland dysfunction, *J. Dent. Res.,* 66, (Sp. Issue), 680, 1987.
6. **Henkin, R. I., Talal, N., Larson, A. L., and Mattern, C. F.,** Abnormalities of taste and smell in Sjögren's syndrome, *Ann. Intern. Med.,* 76, 375, 1972.
7. **Bertram, U.,** Xerostomia: Clinical Aspects, Pathology and Pathogenesis, Aarhuus Stifts Bogtrykkerie, Copenhagen, 1976.
8. **Navezesh, M. and Ship, I.,** Xerostomia: diagnosis and treatment, *Am. J. Otolaryngol.,* 4, 283, 1983.
9. **Saunders, J. R., Mirata, R. M., and Jaques, D. A.,** Salivary glands, *Surg. Clin. North Am.,* 66, 59, 1986.
10. **Levine, M. J., Jones, P. C., Loomis, R. E., Reddy, M. S., Al-Hashimi, I., Bergey, E. J., Bradway, S. D., Cohen, R. E., and Tabak, L. A.,** Functions of human saliva and salivary mucins. An overview in Oral Mucosal Diseases: Biology, Etiology, and Therapy, MacKenzie, I.C., Squier, C.A., and Dabelsteen, E., Eds., Laegeforeningens Forlag, 1987, 24.
11. **Levine, M. J., Reddy, M. S., Tabak, L. A., Loomis, R. E., Bergey, E. J., Jones, P. C., Cohen, R. E., Stinson, M. W., and Al-Hashimi, I.,** Structural aspects of salivary glycoproteins, *J. Dent. Res.,* 66, (Sp. Issue), 436, 1987.
12. **Levine, M. J., Aguirre, A., Hatton, M. N., and Tabak, L. A.,** Artificial salivas: present and future, *J. Dent. Res.,* 66, (Sp. Issue), 693, 1987.
13. **Loomis, R. E., Prakobphol, A., Levine, M. J., Reddy, M. S., and Jones, P. C.,** Biochemical and biophysical comparison of two mucins from human submandibular-sublingual saliva, *Arch. Biochem. Biophys.,* 258, 452, 1987.
14. **Prakobphol, A., Levine, M. J., Tabak, L. A., and Reddy, M. S.,** Purification of a low molecular-weight, mucin-type glycoprotein from human submandibular-sublingual saliva, *Carbohydr. Res.,* 108, 111, 1982.
15. **Kauffman, D. L., Bennick, A., and Keller, P. J.,** Basic proline-rich phospho-glycoproteins of human parotid saliva, *J. Dent. Res.,* 65(Sp. Issue), Abstr. 86, 1985.
16. **Bennick, A.,** Structural and genetic aspects of proline-rich proteins, *J. Dent. Res.,* 66, 457, 1987.
17. **Oppenheim, F. G., Hay, D. I., Smith, D. J., Offner, G. D., and Troxler, R. F.,** Molecular basis of salivary proline-rich protein and peptide synthesis: cell-free translations and processing of human and macaque statherin mRNAs and partial amino acid sequence of their signal peptides, *J. Dent. Res.,* 66, 462, 1987.
18. **Ellison, S. A.,** The identification of salivary components, in *Saliva and Dental Caries,* Kleinberg, I., Ellison, S. A., and Mandel, I. D., Eds., Information Retrieval, New York, 1979, 13.
19. **Bennick, A.,** Salivary proline-rich proteins, *Mol. Cell. Biochem.,* 45, 83, 1982.
20. **Mandel, I. D.,** The functions of saliva, *J. Dent. Res.,* 66, 623, 1987.
21. **Maeda, N., Kin, H.-S., Azen, E. A., and Smithies, O.,** Differential RNA splicing and post-translational cleavages in the human salivary proline-rich protein gene system, *J. Biol. Chem.,* 260, 11123, 1985.
22. **Dickinson, D. P., Ridall, A. L., and Levine, M. J.,** Human submandibular gland statherin and basic histidine-rich peptide are encoded by highly abundant mRNAs derived from a common ancestral sequence, *Biochem. Biophys. Res. Commun.,* 149, 784, 1987.
23. **Merritt, A. D. and Karn, R. C.,** The human $\alpha$-amylases, in *Advances in Human Genetics,* Vol. 8., Harris, H. and Hirshhorn, K., Eds., Plenum Press, New York, 1977, 435.

24. **Cohen, R. E., Jones, P. C., Neiders, M. E., Aguirre, A., and Levine, M. J.**, Monoclonal antibodies to human salivary mucins: immunogenicity, characterization, and application, *J. Dent. Res., 65*(Sp. Issue), Abstr. 1408, 1986.

25. **Cohen, R. E., Aguirre, A., Jones, P. C., Reddy, M. S., Neiders, M. E., and Levine, M. J.**, Immunocytochemistry of human salivary mucins, *J. Dent. Res.,* 66 (Sp. Issue), Abstr. 302, 1987.

26. **Baig, M. M., Winzler, R. J., and Rennert, O. M.**, Isolation of mucin from human submaxillary secretions, *J. Immunol.,* 111, 1826, 1973.

27. **Oemrawsingh, I. and Roukema, P. A.**, Isolation, purification and chemical characterization of human submandibular mucins, *Arch. Oral Biol.,* 19, 613, 1974.

28. **Oemrawsingh, I. and Roukema, P. A.**, Composition and biological properties of mucins, isolated from human submandibular glands, *Arch. Oral Biol.,* 19, 753, 1974.

29. **Hogg, S. D. and Embery, G.**, The isolation and partial characterization of a sulphated glycoprotein from human whole saliva which aggregates strains of *Streptococcus sanguis* but not *Streptococcus mutans, Arch. Oral Biol.,* 24, 791, 1979.

30. **Green, D. R. and Embery, G.**, Structural studies on a sulphated glycoprotein preparation isolated from human saliva, *Arch. Oral. Biol.,* 30, 859, 1985.

31. **Slomiany, B. L., Murty, V. L., Slomiany, A., Zielsnski, J., and Mandel, I. D.**, Mucus glycoprotein of human saliva: differences in the associated and covalently bound lipids with caries, *Biochim. Biophys. Acta,* 882, 18, 1986.

32. **Wagh, P. V. and Bahl, O. P.**, Sugar residues on proteins, *Crit. Rev. Biochem.,* 10, 307, 1981.

33. **Cohen, R. E., Reddy, M. S., and Levine, M. J.**, Human low molecular weight salivary mucin contains both N- and O-glycosidically linked oligosaccharides, *J. Dent. Res.,* 67 (Sp. Issue), Abstr. p. 2243, 1988.

34. **Loomis, R. E., Bergey, E. J., Levine, M. J., and Tabuk, L. A.**, Circular dichroism and fluorescence spectroscopic analyses of a proline-rich glycoprotein from human parotid saliva, *Int. J. Pept. Protein Res.,* 26, 621, 1985.

35. **Reddy, M. S., Levine, M. J., and Tabuk, L. A.**, Structure of the carbohydrate chains of the proline-rich glycoprotein from human parotid saliva, *Biochem. Biophys. Res. Commun.,* 104, 882, 1982.

36. **Loomis, R. E., Bhandary, K. K., Tseng, C.-C., Bergey, E. J., and Levine, M. J.**, Nuclear magnetic resonance spectroscopic and computer-simulated structural analyses of a heptapeptide sequence found around the N-glycosylation site of a proline-rich glycoprotein from human parotid saliva, *Biophys. J.,* 51, 193, 1987.

37. **Fischer, E. H. and Stein, E. A., Alpha-amylases.**, in *The Enzymes,* Vol. 4., 2nd ed., Boyer, P. O., Ed., Academic Press, New York, 1960, 313.

38. **Berfeld, P.**, Amylases, alpha and beta, in *Methods in Enzymology,* Vol. 1, Colowick, S. P. and Kaplan, N. O., Eds., Academic Press, New York, 1955, 149.

39. **Karn, R. C.**, The comparative biochemistry, physiology, and genetics of animal α-amylases, *Adv. Comp. Physiol. Biochem.,* 7, 1, 1978.

40. **Zakowski, J. J. and Bruns, E. E.**, Biochemistry of human alpha amylase isoenzymes, *Crit. Rev. Clin. Lab. Sci.,* 21, 283, 1986.

41. **Korsrud, F. R. and Brandtzaeg, P.**, Characterization of epithelial elements in human major salivary glands by functional markers: localization of amylase, lactoferrin, lysozyme, secretory component, and secretory immunoglobulins by paired immunofluorescence staining, *J. Histochem. Cytochem.,* 30, 657, 1982.

42. **Warner, T. F. C. S., Seo, I. S., Azen, E. A., Hafez, G. R., and Zarling T. A.**, Immunocytochemistry of acinic cell carcinomas and mixed tumors of salivary glands, *Cancer,* 56, 2221, 1985.

43. **Kraus, F. W. and Mestecky, J.**, Immunohistochemical localization of amylase, lysosyme, and immunoglobulins in the human parotid gland, *Arch. Oral Biol.,* 16, 781, 1971.

44. **Stieffel, D. J. and Keller, P. J.**, Preparation and some properties of human pancreatic amylase including a comparison with human parotid amylase, *Biochim. Biophys. Acta,* 302, 345, 1973.

45. **Mayo, J. W. and Carlson, D. M.**, Isolation and properties of four α-amylase isoenzymes from human submandibular saliva, *Arch. Biochem. Biophys.,* 163, 498, 1974.

46. **Aguirre, A., Levine, M. J., Cohen, R. E., and Tabak, L. A.**, Immunochemical quantitation of α-amylase and secretory IgA in parotid saliva from people of various ages, *Arch. Oral Biol.,* 32, 297, 1987.

47. **Takeuchi, T.**, Human amylase isoenzymes separated on concanavalin A-sepharose, *Clin. Chem.,* 25, 1406, 1979.

48. **Keller, P. J., Kauffman, D. L., Allan, B. J., and Williams, B. L.**, Further studies on the structural differences between the isoenzymes of human parotid α-amylase, *Biochem.,* 10, 4867, 1971.

49. **Kauffman, D. L., Zager, N. I., Cohen, E., and Keller, P. J.**, The isoenzymes of human parotid amylase, *Arch. Biochem. Biophys.,* 137, 325, 1970.

50. **Yamashita, K., Yachibana, Y., Nakayama, T., Kitamura, M., Endo, Y., and Kobata, A.**, Structural studies of the sugar chains of human parotid α-amylase, *J. Biol. Chem.,* 225, 5635, 1980.

51. **Nakamura, Y., Ogawa, M., Emi, M., Kosaki, G., Himeno, S., and Matsubara, K.,** Sequences of cDNAs for human salivary and pancreatic α-amylase, *Gene,* 28, 263, 1984.

52. **Nishide, T., Nakamura, Y., Emi, M., Yamamoto, T., Ogawa, M., Mori, T., and Matsubara, K.,** Primary structure of human salivary α-amylase gene, *Gene,* 41, 299, 1986.

53. **Karn, R. C., Rosenblum, B. B., Ward, J. C., Merritt, A. D., and Shulkin, J. D.,** Immunological relationships and posttranslational modifications of human salivary amylase (Amy 1) and pancreatic amylase (Amy 2) isoenzymes, *Biochem. Genet.,* 12, 485, 1974.

54. **Carney, J. A.,** Antiserum raised against human pancreatic α-amylase, *Clin. Chim. Acta,* 67, 153, 1976.

55. **Ogawa, M., Takatsuka, Y., Kitahara, T., Matsuura, K., and Kosaki, G.,** Radioimmunoassay of human pancreatic amylase, in *Methods in Enzymology,* Vol. 74, Langone, J. and Van Vunakis, H., Eds., Academic Press, New York, 1981, 290.

56. **Morrison, M. and Allen, P. Z.,** The identification and isolation of lactoperoxidase from salivary gland, *Biochem. Biophys. Res. Commun.,* 13, 490, 1963.

57. **Morrison, M., Allen, P. Z., Bright, J., and Jayasinghe, W.,** Lactoperoxidase. V. Identification and isolation of lactoperoxidase from salivary gland, *Arch. Biochem. Biophys.,* 111, 126, 1965.

58. **Mansson-Rahemtulla, B.,** Human salivary peroxidase. Characterization of some of the system components and their activity, in Umea University Odontological Dissertations, Departments of Pedodontics and Cariology, University of Umea, Sweden, 1987.

59. **Tashian, R. E., Hewett-Emmett, D., Dodgson, S. J., Foster, R. E., II, and Sly, W. S.,** The value of inherited deficiencies of human carbonic anhydrase isozymes in understanding their cellular roles, *Ann. N.Y. Acad. Sci.,* 429, 262, 1984.

60. **Sundaram, V., Rumbolo, P., Grubb, J., Strisciuglio, P., and Sly, W. S.,** Carbonic anhydrase II deficiency: diagnosis and carrier detection using differential enzyme and inhibition and inactivation, *Am. J. Hum. Genet.,* 38, 125, 1986.

61. **Tashian, R. E. and Carter, N. D.,** Biochemical genetics of carbonic anhydrase, in Advances in Human Genetics, Vol. 7, Hirschhorn, K. and Harris, H., Eds., Plenum Press, New York, 1976, 1.

62. **Heath, R., Jeffrey, S., and Carter, N.,** Radioimmunoassay of human muscle carbonic anhydrase III in dystrophic states, *Clin. Chim. Acta,* 119, 299, 1982.

63. **Lewinson, D., Rosenberg, M., Goldenberg, S., and Warburg, M. R.,** Carbonic anhydrase cytochemistry in mitochondria-rich cells of salamander larvae gill epithelium as related to age and H$^+$ and Na$^+$ concentrations, *J. Cell Physiol.,* 130, 125, 1987.

64. **Vaananen, H. H., Takala, T., and Morris, D. C.,** Immunoelectron microscopic localization of carbonic anhydrase III in rat skeletal muscle, *Histochemistry,* 86, 175, 1986.

65. **Bruns, W., Dermietzel, R., and Gros, G.,** Carbonic anhydrase in the sarcoplasmic reticulum of rabbit skeletal muscle, *J. Physiol. (London),* 371, 351, 1986.

66. **Dodgson, S. J. and Forster, R. E.,** Carbonic anhydrase: inhibition results in decreased urea production by hepatocytes, *J. Appl. Physiol.,* 60, 646, 1986.

67. **Engstron, F. L., Kemp, J. W., and Woodbury, D. M.,** Subcellular distribution of carbonic anhydrase and Na$^+$, K$^+$ and HCO$_3$$^-$-ATPases in brains of DBA and C57 mice, *Epilepsia,* 25, 759, 1984.

68. **Whitney, P. L. and Briggle, T. V.,** Membrane-associated carbonic anhydrase purified from bovine lung, *J. Biol. Chem.,* 257, 12056, 1982.

69. **Wistrand, P. J.,** Properties of membrane-bound carbonic anhydrase, *Ann. N.Y. Acad. Sci.,* 429, 195, 1984.

70. **Sanyal, G., Pessah, N. I., and Maren, T. H.,** Kinetics and inhibition of membrane-bound carbonic anhydrase from canine renal cortex,. *Biochim. Biophys. Acta,* 657, 128, 1981.

71. **McKinley, D. N. and Whitney, P. L.,** Particulate carbonic anhydrase in homogenates of human kidney, *Biochim. Biophys. Acta,* 445, 780, 1976.

72. **Ikejima, T. and Ito, S.,** Carbonic anhydrase in mouse salivary glands and saliva: a histochemical, immunohistochemical, and enzyme activity study, *J. Histochem. Cytochem.,* 32, 625, 1984.

73. **Murakami, H. and Sly, W. S.,** Purification and characterization of human salivary carbonic anhydrase, *J. Biol. Chem.,* 262, 1382, 1987.

74. **Rundegren, J. and Ericson, T.,** Effect of calcium on reactions between a salivary agglutinin and a serotype *c* strain of *Streptococcus mutans, J. Oral Pathol.,* 10, 269, 1981.

75. **Ericson, T. and Rundegren, J.,** Characterization of a salivary agglutinin reacting with a serotype *c* strain of *Streptococcus mutans, Eur. J. Biochem.,* 133, 255, 1983.

76. **Moro, I., Umemura, S., Crago, S. S., and Mestecky, J.,** Immunohistochemical distribution of immunoglobulins, lactoferrin, and lysozyme in human minor salivary glands, *J. Oral Pathol.,* 13, 97, 1984.

77. **Flanagan, J. G., Lefranc, M. P., and Rabbitts, T. H.,** Mechanisms of divergence and convergence of the human immunoglobulin α1 and α2 constant region gene sequences, *Cell,* 38, 681, 1984.

78. **Liu, Y. S. V., Low, T. L. K., Infante, A., and Putnam, F.,** Complete covalent structure of a human IgA1 immunoglobulin, *Science,* 193, 1017, 1976.

79. **Baenziger J. and Kornfeld, S.,** Structure of the carbohydrate units of IgA1 immunoglobulin. I. Structure of the O-glycosidically linked oligosaccharide units, *J. Biol. Chem.,* 249, 7270, 1974.

80. **Tsuzukida, Y., Wang, C.-C., and Putnam, F. W.,** Structure of the A2m(1) allotype of human IgA-a recombinant molecule, *Proc. Natl. Acad. Sci. U.S.A.,* 76, 1104, 1979.

81. **Tomasi, T. B. and McNabb, P. C.,** The secretory immune system, in *Basic and Clinical Immunology,* 3rd ed., Fudenberg, H. H., Stites, D. P., and Caldwell, J. L., Eds., Lange, Los Altos, CA, 1980, 240.

82. **Delacroix, D. L., Dive, C., Rambaud, J. C., and Vaerman, J. P.,** IgA subclasses in various secretions and in serum, *Immunology,* 47, 383, 1983.

83. **Liu, Y.-S. and Putnam, F. W.,** Primary structure of a human IgA1 immunoglobulin, *J. Biol. Chem.,* 254, 2839, 1979.

84. **Purkayastha, S., Rao, C. V. N., and Lamm, M. E.,** Structure of the carbohydrate chain of free secretory component from human milk, *J. Biol. Chem.,* 254, 6583, 1979.

85. **Eiffert, H., Quentin, E., Decker, J., Hillemeir, S., Hufschmidt, M., Klingmuller, D., Weber, M. H., and Hilschmann, N.,** Die Primarstrucktur der menschlichen freinen Sekretkomponente und die Anordnung der Disulfidbrucken, *Hoppe-Seyler's Z. Physiol. Chem.,* 365, 1489, 1984.

86. **Koshland, M. E.,** The coming of age of the immunoglobulin J chain, *Ann. Rev. Immunol.,* 3, 425, 1985.

87. **Simson, J. A. V., Spicer, S. S., Chao, J., Grimm, L., and Margolius, H. S.,** Kallikrein localization in rodent salivary glands and kidney with the immunoglobulin-enzyme bridge technique, *J. Histochem. Cytochem.,* 27, 1567, 1979.

88. **Coghlan, J. P., Penschow, J. D., Hudson, P. J., and Niall, H. D.,** Hybridization histochemistry: use of recombinant DNA for tissue localizations of specific mRNA populations, *Clin. Exper. Hyper.,* Suppl. A6, 63, 1984.

89. **Schachter, M.,** Kallikreins (kininogenases) — a group of serine proteases with bioregulatory actions, *Pharmacol., Rev.,* 31, 1, 1980.

90. **Orstavik, T. B., Brandtzaeg, P., Nustad, K., and Pierce, J. B.,** Immunohistochemical localization of kallikrein in human pancreas and salivary gland, *J. Histochem. Cytochem.,* 28, 557, 1980.

91. **Colman, R. W. and Bagdasarian, A.,** Human kallikrein and prekallikrein, in *Methods in Enzymology,* Vol. 45, Lorand, L., Ed., Academic Press, New York, 1976.

92. **Colman, R. W. and Wong, P. Y.,** Participation of Hageman factor dependent pathways in human disease states, *Thromb. Haemost.,* 38, 751, 1977.

93. **Takaoka, M., Akiyama, H., Ito, K., Okamura, H., and Morimoto, S.,** Isolation of inactive kallikrein from rat urine, *Biochem. Biophys. Res. Commun.,* 109, 841, 1982.

94. **Nustad, K. and Pierce, J. B.,** Purification of rat urinary kallikreins and their specific antibody, *Biochem.,* 13, 2312, 1974.

95. **Oza, N. B., Amin, V. M., McGregor, R. K., Scicli, A. F., and Carretero, O. A.,** Isolation of rat urinary kallikrein and properties of its antibodies, *Biochem. Pharmacol.,* 25, 1607, 1976.

96. **Moriya, H., Ikekita, M., and Kizuki, K.,** Studies on carbohydrate structure and immunological properties of human urinary kallikreins, *Adv. Exp. Med. Biol.,* 198, 35, 1986.

97. **Takahashi, S., Irie, A., Katayama, Y., Ito, K., and Miyake, Y.,** N-terminal amino acid sequence of human urinary prokallikrein, *J. Biochem.,* 99, 989, 1986.

98. **Masson, P. L., Heremans, J. F., Prignot, J. J., and Wanters, G.,** Immunohistochemical localization and bacteriostatic properties of an iron-binding protein from bronchial mucus, *Thorax,* 21, 538, 1966.

99. **Masson, P. L., Heremans, J. F., and Dive, C.,** An iron-binding protein common to many external secretions, *Clin. Chim. Acta,* 14, 735, 1966.

100. **Spitznagel, J. K., Daldorf, F. G., Leffell, M. S., Folds, J. D., Welsh, I. R., Cooney, M. H., and Martin, L. E.,** Character of azurophil and specific granules purifed from human polymorphonuclear leukocytes, *Lab. Invest.,* 30, 774, 1974.

101. **Arnold, R. R., Cole, M. G., and McGhee, J. R.,** A bacteriocidal effect for human lactoferrin, *Science,* 197, 263, 1977.

102. **Tabak, L. A., Mandel, I. D., Karlan, D., and Baurmash, H.,** Alterations in lactoferrin in salivary gland disease, *J. Dent. Res.,* 57, 43, 1977.

103. **Imber, M. J. and Pizzo, S. V.,** Clearance and binding of native and defucosylated lactoferrin, *Biochem. J.,* 212, 249, 1983.

104. **Legrand, D., Mazurier, J., Metz-Boutigue, M., Jolles, J., Joles, P., Montreuil, J., and Spik, G.,** Characterization and localization of an iron-binding 18 kDa glycopeptide isolated from the N-terminal half of human lactotransferrin, *Biochim. Biophys. Acta,* 787, 90, 1984.

105. **Moguilevsky, M., Retegui, L. A., and Masson, P. L.,** Comparison of human lactoferrins from milk and neutrophilic leucocytes. Relative molecular mass, isoelectric point, iron-binding properties and uptake by the liver, *Biochem. J.,* 229, 353, 1985.

106. **Mazurier, J., Metz-Boutigue, M. H., Jolles, J., Spik, G., Montreuil, J., and Jolles, P.,** Human lactotransferrin: molecular, functional, and evolutionary comparisons with human serum transferrin and hen ovotransferrin, *Experientia,* 39, 135, 1983.

107. **Montreuil, J., Tonnelat, J., and Mullet, S.,** Preparation et properties de la lactosiderophiline (lactotransferrine) du lait de femme, *Biochim. Biophys. Acta.,* 45, 413, 1960.
108. **Spik, G., Strecker, G., Fournet, B., Bouquelet, S., and Montreuil, J.,** Primary structure of the glycans from human lactotransferrin, *Eur. J. Biochem.,* 121, 1982.
109. **Metz-Boutigue, M. H., Jolles, J., Mazurier, J., Spik, G., Montreuil, J., and Jolles, P.,** An 88 amino acid long C-terminal sequence of human lactotransferrin, *FEBS Lett.,* 142, 107, 1982.
110. **Metz-Boutigue, M. H., Jolles, J., Mazurier, J., Spik, G. Montreuil, J., and Jolles, P.,** Structural studies concerning human lactotransferrin: its relatedness with human serum transferrin and evidence for internal homology, *Biochimie,* 60, 557, 1978.
111. **Gorinsky, B., Horsbargh, C., Lindley, P. F., Moss, D. S., Parkar, M., and Watson, J. L.,** Evidence for the bilobal nature of diferric rabbit plasma transferrin, *Nature (London),* 281, 157, 1979.
112. **Bluard-Deconinck, J., Williams, J., Evans, R. W., Van Snick, J., Osinski, P. A., and Masson, P. L.,** Iron-binding fragments from the N-terminal and C-terminal regions of human lactoferrin, *Biochem. J.,* 171, 321, 1978.
113. **Hynes, R. O.,** Fibronectins, *Sci. Am.,* 254, 42, 1986.
114. **Tynelius-Bratthall, G., Ericson, D., and Araujo, H. M.,** Fibronectin in saliva and gingival crevices, *J. Periodontal Res.,* 21, 563, 1986.
115. **Linde, A., Berghem, L. E., Hansson, H. A., Jonsson, R., and Redfors, Y.,** Ultrastructural localization of fibronectin in duct cells of human minor salivary glands and its immunochemical detection in minor salivary gland secretion, *Arch. Oral Biol.,* 29, 921, 1984.
116. **Linde, A. and Jonsson, R.,** Immunofluorescent localization of fibronectin in human oral mucosa, *Arch. Oral Biol.,* 27, 1047, 1982.
117. **Babu, J. P. and Dabbous, M. K.,** Interaction of salivary fibronectin with oral streptococci, *J. Dent. Res.,* 65, 1094, 1986.
118. **Akiyama, S. K. and Yamada, K. M.,** Fibronectin, *Adv. Enzymol.,* 59, 1, 1987.
119. **Yamada, K. M. and Kennedy, D. W.,** Fibroblast cellular and plasma fibronectins are similar but not identical, *J. Cell Biol.,* 80, 492, 1979.
120. **Yamada, K. M., Schlesinger, D. H., Kennedy, D. W., and Pastan, I.,** Characterization of a major fibroblast cell surface glycoprotein, *Biochemistry,* 16, 5552, 1977.
121. **Colonna, G., Alexander, S. S., Jr., Yamada, K. M., Pastan, I., and Edelhoch, H.,** The stability of cell surface proteins to surfactants and denaturants, *J. Biol. Chem.,* 253, 7787, 1978.
122. **Alexander, S. S., Jr., Colonna, G., and Edelhoch, H.,** The structure and stability of human plasma cold-insoluble globulin, *J. Biol. Chem.,* 254, 1501, 1979.
123. **Moseson, M. W., Chen, A. B., and Huseby, R. M.,** The cold-insoluble globulin of human plasma: studies of its essential structural features, *Biochim. Biophys. Acta,* 386, 509, 1975.
124. **Hynes, R.,** Molecular biology of fibronectin, *Ann. Rev. Cell. Biol.,* 1, 67, 1985.
125. **Tamkun, J. W., Schwarzbauer, J. E., and Hynes, R. O.,** A single rat fibronectin gene generates three different mRNAs by alternative splicing of a complete exon, *Proc. Natl. Acad. Sci. U.S.A.,* 81, 5140, 1984.
126. **Skorstengaard, K., Thgersen, H. C., Vibe-Pedersen, K., Petersen, T. E., and Magnusson, S.,** Purification of twelve cyanogen bromide fragments from bovine plasma fibronectin and the amino acid sequence of eight of them, *Eur. J. Biochem.,* 128, 605, 1982.
127. **Skorstengaard, K., Thgersen, H. C., and Petersen, T. E.,** Complete primary structure of the collagen-binding domain of bovine fibronectin, *Eur. J. Biochem.,* 140, 235, 1984.
128. **Rocco, M., Carson, M., Hantgan, R. McDonagh, J., and Dermans, J.,** Dependence on the shape of the plasma fibronectin molecule on solvent composition. Ionic strength and glycerol content, *J. Biol. Chem.,* 258, 14545, 1983.
129. **Holly, F. J., Dolowy, K., and Yamada, K. M.,** Comparative surface chemical studies of cellular fibronectin and submaxillary mucin monolayers: effects of pH, ionic strength, and presence of calcium ions, *J. Colloid Interface Sci.,* 100, 210, 1984.
130. **Alexander, S. S., Jr., Colonna, G., Yamada, K. M., Pastan, I., and Edelhoch, H.,** Molecular properties of a major cell surface protein from chick embryo fibroblasts, *J. Biol. Chem.,* 253, 5820, 1978.
131. **Williams, E. C., Janney, P. A., Ferry, J. D., and Mosher, D. F.,** Conformational states of fibronectin. Effects of pH, ionic strength, and collagen binding, *J. Biol. Chem.,* 257, 14973, 1982.
132. **Williams, E. C., Janney, P. A., Johnson, R. B., and Mosher, D. F.,** Fibronectin. Effect of disulfide bond reduction on its physical and functional properties, *J. Biol. Chem.,* 258, 5911, 1982.
133. **Hubbard, S. C. and Ivatt, R. J.,** Synthesis and processing of asparagine-linked oligosaccharides, *Ann. Rev. Biochem.,* 50, 555, 1981.
134. **Staneloni, R. J. and Leloir, L. F.,** The biosynthetic pathway of the asparagine-linked oligosaccharides of glycoproteins, *Crit. Rev. Biochem.,* 12, 289, 1982.
135. **Kornfeld, R. and Kornfeld, S.,** Assembly of asparagine-linked oligosaccharides, *Ann. Rev. Biochem.,* 54, 631, 1985.

136. **Blobel, G. and Dobberstein, B.,** Transfer of proteins across membranes. I. Presence of proteolytically processed and unprocessed nascent immunoglobulin light chains on membrane-bound ribosomes of murine myleoma, *J. Cell Biol.,* 67, 835, 1975.

137. **Unwin, P. N. T.,** Attachment of ribosome crystals to intracellular membranes, *J. Mol. Biol.,* 132, 69, 1979.

138. **Palade, G.,** Intracellular aspects of the process of protein synthesis, *Science,* 189, 347, 1975.

139. **Kreibich, G., Ulrich, B. L., and Sabatini, D. D.,** Proteins of rough microsomal membranes related to ribosome binding. I. Identification of ribophorins I and II, membrane proteins characteristic of rough microsomes, *J. Cell Biol.,* 77, 464, 1978.

140. **Kreibich, G., Czako-Graham, M., Grebenau, R. Mok, W., Rodriguez-Boulan, E., and Sabatini, D. D.,** Characterization of the ribosomal binding site on rat liver rough microsomes: Ribophorins I and II, two integral membrane proteins related to ribosomal binding, *J. Supramol. Struct.,* 8, 279, 1978.

141. **Thibodeau, S. N. and Walsh, K. A.,** Processing of precursor proteins by preparation of oviduct microsomes, *Ann. N.Y. Acad. Sci.,* 343, 180, 1980.

142. **Jackson, R. G. and Blobel, G.,** Post-translational processing of full-length presecretory proteins with canine pancreatic signal peptidase, *Ann. N.Y. Acad. Sci.,* 343, 391, 1980.

143. **Rosenblatt, M., Beaudette, N. V., and Fasman, G. D.,** Conformational studies of the synthetic precursor-specific region of preproparathyroid hormone, *Proc. Natl. Acad. Sci. U.S.A.,* 77, 3983, 1980.

144. **Reddy, G. L. and Nagaraj, J.,** Circular dichroism studies on synthetic peptides corresponding to the cleavage site region of precursor proteins, *Int. J. Pept. Protein Res.,* 29, 497, 1987.

145. **Laxma-Reddy, G. and Nagaraj, R.,** Circular dichroism studies on the signal sequence of *E. coli* alkaline phosphatase indicate the presence of both alpha-helix and beta structure in hydrophobic environments, *FEBS Lett.,* 202, 349, 1986.

146. **Kreil, G.,** Transfer of proteins across membranes, *Ann. Rev. Biochem.,* 50, 317, 1981.

147. **Ronnett, G. O. and Lane, M. D.,** Post-translational glycosylation-induced activation of aglycoinsulin receptor accumulated during tunicamycin treatment, *J. Biol. Chem.,* 256, 4704, 1981.

148. **Hanover, J. A. and Lennarz, W. J.,** N-linked glycoprotein assembly. Evidence that oligosaccharide attachment occurs within the lumen of the endoplasmic reticulum, *J. Biol. Chem.,* 255, 3600, 1980.

149. **Lingappa, V. R., Lingappa, J. R., Prasad, R., Ebner, K. E., and Blobel, G.,** Coupled cell free synthesis, segregation, and core glycosylation of a secretory protein, *Proc. Natl. Acad. Sci. U.S.A.,* 75, 2338, 1978.

150. **Schlesinger, S., Malfer, C., and Schlesinger, M. J.,** The formation of vesicular stomatitis virus (San Juan strain) becomes temperature-sensitive when glucose residues are retained on the oligosaccharides of the glycoprotein, *J. Biol. Chem.,* 259, 7597, 1984.

151. **Lodish, H. F. and Kong, N. J.,** Glucose removal from N-linked oligosaccharides is required for efficient maturation of certain secretory glycoproteins from the rough endoplasmic reticulum to the Golgi complex, *Cell Biol.,* 98, 1720, 1984.

152. **Hanover, J. A., Lennarz, W. J., and Young, J. D.,** Synthesis of N- and O-linked glycopeptides in oviduct membrane preparations, *J. Biol. Chem.,* 255, 6713, 1980.

153. **Williams, D. and Schachter, H.,** Mucin synthesis. I. Detection in canine submaxillary glands of an *N*-acetylglucosaminyl transferase which acts on mucin substrates, *J. Biol. Chem.,* 255, 11247, 1980.

154. **Gallager, J. T. and Corfield, A. P.,** Mucin-type glycoproteins — new perspectives on their structure and synthesis, *Trends Biochem. Sci.,* 38, 1978.

155. **Tabak, L. A., Levine, M. J., Mandel, I. D., and Ellison, S. A.,** Role of salivary mucins in the protection of the oral cavity, *J. Oral Pathol.,* 11, 1, 1982.

156. **Porter, R. R.,** The hydrolysis of rabbit gamma globulin and antibodies with crystalline papain, *Biochem. J.,* 73, 119, 1959.

157. **Porter, R. R.,** Structural studies of immunoglobulins, *Science,* 180, 713, 1973.

158. **Ruoslahti, E., Pierschbacher, M., Hayman, E. G., and Engvall, E.,** Fibronectin: a molecule with remarkable structural and functional diversity, *Trends Biol. Sci.,* 7, 188, 1982.

159. **Ruoslahti, E.,** Fibronectin, *J. Oral Pathol.,* 10, 3, 1981.

160. **Rouslahti, E., Engvall, E., and Hayman, E. G.,** Fibronectin: current concepts of its structure and function, *Collagen Res.,* 1, 95, 1981.

161. **Rouslahti, E., Hayman, E. G., Kuusela, P., Shively, J. E., and Engvall, E.,** Isolation of a tryptic fragment containing the collagen-binding site of plasma fibronectin., *J. Biol. Chem.,* 254, 6054, 1979.

162. **Miller, E. J.,** Biochemical characteristics and biological significance of the genetically-distinct collagens., *Mol. Cell. Biochem.,* 13, 165, 1976.

163. **Eyre, D. R.,** Collagen: molecular diversity in the body's protein scaffold, *Science* 207, 1315, 1980.

164. **Villar, E., Schuster, B., Peterson, D., and Schirch, V.,** C1-tetrahydrofolate synthase from rabbit liver. Structural and kinetic properties of the enzyme and its two domains., *J. Biol. Chem.,* 260, 2245, 1985.

165. **Weldon, S. L. and Taylor, S. S.,** Monoclonal antibodies as probes for functional domains in cAMP-dependent protein kinase II., *J. Biol. Chem.,* 260, 4203, 1985.

166. **Huang, K.-P. and Huang, F. L.,** Immunochemical characterization of rat brain protein kinase c, *J. Biol. Chem.,* 261, 14781, 1986.

167. **Hill, R. L., Delaney, R., Fellows, R. E., and Lebovitz, H. E.,** The evolutionary origins of the immunoglobulins, *Proc. Natl. Acad. Sci. U.S.A.,* 56, 1762, 1966.

168. **Edelman, G. M.,** The covalent structure of human gamma G-immunoglobulin. XI. Functional implications, *Biochemistry,* 9, 3197, 1970.

169. **Coggins, J. R. and Hardie, D. G.,** The domain as the fundamental unit of protein structure and evolution, in *Multidomain Proteins — Structure and Evolution,* Coggins, J. R. and Hardie, D. G., Eds., Elsevier, Amsterdam, 1986, 1.

170. **Kousvelari, E. E., Baratz, R. S., Burke, B., and Oppenheim, F. G.,** Immunological identification and determination of proline-rich proteins in salivary secretions, enamel pellicle and glandular tissue specimens, *J. Dent. Res.,* 59, 1430, 1980.

171. **Tabak, L. A., Levine, M. J., Jain, N. K., Bryan, A. R., Cohen, R. E., Monte, L. D., Zawacki, S., Nancollas, G. H., Slomiany, A., and Slomiany, B. L.,** Adsorption of human salivary mucins to hydroxyapatite, *Arch. Oral Biol.,* 30, 423, 1985.

172. **Al-Hashimi, I., Levine, M. J., and Mandel, I. D.,** Studies on acquired human enamel pellicle, *J. Dent. Res.,* 64 (Sp. Issue), Abst. 718, 1985.

173. **Fisher, S. J., Prakobphol, A., Kajisa, L., and Murray, P. A.,** External radiolabelling of components of pellicle on human enamel, *Arch. Oral Biol.,* 32, 509, 1987.

174. **Orstavik, D. and Kraus, F. W.,** The acquired pellicle: Immunofluorescent demonstration of specific proteins, *J. Oral Pathol.,* 2, 68, 1973.

175. **Kraus, F. W., Orstavik, D., Hurst, D. C., and Cook, C. H.,** The acquired pellicle: variability and subject-dependence of specific proteins, *J. Oral Pathol.,* 2, 165, 1973.

176. **Armstrong, W. G. and Hayward, A. F.,** Acquired organic integuments of human enamel: a comparison of analytical studies with optical, phase-contrast, and electron microscope examinations, *Caries Res.,* 2, 294, 1968.

177. **Levine, M. J., Tabak, L. A., Reddy, M. S., and Mandel, I. D.,** Nature of salivary pellicles in microbial adherence: role of salivary mucins, in *Molecular Basis of Oral Microbial Adhesion,* Mergenhagen, S. E. and Rosan, B., Eds., American Society Microbiologists, Washington, D. C., 1985, 125.

178. **Koutsoukos, P. G., Al-Hashimi, I., Nancollas, G. H., and Levine, M. J.,** Influence of salivary proteins on the crystallization of hydroxyapatite, *J. Dent. Res.,* 74 (Sp. Issue), Abstr. 146, 1985.

179. **Sabin, A. B. and Ward, R.,** The natural history of poliomyelitis. I. Distribution of virus in nervous and non-nervous tissues, *J. Exp. Med.,* 73, 771, 1941.

180. **McNabb, P. C. and Tomasi, T. B.,** Host defense mechanisms at mucosal surfaces, *Ann. Rev. Microbiol.,* 35, 477, 1981.

181. **Carlsson, B., Grahnen, H., and Jonsson, G.,** Lactobacilli and streptococci in the mouth of children, *Caries Res.,* 9, 333, 1975.

182. **Tenovuo, J., Mansson-Rahemtulla, B., Pruitt, K. M., and Arnold, R. R.,** Inhibition of dental plaque acid production by the salivary lactoperoxidase system, *Infect. Immun.,* 34, 208, 1981.

183. **Terranova, V. and Martin, G.,** Molecular factors determining gingival tissue interaction with tooth surface, *J. Periodontal Res.,* 17, 530, 1982.

184. **Woods, D. E., Strauss, D. C., Johanson, W. G., Jr., and Bass, J. A.,** Role of salivary protease activity in adherence of Gram-negative bacilli to mammalian buccal epithelial cells *in vivo, J. Clin. Invest.,* 68, 1435, 1981.

185. **Woods, D. E., Bass, J. A., Johanson, W. G., Jr., and Strauss, D. C.,** Role of adherence in the pathogenesis of *Pseudomonas aeruginosa* lung infection in cystic fibrosis patients, *Infect. Immun.,* 30, 694, 1980.

186. **Woods, D. E., Strauss, D. C., Johanson, W. G., Jr., and Bass, J. A.,** Role of fibronectin in the prevention of adherence of *Pseudomonas aeruginosa* to buccal cells, *J. Infect. Dis.,* 143, 784, 1981.

187. **Hasty, D. L. and Simpson, W. A.,** Effects of fibronectin and other salivary macromolecules on the adherence of *Escherichia coli* to buccal epithelium, *Infect. Immun.,* 55, 2103, 1987.

188. **Hatton, M. N., Loomis, R. E., Levine, M. J., and Tabak, L. A.,** Masticatory lubrication. The role of carbohydrate in the lubricating property of a salivary glycoprotein-albumin complex, *Biochem. J.,* 230, 817, 1985.

189. **Hatton, M. N., Levine, M. J., Margarone, J. E., and Aguirre, A.,** Lubrication and viscosity features of human saliva and commercially available saliva substitutes, *J. Oral Maxilliofac. Surg.,* 45, 496, 1987.

190. **Levine, M. J., Aguirre, A., Hatton, M. N., and Tabak, L. A.,** Artificial salivas: present and future, *J. Dent. Res.,* 66 (Sp. Issue), 693, 1987.

191. **Aguirre, A., Vecchio, C., Hatton, M. N., Cohen, R. E., and Levine, M. J.,** Correlation between salivary viscosity and lubrication, *J. Dent. Res.,* 65 (Sp. Issue), Abstr. 1407, 1986.

192. **Swann, D. A., Bloch, K. J., Swindell, D., and Shore, E.,** The lubricating activity of human synovial fluids, *Arthritis Rheum.,* 27, 552, 1984.

193. **Swann, D. A., Hendren, R. B., Radin, E. L., Sothman, S. L., and Duda, E. A.,** The lubricating activity of synovial fluid glycoproteins, *Arthritis Rheum.,* 24, 22, 1981.

194. **Douglas, C. W. I.,** The binding of human salivary α-amylase by oral strains of streptococcal bacteria, *Arch. Oral Biol.,* 28, 567, 1983.

195. **Bergey, E. J., Levine, M. J., Reddy, M. S., Bradway, S. D., and Al-Hashimi, I.,** Use of the photoaffinity crosslinking agent, *N*-hydroxsuccinididyl-4-azidosalicylic acid, to characterize salivary-bacterial interactions, *Biochem. J.,* 234, 43, 1986.

196. **Nagata, K., Nakao, M., Shibata, S., Shizukuishi, S., Nakamura, R., and Tsunemitsu, A.,** Purification and characterization of a galactosephilic component present of the cell surface of *Streptococcus sanguis, J. Periodontol.,* 54, 163, 1983.

197. **Shibata, S., Nagata, K., Nakamura, R., Tsunemitsu, A., and Misaki, A.,** Effect of some factors on binding of parotid saliva basic glycoprotein to oral streptococci, *J. Periodontol.,* 51, 499, 1980.

198. **Stinson, M. W., Levine, M. J., Cavese, J. M., Prakobphol, A., Murray, P. A., Tabak, L. A., and Reddy, M. S.,** Adherence of *Streptococcus sanguis* to salivary mucin bound to glass, *J. Dent. Res.,* 61, 1390, 1982.

199. **Gibbons, R. J., Etherden, I., and Moreno, E. C.,** Association of neuraminidase-sensitive receptors and putative hydrophobic interactions with high affinity binding sites for *Streptococcus sanguis* C5 in salivary pellicles, *Infect. Immun.,* 42, 1006, 1983.

200. **Gibbons, R. J. and Qureshi, J. V.,** Interactions of *Streptococcus mutans* and other oral bacteria with blood group reactive substances, in *Microbial Aspects of Dental Caries,* Stiles, H. M., Loeshe, W. J., and O'Brien, T. C., Eds., Information Retrieval, Washington, D.C., 1976, 163.

201. **Gibbons, R. J. and Qureshi, J. V.,** Selective binding of blood group reactive salivary mucins by *Streptococcus mutans* and other oral organisms, *Infect. Immunc.,* 22, 665, 1978.

202. **Hay, D. I., Gibbons, R. J. and Spinell, D. M.,** Characteristics of some high molecular weight constituents with bacterial aggregating activity from whole saliva and dental plaque, *Caries Res.,* 5, 111, 1971.

203. **McBride, B. C. and Gisslow, M. T.,** Role of sialic acid in induced aggregation of *Streptococcus sanguis, Infect. Immun.,* 18, 35, 1977.

204. **Morris, E. J. and McBride, B. C.,** Adherence of *Streptococcus sanguis* to saliva-coated hydroxyapatite: evidence for two binding sites, *Infect. Immun.,* 43, 656, 1984.

205. **Levine, M. J., Herzberg, M. C., Levine, M. S., Ellison, S. A., Stinson, M. W., Li, H. C., and Van Dyke, T.,** Specificity of salivary-bacterial interactions: role of terminal sialic acid residues in the interaction of salivary glycoproteins with *Streptococcus sanguis* and *Streptococcus mutans, Infect. Immun.,* 19, 107, 1978.

206. **Murray, P. A., Levine, M. J., Tabak, L. A., and Reddy, M. S.,** Specificity of salivary-bacterial interactions. I. Evidence for a lectin on *Streptococcus sanguis* with specificity for a NeuAcα2,3Galβ1,3GalNAc sequence, *Biochem. Biophys. Res. Commun.,* 106, 390, 1982.

207. **Reddy, M. S., Levine, M. J., and Prakobphol, A.,** Characterization of oligosaccharides from the lower molecular weight salivary mucin of a normal individual and one with cystic fibrosis, *J. Dent. Res.,* 64, 33, 1985.

208. **Murray, P. A., Levine, M. J., Reddy, M. S., Tabak, L. A., and Bergey, E. J.,** Preparation of a sialic acid binding protein from *Streptococcus mitis* strain KS32AR *Infect. Immun.,* 53, 359, 1986.

209. **Jones, P. C., Cohen, R. E., and Levine, M. J.** Streptococcal agglutination by human submandibular-sublingual saliva depleted of mucin glycoproteins, *J. Dent. Res.,* 66, (Sp. Issue), Abstr. 1431, 1987.

210. **McNabb, P. C. and Tomasi, T. B.,** Host defense mechanisms at mucosal surfaces, *Ann. Rev. Microbiol.,* 35, 477, 1981.

211. **Underdown, B. J. and Schiff, J. M.,** Immunoglobulin A: strategic defense initiative at the mucosal surface, *Ann. Rev. Immunol.,* 4, 389, 1986.

212. **Williams, R. C. and Gibbons, R. J.,** Inhibition of bacterial adherence by secretory immunoglobulin A: a mechanism of antigen disposal, *Science,* 177, 697, 1972.

213. **Genco, R. J., Evans, R. T., and Taubman, M. A.,** Specificity of antibodies to *Streptococcus mutans;* significance in inhibition of adherence, *Adv. Exp. Med. Biol.,* 45, 327, 1974.

214. **McGhee, J. R., Michalek, S. M., Webb, J., Navia, J. M., Rahman, A. F., and Legler, D. W.,** Effective immunity to dental caries: protection of gnotobiotic rats by local immunization with *Streptococcus mutans, J. Immunol.,* 114, 300, 1975.

215. **Michalek, S. M., McGhee, J. R., Mestecky, J., Arnold, R. R., and Bozzo, L.,** Ingestion of *Streptococcus mutans* induces secretory immunoglobulin A and caries immunity, *Science,* 192, 1238, 1976.

216. **Gahnberg, L., Olsson, J., Krasse, B., and Carlen, A.,** Interference of salivary immunoglobulin A antibodies and other salivary fractions with adherence of *Streptococcus mutans* to hydroxyapatitie, *Infect. Immun.,* 37, 401, 1982.

217. **Taylor, H. and Dimmock, N. J.,** Mechanism of neutralization of influenza virus by secretory IgA is different from that on monomeric IgA or IgG, *J. Exp. Med.,* 161, 198, 1985.

218. **Abraham, S. N., Beachey, E. H., and Simpson, W. A.,** Adherence of *Streptococcus pyogenes, Escherichia coli,* and *Pseudomonas aeruginosa* to fibronectin-coated and uncoated epithelial cells, *Infect. Immun.,* 41, 1261, 1983.

219. **Simpson, W. A. and Beachey, E. H.,** Adherence of group A streptococci to fibronectin on oral epithelial cells, *Infect. Immun.,* 39, 275, 1983.

220. **Scannapieco, F. A., Bergey, E. J., and Levine, M. J.,** Specific binding of a non-glycosylated isoenzyme of human parotid α-amylase to *Streptococcus sanguis, J. Dent. Res.,* 67 (Sp. Issue), Abstr., p. 832, 1988.

221. **Douglas, C. W. I. and Russell, R. R. B.,** The adsorption of human salivary components to strains of the bacterium *Streptococcus mutans, Arch. Oral Biol.,* 29, 751, 1984.

222. **Mellersh, A., Clark, A., and Hafiz, S.,** Inhibition of *Neisseria gonorrhoeae* by normal human saliva, *Br. J. Vener. Dis.,* 55, 20, 1979.

223. **Pruitt, K. M., Mansson-Rahemtulla, B., and Tenovuo, J.,** Detection of the hypothiocyanite (OSCN⁻ ion in human parotid saliva and the effect of pH on OSCN⁻ generation in the salivary peroxidase antimicrobial system, *Arch. Oral Biol.,* 28, 517, 1983.

224. **Aune, T. M. and Thomas, E. L.,** Accumulation of hypothiocyanate ion during peroxidase catalyzed oxidation of thiocyanate ion, *Eur. J. Biochem.,* 80, 209, 1977.

225. **Klebanoff, S. J. and Luebke, R. G.,** The antilactobacillus system of saliva. Role of salivary peroxidase, *Proc. Soc. Exp. Biol. Med.,* 118, 483, 1965.

226. **Slowey, R. R., Eidelman, S., and Klebanoff, S. J.,** Antibacterial activity of the purified peroxidase from human parotid saliva, *J. Bacteriol.,* 96, 575, 1968.

227. **Tenovuo, J. and Knuuttila, M. L. E.,** Antibacterial effect of salivary peroxidases on a cariogenic strain of *Streptococcus mutans, J. Dent. Res.,* 56, 1608, 1977.

228. **Donoghue, H. D., Hudson, D. E., and Perrons, C. J.,** Effect of lactoperoxidase system on streptococcal acid production and growth, *J. Dent. Res.,* 66, 616, 1987.

229. **Mansson-Rahemtulla, B., Baldone, D. C., Pruitt, K. M., and Rahemtulla, F.,** Effects of variations in pH and hypothiocyanite concentrations on *S. mutans* glucose metabolism, *J. Dent. Res.,* 66, 486, 1987.

230. **Pruitt, K. M. and Reiter, B.,** Biochemistry of peroxidase system: antimicrobial effects, in *The Lactoperoxidase System,* Pruitt, K. M. and Tenovuo, J. O., Eds., Marcel Dekker, New York, 1985, 143.

231. **Hanstrom, L., Johansson, A., and Carlsson, J.,** Lactoperoxidase and thiocyanate protect cultured mammalian cells against hydrogen peroxide toxicity, *Med. Biol.,* 61, 268, 1983.

232. **Tenovuo, J. and Larjava, H.,** The protective effect of peroxidase and thiocyanate against hydrogen peroxide toxicity assessed by the uptake of [³H]-thymidine by human gingival fibroblasts cultured *in-vitro, Arch. Oral Biol.,* 29, 445, 1984.

233. **Weinberg, E. D.,** Iron and Infection, *Microbiol. Rev.,* 42, 45, 1978.

234. **Bullen, J. J., Rogers, H. J., and Griffiths, E.,** Role of iron in bacterial infection, *Curr. Top. Microbiol. Immunol.,* 80, 1, 1978.

235. **Arnold, R. R., Brewer, M., and Gauthier, J. J.,** Bactericidal activity of human lactoferrin: sensitivity of a variety of microorganisms, *Infect. Immun.,* 28, 893, 1980.

236. **Lassiter, M. O., Newsome, A. L., Sams, L. D., and Arnold, R. R.,** Characterization of lactoferrin interaction with *Streptococcus mutans, J. Dent. Res.,* 66, 480, 1987.

237. **Cole, M. F., Arnold, R. R., Mestecky, J., Prince, S., Kulhavy, R., and McGhee, J. R.,** Studies with human lactoferrin and *S. mutans,* in *Microbial Aspects of Dental Caries,* Vol. 2, Information Retrieval, Washington, D. C., 1977, 359.

238. **Arnold, R. R., Russell, J. E., Champion, W. J., Brewer, M., and Gauthier, J. J.,** Bactericidal activity of human lactoferrin: differentiation from the stasis of iron deprivation, *Infect. Immun.,* 36, 792, 1982.

239. **Gauldie, J., Richards, C., and Lamontage, L.,** Fc receptors for IgA and other immunoglobulins on resident and activated alveolar macrophages, *Mol. Immunol.,* 20, 1029, 1983.

240. **Fanger, M. W., Goldstine, S. N., and Shen, L.,** The properties and role of receptors for IgA on human leukocytes, *Ann. N.Y. Acad. Sci.,* 409, 552, 1983.

241. **Tagliabue, A., Boraschi, D., Villa, L., Keren, D. F., Lowell, G. H., Rappuoli, R., and Nencioni, L.,** IgA-dependent cell-mediated activity against enteropathogenic bacteria: distribution, specificity and characterization of the effector cell. *J. Immunol.,* 133, 988, 1984.

242. **Boackle, R. J., Pruitt, K. M., and Mestecky, J.,** The interactions of human complement with interfacially aggregated preparations of human secretory IgA, *Immunochemistry,* 11, 543, 1974.

243. **Romer, W., Rother, V., and Roelcke, D.,** Failure of IgA cold agglutinin to activate complement, *Immunobiology,* 157, 41, 1980.

244. **DeJong, M. H. and Van Der Hoeven, J. S.,** The growth of oral bacterial on saliva, *J. Dent. Res.,* 66, 498, 1987.

245. **Bothwell, M. A., Wilson, W. H., and Shooter, E. M.,** The relationship between glandular kallikrein and growth factor-processing proteases of mouse submaxillary gland, *J. Biol. Chem.,* 254, 7287, 1979.

246. **Wong, R. S. C., Madapallimattam, G., and Bennick, A.,** The role of glandular kallikrein in the formation of a salivary proline-rich protein A by cleavage of a single bond in salivary protein C, *Biochem. J.,* 211, 35, 1983.

247. **Hamosh, M. and Burns, W. A.,** Lipolytic activity of human lingual glands (ebner), *Lab. Invest.,* 37, 603, 1977.

248. **Helm, J. F., Dodds, W. J., Hogan, W. J., Suergel, K. H., Egide, M. S., and Wood, C. M.,** Acid neutralizing capacity of human saliva, *Gastroenterology,* 83, 69, 1982.

249. **Allen, A. and Garner, A.,** Mucus and bicarbonate secretion in the stomach and their possible role in mucosal protection, *Gut,* 21, 249, 1980.

250. **Rees, W. D. W. and Turnberg, L. A.,** Mechanisms of gastric mucosal protection: a role for the "mucus-bicarbonate" barrier, *Clin. Sci.,* 62, 343, 1982.

251. **Shomers, J. P., Tabak, L. A., Levine, M. J., Mandel, I. D., and Ellison, S. A.,** The isolation of a family of cysteine-containing phosphoproteins from human submandibular-sublingual saliva, *J. Dent. Res.,* 61, 973, 1982.

252. **Reinholdt, J. and Kilian, M.,** Association between IgA and salivary mucin: nature and site of binding, *J. Dent. Res.,* 63, 227(Abstr. 513), 1984.

253. **Cohen, R. E., Neiders, M. E., and Levine, M. J.,** Monoclonal antibodies against salivary glycoproteins, *J. Dent. Res.,* 64, 328(Abstr.1377), 1985.

254. **Murray, P. A., Levine, M. J., Tabak, L. A., and Reddy, M. S.,** Neuraminidase activity: a biochemical market to distinguish *Streptococcus mitis* from *Streptococcus sanguis, J. Dent. Res.,* 63, 111, 1984.

255. **Gibbons, R. J. and van Houte, J.,** Bacterial adherence and the formation of dental plaque, in *Bacterial Adherence,* Beachey, E. H., Ed., Chapman and Hall, New York, 1980, 62.

256. **Gibbons, R. J. Etherden, I., and Peros, W.,** Aspects of the attachment of oral streptococci to experimental pellicles, in *Molecular Basis of Oral Microbial Adhesion,* Mergenhagen, S. E. and Rosan, B., Eds., American Society for Microbiology, Washington, D. C., 1985, 77.

257. **Fujiyama, Y., Kobayashi, K., Senda, S., Benno, Y., Bamba, T., and Hosoda, S.,** A novel IgA protease from *Clostridium* sp. capable of cleaving IgA1 and IgA2 A2m(1) allotype but not IgA2 A2m(2) allotype paraproteins, *J. Immunol.,* 134, 573, 1985.

258. **Plaut, A. G.,** The IgA1 proteases of pathogenic bacteria, *Ann. Rev. Microbiol.,* 37, 603, 1983.

259. **Reinholdt, J. and Kilian, M.,** Interference of IgA protease with the effect of secretory IgA on adherence of oral streptococci to saliva-coated hydroxyapatite, *J. Dent. Res.,* 65 (Sp. Issue), 492, 1987.

260. **Karn, R. C., Shulkin, J. D., Merritt, A. D., and Newell, R. C.,** Evidence for posttranscriptional modification of human salivary amylase (Amy 1) isoenzymes, *Biochem. Genet.,* 10, 341, 1973.

261. **Midelfort, C. F. and Mehler, A. H.,** Deamidation *in vivo* of an asparagine residue of rabbit muscle aldolase, *Proc. Natl. Acad. Sci. U.S.A.,* 69, 1816, 1972.

262. **Robinson, A. B. and Rudd, C. J.,** Deamidation of glutaminyl and asparaginyl residues in peptides and proteins, in *Current Topics in Cellular Regulation,* Vol. 8, Horecker, B. L. and Stadtman, E. R., Eds., Dekker and Nordeman, Amsterdam, 1974, 247.

263. **Van Kleef, F. S. M., de Jong, W. W., and Hoenders, H. J.,** Stepwise degradations and deamidation of the eye lens protein α-crystallin in ageing, *Nature (London),* 258, 264, 1975.

264. **Wikstrom, M. and Linde, A.,** Ability of oral bacteria to degrade fibronectin, *Infect. Immun.,* 51, 707, 1986.

265. **Ericson, T. and Adamson, M.,** Lactoperoxidase protects sialic acid from oxidative decarboxylation by $H_2O_2$, *J. Dent. Res.,* 61 (Sp. Issue), Abstr. 4, 1982.

266. **Ciancio, S. J., Cohen, R. E., Bergey, E. J., Tseng, C. C., and Levine, M. J.,** Monoclonal antibodies to human salivary proline-rich glycoprotein, *J. Dent. Res.,* 66 (Sp. Issue), Abstr. 1589, 1987.

267. **Aguirre, A., Cohen, R. E., Majewski, P., and Levine, M. J.,** Immunoquantitation of low molecular weight salivary mucin within human submandibular-sublingual saliva, *J. Dent. Res.,* 66 (Special Issue), Abstr. 923, 1987.

268. **Rudney, J. D., Kajander, K. C., and Smith, Q. T.,** Correlations between human salivary levels of lysozyme, lactoferrin, salivary peroxidase, and secretory immunoglobulin A with different stimulatory states over time, *Arch. Oral Biol.,* 30, 765, 1985.

Chapter 5

# STATHERIN AND THE ACIDIC PROLINE-RICH PROTEINS

**Donald I. Hay and Edgard C. Moreno**

## I. INTRODUCTION

The purpose of this chapter is to describe the properties and proposed functions of statherin and the acidic proline-rich proteins (PRP). These two types of phosphoproteins are present in the human parotid and submandibular salivary secretions and possess the unusual property of inhibiting primary (spontaneous) and secondary precipitation (crystal growth) of calcium phosphate salts. This appears to be a necessary and important activity in the oral cavity, because human salivary secretions are supersaturated with respect to most calcium phosphate salts. Consequently, it has been proposed that the biological function of statherin and the PRP is to inhibit precipitation of calcium phosphate salts in the salivary glands, in the oral fluid, and onto tooth surfaces. The resulting stable but supersaturated state of the salivary secretions, with respect to calcium phosphate salts, constitutes a protective and reparative environment which is important for the integrity of the teeth.

To understand the mechanims involved in this tooth-protective system and to define the system in quantitative terms, it is necessary to consider the following points, each of which will be discussed in turn in this chapter. First, the calculation of the degree of saturation of salivary secretions with respect to calcium phosphate salts will be described. This requires knowledge of the concentrations of calcium and phosphate ions in the salivary secretions (which, in turn, requires knowledge of all complexes involving these constituents) and the calculation of their ionic activities. From these values, and other analytical data, the degree of saturation of salivary secretions with respect to calcium phosphate salts can be calculated. Second, the clinical significance of supersaturation of saliva with respect to the calcium phosphate salts which form the tooth mineral will be discussed. From this it will be apparent that the beneficial consequences of salivary supersaturation with respect to calcium phosphate salts are selectively expressed in the oral cavity — that is, protection is provided for the dental enamel — while undesirable consequences, for example, precipitation of calcium phosphates in the salivary glands and onto the teeth, do not occur. Third, the role played by statherin and the PRP in this system will be considered. Their identification as inhibitors of calcium phosphate precipitation will be described, and their inhibitory activities explained in terms of their molecular structures. Fourth, the quantitative relationship between the degree of supersaturation of salivary secretions, the specific inhibitory activities of the proteins, and their normal concentrations in saliva will be discussed. Finally, the failure of the inhibitory activities of the proteins in formation of salivary gland and dental calculi will be considered.

## II. SUPERSATURATION OF HUMAN SALIVARY SECRETIONS WITH RESPECT TO CALCIUM PHOSPHATE SALTS

### A. State of Calcium and Phosphate in Saliva and Calculation of the Degree of Saturation with Respect to Calcium Phosphates

Several steps are required to calculate the state of saturation of a solution with respect to a given salt. First, the total concentrations in the solution of the constituents of the salt of interest must be known. Second, from these values, and from knowledge of the concentrations of other solution constituents, such as compounds which may form complexes with the ions of interest, and of solution conditions, such as pH, which strongly influence the concentration of ions such as $PO_4^{3-}$, for example, concentrations of free ions in solution are calculated. These values are then used to calculate ionic activities, quantities which may be considered to represent the effective concentrations of the ions of interest and which take into account the effect of ionic strength and temperature of the solution. From the ionic activities a degree of saturation (DS) value is obtained. This may be calculated as the ratio of the product of the solution ionic activities of the ions present in the salt of interest, and the solubility product of the salt, as described later for calcium phosphate salts. The DS value represents the extent to which a solution is undersaturated (DS <1) or supersaturated (DS >1) with respect to a given salt and indicates the extent of departure from the state of equilibrium (saturation) of a system under the conditions considered. The DS value is important because it represents the thermodynamic driving force for dissolution and precipitation processes.

Determination of DS values in biological fluids often involves some extra steps in addition to those required in the conventional procedure. Thus, to calculate the degree of saturation of saliva samples with respect to calcium phosphate salts, the following steps are necessary. First, the pH values of the saliva samples are determined under conditions of constant $PCO_2$, selected to mimic conditions at the time of secretion. Second, the samples are analyzed for their major constituents such as sodium, potassium, calcium, chloride, bicarbonate, and phosphate, and, for complete and accurate results, for minor constituents such as magnesium, thiocyanate, lactate, citrate, and fluoride. Third, the presence of calcium bound by protein and phosphate ions in various complexes has to be considered. Calcium ion binding by salivary proteins[1] ranges from 3% (0.02mM, unstimulated parotid) to 11% (0.13mM, stimulated parotid) of the total calcium present. Calcium also forms complexes with phosphate i.e., $CaHPO_4^\circ$ and $CaH_2PO_4^+$, bicarbonate i.e., $CaHCO_3^-$, and lactate and citrate ions. Formation of these complexes reduces the concentrations of free calcium and phosphate ions in saliva to a significant extent and must be allowed for in calculating the concentrations of the free ions. These calculations are made using computer programs written for this purpose, which also give values for the ionic strength of the samples[1-3] required for the calculation of ionic activities. A more direct approach for determining calcium ion activities is to use a specific calcium ion electrode,[4,5] though concentrations of free and complexed phosphate must be calculated. These two approaches gave similar results for stimulated parotid saliva[1,4,5] and indicated for the parotid saliva that about 45% of the total calcium is involved in complexes over pH 6 to 7.5, though considerable variation between individuals is observed. The only complexes of phosphate ions in saliva, important in this context, are the soluble calcium phosphate complexes, noted earlier. The previously reported complexing of phosphate by salivary proteins[6] has been shown to be an artifact of the ultrafiltration technique used.[1]

By following the foregoing steps, it is possible to calculate the degree of saturation of saliva with respect to calcium phosphate salts. Several such salts must be considered, as follows:

| | | |
|---|---|---|
| Dicalcium phosphate dihydrate | (DCPD) | $CaHPO_4 \cdot 2H_2O$ |
| Octacalcium phosphate | (OCP) | $Ca_4H(PO_4)_3 \cdot 2\frac{1}{2}H_2O$ |
| Beta-tricalcium phosphate | (TCP) | $\beta\text{-}Ca_3(PO_4)_2$ |
| Hydroxyapatite | (HA) | $Ca_5(OH)(PO_4)_3$ |
| Fluorapatite | (FA) | $Ca_5F(PO_4)_3$ |

The degree of saturation of a solution with respect to a given calcium phosphate such as $Ca_5(OH)(PO_4)_3$, HA, for example, may be defined by the ratio:

$$\text{Degree of saturation (DS)} = \frac{(Ca^{2+})^5(OH^-)(PO_4^{3-})^3}{K_{HA}}$$

where the parentheses denote the activities of the ionic species enclosed, calculated for the solution being considered, and $K_{HA}$ is the solubility product constant of HA. The numerator in the preceding expression is the ionic activity product for HA in the solution, and $K_{HA}$ is also the ionic activity product, when the solution is saturated (in equilibrium) with HA. Similar expressions, using the relevant values for ionic activities raised to the appropriate power and the appropriate solubility product constant, are used to calculate the degree of

**Table 1**
## STATE OF SATURATION OF STIMULATED HUMAN SALIVARY SECRETIONS WITH RESPECT TO DCPD AND HA EXPRESSED IN TERMS OF DS[1]

| Secretion | N | DCPD | | HA | |
|---|---|---|---|---|---|
| | | Mean | Range | Mean ($\times 10^{12}$) | Range ($\times 10^{12}$) |
| Parotid | 22 | 1.27 | 0.49—2.50 | 0.69 | 0.003—6.13 |
| Submandibular | 18 | 2.14 | 1.03—3.54 | 5.62 | 0.033—78.3 |
| | | | | (1.35 | 0.033—4.87) |
| Whole | 31 | 1.58 | 0.78—3.48 | 0.44 | 0.001—3.35 |
| Assay system | | 5.66 | | 3.56 | |

*Note:*  If the most supersaturated submandibular sample (DS = 78.3 $\times$ $10^{12}$) is not
included, the values given in parentheses are obtained.

saturation with respect to other calcium phosphates. A DS value of less than 1 indicates a state of undersaturation with respect to the salt considered; a value greater than 1 indicates a states of supersaturation. Table 1 summarizes DS values obtained for samples of parotid, submandibular and whole salivas with respect to DCPD and HA[7] using this approach. DCPD and HA are the most and least soluble, respectively, of the calcium phosphate salts considered. Fluorapatite, which is less soluble than HA, is not considered here because fluoride concentrations were not determined in the samples used in these studies. The original analytical data used for these calculations were those reported by Gron,[6] but the values in Table 1 were calculated taking into account the binding of calcium by salivary proteins,[1] lactate, and citrate in addition to the calcium-phosphate complexes. A value of 7.35 $\times$ $10^{-6}$ was used for the solubility product constant of HA at 37°C,[8] and a value of 2.37 $\times$ $10^{-7}$ was used for the corresponding constant for DCPD.[2]

Table 1 shows that the saliva samples considered range from undersaturated to significantly supersaturated with respect to DCPD. The DS values range from 0.49 to 3.54, and more samples are supersaturated than undersaturated with respect to this relatively soluble salt. The mean DS value of 1.27 (0.49 to 2.50) for parotid salivas from 22 subjects is not greatly different from the corresponding values reported by Lagerlof[5] for parotid saliva from 5 subjects. With respect to HA, the salivary secretions display a substantial supersaturation. The DS values given in Table 1, however, should be interpreted with caution: the high values stem from the chosen definition of DS. An equally valid definition is the ratio of the mean activity for the calcium phosphate under consideration in saliva to the mean activity of the same salt at saturation. If the value obtained according to the latter definition is called ds, then ds = $(DS)^{1/n}$ where n is the number of ions into which the salt dissociates upon dissolution (e.g., n has a value for 2 for DCPD and a value of 9 for HA). Using this definition, the range of ds values for DCPD in Table 1 is from 0.7 to 1.9, and for HA from 10.0 to 35.0. Similarly, the mean ds values for parotid saliva with respect to DCPD and HA are 1.1 and 20.7, respectively. The advantage of using DS values is that it can be said correctly that parotid saliva is about 20 times more supersaturated with respect to HA than with respect to DCPD. Such an assertion is not obvious when the degree of supersaturation is expressed as the ratio of ionic activity products, or DS values.

## B. Clinical Implications of Supersaturation of Saliva with Respect to Calcium Phosphate Salts of Dental Enamel

The teeth exist in a fluid environment and are exposed to a constant flow of saliva, estimated at 500 ml/d. Although dental enamel is considered to be formed from the relatively insoluble HA, 500 ml of a solution with the ionic strength and pH of saliva, but lacking calcium and phosphate, would dissolve approximately 50 mg of HA to reach saturation. Although relatively slow dissolution rates of enamel would be expected under salivary conditions, so that losses of this scale would not occur, loss of mineral over years and decades would still be substantial. This loss would be greatly increased during reduction of the pH of the oral fluid, as occurs during ingestion of fermentable carbohydrate and acid foods and drinks. In spite of this considerable potential for enamel demineralization, teeth do not readily lose mineral and normally retain their form for many decades. Also, it is a well-established clinical phenomenon that many early carious lesions recalcify, given appropriate conditions. Thus, Backer-Dirks[9] observed that nearly half the "white-spot" or early carious lesions identified on the erupting first molars of children 8 years old had recalcified and become undetectable when these teeth were examined 5 years later. A similar phenomenon has been observed in adults,[10] where early carious lesions were induced and recalcified at will by adjusting diet and oral hygiene procedures. A similar effect has been shown with artifically demineralized enamel placed in the mouth.[11]

These effects are critically dependent on the state of saturation of the fluid surrounding the teeth with respect to the tooth mineral. Physical chemical evidence (Table 1) shows that the salivary secretions are normally highly supersaturated with respect to tooth mineral. Given this condition, the stability of the enamel mineral becomes understandable. The salivary supersaturation constitutes a thermodynamic driving force for the formation of calcium phosphate salts, and, therefore, under normal conditions dissolution of enamel will not occur. Substantial reductions in pH or large changes in other salivary conditions will be required to attain a state of undersaturation, thereby inducing enamel dissolution. The high degree of supersaturation of saliva with respect to enamel mineral thus provides significant protection against enamel demineralization. Recalcification of early carious lesions can be understood in similar terms. Loss of mineral from carious lesions occurs as a consequence of lowered plaque pH from microbial activity, which brings about undersaturation of plaque fluid with respect to enamel mineral. Removal of plaque makes the lesion accessible to the supersaturated saliva, and, within certain limitations, discussed later, recalcification of lesions[9,10] will occur. The presence of fluoride evidently accelerates such recalcification, an effect consistent with the increase in the rate of crystal growth of HA induced by low concentrations of fluoride ions.[12] Similar effects may be important in the posteruptive mineralization of teeth in rodents and in the protection of exposed tooth roots in humans.

## C. Anomalies Associated with Supersaturation of Saliva with Respect to Dental Enamel Mineral

The previously noted activities, attributable to the supersaturated state of the salivary secretions, represent an important protective mechanism. They emphasize the dynamic state of dental enamel in the oral cavity under normal conditions, and the results of studies of remineralization of natural[9] and artifically induced[10] carious lesions strongly suggest that dental caries would be considerably more damaging if these protective and reparative activities were absent from saliva. These activities, however, depend on the potential of the supersaturated saliva to form mineral, and in the case of the repair of early carious lesions, mineral is actually formed. This represents a remarkable anomaly. The supersaturated state is unstable, by definition. It is often characterized by the tendency for dissolved material to precipitate spontaneously from solution. Even if the degree of supersaturation is insufficient to initiate primary precipitation, secondary precipitation, or crystal growth of calcium phosphates on preexisting mineral, is inevitable. Thus, dental enamel or seed crystals of HA added to saliva or tooth surfaces in the mouth should provide sites for crystal growth. This implies that there is the potential for spontaneous precipitation of calcium phosphate salts in the salivary gland acini, ducts, and in the oral fluid, and that crystal growth of mineral on tooth surfaces should occur.

These highly undesirable and potentially harmful processes do not normally occur. Precipitation of calcium phosphate salts is not seen in normal salivas, though it has been reported in some pathological states, such as cystic fibrosis.[13] Salivary gland calculi are rare and are usually associated with infection or injury. The prior formation of dental plaque appears to be necessary for the formation of dental calculi, an important topic discussed later. Tooth surfaces which are kept clean, a state which might be expected to favor calcium phosphate crystal growth, do not accumulate mineral. Consequently, it would seem that saliva, supersaturated with respect to dental enamel, can remain in contact with this mineral for long periods of time with no evidence of significant precipitation. This situation appears to contravene basic physical chemical principles, a contravention which is particularly striking considering that many early carious lesions are seen to recalcify, but on completion of repair, mineral formation evidently ceases. Also, dental enamel, in *in vitro* experiments, effectively seeds synthetic solutions which are supersaturated with respect to HA,[14] showing that the absence of crystal growth on dental enamel *in vivo* is not related to some unusual property of this mineral.

Investigators who considered this problem concluded that although saliva possesses certain properties indicating a state of supersaturation with respect to most calcium phosphate salts, this did not represent true supersaturation, since fundamental properties associated with this state were lacking. Rather, it was considered that the saliva was in a "potential state of supersaturation" with respect to dental enamel. No mechanisms were proposed to explain this state, but recent studies have shown that this proposal is, in a general sense, correct. A particularly striking aspect of this situation is the selective way in which these effects operate, with the beneficial effects being expressed and the undesirable effects evidently being suppressed in the oral environment. This biologically advantageous selective control of salivary supersaturation has recently been explained in terms of the activities of specific inhibitors of calcium phosphate precipitation present in the glandular salivary secretions.

The presence of inhibitors of precipitation in biological systems has been reported for several body fluids. Thus, consideration of the state of saturation of plasma with respect to HA led to the conclusion that this fluid may be marginally supersaturated with respect to this salt and that absence of precipitation may be associated with the presence of inhibitors such as pyrophosphate and other ions.[15,16] The importance of this inhibitory activity is evident when problems such as calcification of arterial plaques, injured tissues, and joints are considered, and other dystrophic calcifications and calcinoses of the skin. Similarly, studies of urine[17] and pancreatic fluid,[18,19] for example, have shown that these fluids are supersaturated with respect to various salts, including calcium phosphates, oxalate, and carbonate, and that various inhibitors play important roles in preventing precipitation of these salts. A special situation exists in the oral cavity because of the substantial supersaturation of saliva with respect to HA, indicating a potential for both spontaneous precipitation and crystal growth of calcium phosphates on dental enamel surfaces. Consequently, the presence in saliva of specific molecules which inhibit precipitation of calcium phosphate salts fulfills a biological need.

## III. INHIBITORS OF PRECIPITATION OF CALCIUM PHOSPHATE SALTS IN SALIVA

### A. Human Salivary Statherin

*1. Identification of Statherin as an Inhibitor of Primary Precipitation of Calcium Phosphate Salts*

As noted earlier, it seemed likely that the anomalous chemistry of calcium phosphates observed in saliva could be explained in terms of selective inhibition of calcium phosphate precipitation. Evidence that saliva contained inhibitor(s) capable of this activity was obtained

**Table 2**
**COMPOSITION AND**
**SOME PROPERTIES OF**
**HUMAN SALIVARY**
**STATHERIN**[22]

Residues/minimum mol wt

| | | | |
|-----|----|-----------|---|
| Asp | 1  | Ile       | 1 |
| Glu | 10 | Leu       | 2 |
| Thr | 1  | Phe       | 3 |
| Ser | 2  | Tyr       | 7 |
| Pro | 7  | Arg       | 3 |
| Gly | 4  | Lys       | 1 |
| Val | 1  | Phosphate | 2 |

Isoelectric point at 20° 4.22
Molecular weight (sequence) 5380

by studying inhibition of calcium phosphate precipitation by saliva samples from standard assay systems which were supersaturated with respect to calcium phosphate salts.[20] These assay solutions had degrees of supersaturation with respect to HA similar to saliva but were significantly more supersaturated than saliva with respect to DCPD (Table 1). Although spontaneous precipitation from these systems occurred within 0.5 to 1.0 h, precipitation was readily inhibited by relatively small volumes of glandular salivas (0.05 to 0.2 ml of saliva per milliliter of the assay solution) for periods as long as 24 h. In some experiments, precipitation was delayed for as long as 11 d. It was found that salivary ultrafiltrates (molecular weights less than 1000) had little effect on precipitation behavior, but the protein fractions of saliva samples strongly inhibited precipitation. The protein fractions of individual salivas differed in their effectiveness, with the concentrations required to inhibit precipitation varying from 0.15 to 0.47 mg/ml. Significantly, serum proteins at over ten times these concentrations did not inhibit precipitation, indicating the presence in saliva of potent saliva-specific inhibitor(s) of calcium phosphate precipitation.

The nature of the material in the glandular salivary secretions responsible for this inhibitory activity was identified by chromatographing parotid and submandibular saliva samples on DEAE-Sephadex®, using a chloride gradient for eluting the proteins, assaying the resulting fractions for inhibitory activity, and identifying the proteins present in the fractions by polyacrylamide gel electrophoresis.[21] Only one of the many protein constituents of saliva was found to have significant inhibitory activity under the conditions used. This material was identified from its chromatographic and electrophoretic behavior as a previously described tyrosine-rich peptide or small protein named statherin.[23]

### 2. Isolation, Purification, and Structure Determination

Statherin is present in both parotid and submandibular salivas and was previously isolated from the parotid secretion by ammonium sulfate precipitation, gel filtration, and preparative electrophoresis.[22] A simpler purification protocol involving anion exchange chromatography of saliva on DEAE-Sephadex®, and gel filtration of P6 Biogel®, was reported later.[23] Analysis of the purified material showed it to contain high proportions of acidic amino acids, tyrosine, and proline. Its isoelectric point was 4.2, it contained two phosphate groups per molecule, and the minimum molecular weight calculated from the amino acid sequence (see later) was 5380. These properties are summarized in Table 2.

Figure 1 shows the amino acid sequence of statherin.[23] This molecule is remarkable for its high degree of charge and structural asymmetry. Ten of the 12 charged groups present

$$
\begin{array}{c}
\phantom{NH_3^+-ASP-}\overset{\displaystyle H_2PO_3}{\phantom{SER}}\ \overset{\displaystyle H_2PO_3}{\phantom{SER}}
\end{array}
$$

```
            H2PO3 H2PO3
      1       |     |        5                        10
NH3+-ASP-SER-SER-GLU-GLU-LYS-PHE-LEU-ARG-ARG-ILE-GLY-ARG-PHE-
      -    -    -    -    -    +         +    +              +

     15                20                25
    GLY-TYR-GLY-TYR-GLY-PRO-TYR-GLN-PRO-VAL-PRO-GLU-GLN-PRO-LEU-
                                                   -

     30                35                40            43
    TYR-PRO-GLN-PRO-TYR-GLN-PRO-GLN-TYR-GLN-GLN-TYR-THR-PHE-COO-
```

FIGURE 1.   Primary structure of human statherin.[69]

in statherin occur in the amino-terminal 13 residues, with an exceptional grouping of 5 negatively charged residues at the amino terminus. All the tyrosine, proline, and glutamine residues are confined to the carboxy-terminal two thirds of the molecule, of which they form 75% of the residues present in this segment.

### 3. Mechanism of Action as an Inhibitor of Primary Precipitation
#### a. Nature of Primary Precipitation and Its Inhibition

The mechanism by which salts such as calcium phosphates precipitate spontaneously from solution is not well understood. Consequently, possible mechanisms by which inhibitors of spontaneous precipitation may act are difficult to define. A mechanistic explanation of primary precipitation, however, is available. The first step in spontaneous precipitation is normally considered to be the formation of small aggregates of ions. These clusters have been called nuclei or embryo crystals — that is, they have not reached the level of organization characteristic of a crystal. In the case of calcium phosphates and some other compounds, the formation of nuclei appears to be the rate-determining step in spontaneous precipitation for moderate degrees of supersaturation. The nuclei grow slowly and at some point spontaneously transform and grow rapidly to form a precipitating phase. Inhibitors of this process are considered to act by binding to the nuclei and inhibiting their growth or transformation. The mechanism of action of such inhibitors may, therefore, be somewhat similar to the mechanism by which inhibitors of calcium phosphate crystal growth are considered to act — that is, the inhibitors bind to either a forming solid or a crystalline calcium phosphate phase and prevent or delay further attachment of calcium and phosphate ions from solution to the forming precipitate or to the calcium phosphate crystal surface.

A broad range of compounds has been shown to inhibit crystal growth of calcium phosphate salts. Typically, such inhibitors are anionic, often contain a phosphate group, and preferably a second phosphate group or a carboxyl moiety.[24,25] Anionic polymers, such as polyaspartate, are also highly effective,[26] but factors other than charge, secondary structure, for example,[27,28] are also important, since polyglutamate of the same molecular size is far less active than polyaspartate. Typical inhibitors are compounds such as pyrophosphate,[16,29] polyphosphonates,[30] citrate-metal complexes,[31] phosphocitrate,[32] nucleoside phosphates,[33] and many other compounds.

#### b. Structure-Activity Relationships of Statherin

It is interesting to consider the structure of statherin in relationship to the foregoing generalizations. The acidic amino-terminal pentapeptide of statherin, which consists of acidic residues (Figure 1), fulfills the previously noted compositional and structural requirements for an inhibitor of calcium phosphate precipitation. The rest of the molecule, however, consisting mainly of hydrophobic and uncharged residues, has none of these characteristics. The first step toward investigating the structural basis of the activity of statherin involved

## Table 3
### STATHERIN CONCENTRATIONS IN STIMULATED PAROTID SALIVA MEASURED BY SINGLE RADIAL IMMUNODIFFUSION (SRID)[7]

| No. of subjects | Statherin concentration | | |
| --- | --- | --- | --- |
| | Mean | Range | S.D. |
| 68 | 6.86 mg% | 1.6—14.7 mg% | 2.93 mg% |
| | 12.8 $\mu M$ | 3.0—27.3 $\mu M$ | 5.46 $\mu M$ |

*Note:* The single sample with a statherin concentration outside the range of the SRID was not included in the calculation of the mean.

treating the protein with trypsin, purifying the resulting tryptic peptides, and assaying them for inhibitory activity.[26,34] Trypsin hydrolyzes peptide bonds on the carboxyl side of lysine and arginine residues, to give the segments $Asp_1$-$Lys_6$, $Phe_7$-$Arg_9$, $Arg_{10}$, $Ile_{11}$-$Arg_{13}$, and $Phe_{14}$-$Phe_{43}$ (Figure 1). As might be expected, only the amino-terminal hexapeptide possessed inhibitory activity. Surprisingly, this segment was far less effective as an inhibitor of spontaneous precipitation than intact statherin. Although polymer size is an important determinant in inhibitory activity for compounds such as polyaspartate,[26] it did not seem likely that the removal of an essentially uncharged and relatively hydrophobic segment of the molecule would reduce activity. The hexapeptide, however, had only approximately one tenth the activity of intact statherin. Also, removal of a small carboxy-terminal segment, $Tyr_{38}$-$Phe_{43}$, caused a surprisingly large reduction in activity, about 50%.[35]

These findings suggest a distinctly more complex mechanism for inhibition of calcium phosphate precipitation by statherin than has been advanced for other inhibitors, since it seems to involve the uncharged and relatively hydrophobic segment of the molecule. A possible explanation is that the first interaction between a developing nucleus or embryo crystal, and statherin, involves the negatively charged, phosphoserine-containing, amino-terminal segment of the molecule, followed by folding of the hydrophobic segment around the resulting complex, thus screening it from further interactions with calcium and phosphate ions in the solution. It could also be that statherin exists in solution as a dimer,[22] formed by hydrophobic bonds between the carboxy-terminal segments of two statherin molecules. Possibly, the removal of the segment $Tyr_{38}$-$Phe_{43}$ decreases the ability to form such bonds, with a concomitant reduction of inhibitory activity. Further work, however, is required to characterize such behavior and substantiate these speculative explanations.

### 4. Biological Aspects
#### a. Concentration Range and Activity of Statherin in Saliva

Although statherin is clearly a potent inhibitor of precipitation of calcium phosphate salts, a complete understanding of its role in saliva requires knowledge of (1) the state of saturation of normal saliva samples with respect to calcium phosphate salts, (2) the specific inhibitory activity of statherin, and (3) its normal concentration range in human salivary secretions. These three factors must be related to show that statherin has a sufficiently high specific activity and is present in saliva at sufficiently high concentrations to inhibit precipitation of calcium phosphate salts from solutions as supersaturated as saliva. Table 1 shows saturation values for stimulated salivary secretions,[1,7] and Table 3 shows the concentrations of statherin in 68 parotid saliva samples,[7] determined using a single radial immunodiffusion method.

In this study[7] the activity of statherin was evaluated at two levels. The first level was simply to consider the activity of statherin in a standard assay with a known level of supersaturation, and to consider the state of supersaturation of saliva samples in terms of this activity. From Table 1 it can be seen that the assay system used was more supersaturated with respect to DCPD than the saliva samples, and, with the exception of one unusually supersaturated sample, the assay solution was equivalent to the saliva samples which were most supersaturated with respect to HA. Statherin, at a concentration of 1.25 $\mu M$, inhibited precipitation from this assay system for 24 h. This concentration is derived from detailed studies of the inhibitory activity of statherin using the assay method described previously or similar assays.[7,21,36]

Based on this result, it seems probable that precipitation in virtually all of the saliva samples would be inhibited, because the lowest salivary concentration of statherin found was 3.0 $\mu M$, well above the 1.25 $\mu M$ level required. Also, the 24-h standard inhibition period used was adopted for experimental convenience and is much longer than is required in biological situations. Thus, to fulfill its proposed biological function, statherin is required to inhibit precipitation as long as the saliva remains in the salivary gland acini and ducts and in the mouth. This time period is not known for all locations in the oral cavity, but for most it will be much less than 24 h. According to the foregoing test, all saliva samples examined contained more than adequate concentrations of statherin to prevent precipitation within time periods of biological relevance. The most supersaturated of the saliva samples, however, with a DS value of $78.3 \times 10^{12}$, presents a special problem. It is not known whether this sample would be inhibited by statherin at the standard level of 1.25 $\mu M$. Further information is required in this respect because the relationship between the degree of supersaturation of a sample and its statherin concentration was not determined in the foregoing studies. Thus, even the most supersaturated saliva sample may be inhibited by the highest statherin concentration found, over 27 $\mu M$, but it is not yet known if there is a relationship between the degree of supersaturation and statherin concentration in saliva.

The second level of evaluation was intended to determine if statherin acts without interference from other salivary constituents. The saliva samples used to determine statherin concentrations (Table 3) were sequentially diluted, and the diluted samples assayed for inhibitory activity. Control samples of statherin, with a concentration range similar to that of the saliva samples, were treated in the same way. Essentially identical results were obtained with the saliva and statherin samples, showing that in most cases statherin acted independently and without interference from other salivary constituents. Interestingly, a few samples (5 of 65) showed more activity than anticipated from their statherin concentrations, suggesting the presence in some parotid salivas of other as yet undetected inhibitors or synergistic effects. Other phosphoproteins with inhibitory activity have been identified in human submandibular salivas.[37]

### b. The Function of Statherin and Possible Sites of Its Action

Statherin exhibits a unique activity compared with all other salivary and serum proteins in that, at concentrations at which it occurs naturally, it will inhibit spontaneous precipitation of calcium phosphate salts from an assay system which is as supersaturated as human salivary secretions. This finding is strong presumptive evidence that this inhibitory activity is the actual biological function of statherin, since it seems likely that spontaneous precipitation of calcium phosphate salts could occur in the salivary glands in the absence of statherin. This latter point, however, is difficult to establish with absolute certainty. Generally, it is considered that solutions which are supersaturated with respect to HA, but undersaturated with respect to DCPD, will exhibit metastability at pH values below 7.4 — that is, spontaneous precipitation will not normally occur within time periods of significance to the present problem.[38]

An important point, then, regarding the function of statherin, may be the degree of supersaturation of saliva with respect to DCPD. There are few investigations which deal directly with this point. Hay and co-workers,[1,7] using analytical data previously reported by

Gron,[6] computed calcium and other ionic activities, and states of supersaturation of glandular and whole salivary secretions, and concluded that a significant fraction of the stimulated parotid, submandibular, and whole salivary secretions examined were supersaturated with respect to DCPD. These data are given in Table 1. Lagerlof[5] determined calcium ion activities directly using an electrode and concluded that the parotid saliva samples investigated were slightly undersaturated or just saturated with respect to DCPD. There is probably no disagreement between the two studies, because, as shown in Table 1, the mean value for the degree of supersaturation of parotid saliva with respect to DCPD is 1.27, with a range of 0.49 to 2.50, which would be consistent with the data of Lagerlof.[5] The greater number of samples (71 vs. 5) investigated by Hay et al.[1,7] (Table 1) are more likely to reveal the extent of biological variation. The tendency for unstimulated salivas to be less saturated with respect to calcium phosphate salts than the stimulated secretions[1,5] results from postsecretory processing as the saliva passes down the ducts, particularly with respect to decreases in pH. The fluid in the acinar spaces has properties closer to the stimulated, rather than the unstimulated, secretions.

From this it can be concluded that a significant number of human glandular salivas may be supersaturated with respect to DCPD and that the potential for spontaneous precipitation may exist in the acinar fluid at all times, and also in the stimulated glandular secretions. The consequences of such precipitation would be potential harm to the salivary gland acini and ducts and loss of the state of supersaturation of the saliva with respect to enamel mineral, with loss of the associated protective activities, and potential for harm to the teeth. Since the saliva contains potent inhibitors of calcium phosphate crystal growth (discussed later), particles of precipitated mineral are not likely to grow to a significant size under normal conditions. Consequently, absence of statherin alone may lead to microcrystalline precipitates but not necessarily predispose to formation of more dense precipitates of calcium phosphates or to formation of salivary gland calculi. The loss of the protective effects of the supersaturated saliva would appear to be a more serious matter. A realistic test of this reasoning requires identification of statherin-deficient individuals.

Although there is a clear need for statherin to function in the salivary gland, it is less obvious to what extent this function is needed in the oral cavity. Considering the degree of supersaturation reported for whole salivary secretions (Table 1), inhibitory activity in the oral fluid would appear to be desirable. Statherin in whole saliva, however, is degraded,[39,40] presumably by proteases associated with the oral microflora. The rate of this degradation, however, has not been determined, nor is there adequate information regarding the residence time of saliva in the mouth relevant to this problem. Such information is needed before definitive statements can be made regarding persistence of statherin and its inhibitory activity in oral fluid, although statherin can evidently be recovered from whole saliva by adsorption onto HA.[41] A further point regarding the role of statherin in the oral cavity is related to its ability to adsorb selectively from saliva onto HA and dental enamel[42] and also to act as an inhibitor of calcium phosphate crystal growth. Although the foregoing discussion emphasizes the role of statherin as an inhibitor of spontaneous precipitation, a role for this molecule and its degradation products as inhibitors of crystal growth on tooth surfaces, or a role for these materials in the formation of enamel pellicle, cannot be excluded.

## B. Proline-Rich Proteins (PRP)
### 1. Identification as Inhibitors of Secondary Precipitation
During the studies in which statherin was identified as an inhibitor of primary precipitation of calcium phosphate salts,[21] effects were noted which suggested that material was present in saliva, in addition to statherin, which affected calcium phosphate precipitation. These effects were observed when salivary fractions which contained the PRP were assayed for inhibition of primary precipitation of calcium phosphates. Although inhibition of precipitation

was not observed, the crystal habit of the precipitated calcium phosphate differed, and precipitation did not proceed to the same extent as occurred when assaying inactive fractions or control samples. Since it seemed that the observed effect could be explained in terms of inhibition of crystal growth of the precipitated calcium phosphate, saliva samples, and fractions were assayed for the latter activity, rather than for inhibition of primary precipitation. The method used[6,43] was based on the fact that hydrolysis of DCPD to more basic calcium phosphate, which proceeds spontaneously at pH values greater than 6.2, is inhibited by compounds which inhibit calcium phosphate crystal growth. This provided a highly sensitive method for identification and semiquantitative study of inhibitors of calcium phosphate crystal growth, though better-defined systems[44,45] are required for detailed studies of these inhibitors.

Results of these experiments[26,43] showed that only two groups of fractions possessed the ability to inhibit calcium phosphate crystal growth strongly. As expected, activity was found in the fractions containing statherin and was also found in the fractions containing the PRP. Isolation and assay of the major members of this complex group of proteins showed that the PRP were responsible for the inhibitory activity, though the specific activities of the four major PRP were significantly different.[26]

### 2. Isolation, Purification, and Structure Determination of the PRP

Isolation from human parotid saliva and initial characterization of the PRP were reported in the same year by Oppenheim et al.,[46] who described the four major proteins, PRP-1, -2, -3, and -4, and Bennick and Connell,[47] who described Protein C (PRP-1) and Protein A (PRP-3). The presence of as many as eight additional PRP, and the isolation of some of these were reported.[48] Further characterization[49-52] included studies of calcium binding by the PRP. These initial studies showed the presence in human saliva of an unusually complex family of very closely related proteins, with nearly identical compositions.

Sequences of the amino-terminal regions (residues 1 to 20) of the four major PRP were reported by Schlesinger et al.[53] The partial sequence of PRP-3 was reported by Bennick et al.,[54] who later published its complete sequence.[55] The complete structures of PRP-4[56] and PRP-1[57] were published later, and the determination of the structure of PRP-2 has now been completed.[58] Also, a 44-residue peptide has been isolated from parotid saliva which corresponds to the last 44 residues of PRP-1 and PRP-2,[59] the significance of which will be discussed later. These studies are summarized in the general sequence for the major PRP, shown in Figure 2. According to studies published up to 1984, all four proteins share the same sequence from residues 1 to 106, with the single exception that residue 4, which is ASN in PRP-1 and PRP-3, is ASP in PRP-2 and PRP-4. The larger proteins, PRP-1 and PRP-2, both have the same 44-residue extension, 107 to 150. As more completely described by Azen (Chapter 7), these PRP are inherited in pairs. Thus, two homozygotes — that is, PRP-1 and -3, and PRP-2 and -4 — and heterozygotes with all four proteins have been identified.

With a single exception these structures were recently confirmed by Maeda et al.,[60] who isolated and sequenced the cDNA for the acidic proline-rich proteins from a subject who was homozygous for PRP-1 and -3. It was concluded that the two proteins were coded for by the same gene and that PRP-3 was formed by posttranslational cleavage of PRP-1 at the bond $Arg_{106}$-$Gly_{107}$, a conclusion supported by the presence of what appears to be the derived segment, residues 107 to 150, in human parotid saliva,[59] and by the selective cleavage of PRP-1 at $Arg_{106}$-$Gly_{107}$ by salivary kallikrein.[61] Considering these findings, it seems likely that a similar situation will exist for the protein pair PRP-2 and -4.

The exception regarding these structures, noted previously, concerns the finding that a closely related PRP, called PIF, for parotid isoelectric focusing variant,[62] was copurified with PRP-1 during its isolation[46,47] and was present in the protein preparation used for sequencing. The sequence of PIF has not been determined but can be inferred from the

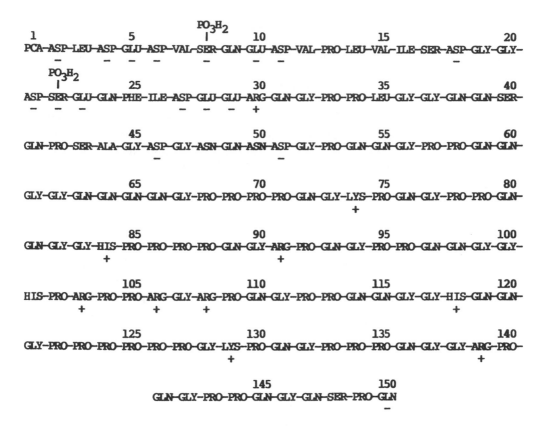

FIGURE 2. Primary structure of a human acidic proline-rich phosphoprotein. The structure shown is designated as PRP-1. Several other closely related PRP differ from PRP-1 either by substitutions at residues 4 and 50 or by posttranslational modification, as follows.

|  | Residue 4 | Residue 50 | Molecular size[a] residues |
|---|---|---|---|
| PRP-1 | ASP | ASN | 150 |
| PIF (slow) | ASN | ASP | 150 |
| PRP-2 | ASP | ASN | 150 |
| PRP-3 | ASN | ASP | 106 |
| PIF (fast) | ASP | ASN | 106 |
| PRP-4 | ASP | ASP | 106 |

[a]   PRP-3, PIF(fast), and PRP-4 are considered to be formed by posttranslational cleavage of the larger proteins at the bond-$ARG_{106}$-$GLY_{107}$. PCA, residue 1, is pyrrolidone carboxylic acid, derived from glutamate by pyrrolidone ring formation, a spontaneous reaction which occurs when glutamate occupies the aminoterminus.

nucleotide sequence of the cDNA reported by Maeda et al.[60] PRP-1 and PIF differ in that residue 4 is ASN and residue 50 is ASP in one protein, and the reverse arrangement in the second protein. Consequently, PRP-1 and PIF have the same net charge and identical compositions, features which make their separation on a preparative scale exceedingly difficult, though they have been separated by isoelectric focusing.[62] In Figure 2, PRP-1 has been assumed to have ASP at residue 4 and ASN at residue 50, but this assignment has to be confirmed (please see Note Added in Proof).

Like statherin, the primary structures of the PRP are remarkable for a high degree of compositional and charge asymmetry. Thus, the amino-terminal 50 residues contain most of the negatively charged residues present, with a particularly marked grouping of negatively charged residues including the two phosphoserines present in these molecules, in the amino-terminal 29-residue segment. The remainder of the molecule is formed primarily from neutral and hydrophobic amino acids, with several positively charged residues in this region. These structural characteristics are important in understanding properties which are pertinent to the biological functions attributed to these molecules. These include (1) a high reactivity for the surfaces of calcium phosphate salts, such as HA and dental enamel, (2) a closely related ability to strongly inhibit crystal growth of calcium phosphate salts, and (3) the ability to bind calcium ions. In addition, the PRP have recently been shown to mediate selective adhesion of bacteria to HA surfaces *in vitro*, an activity which, if confirmed to occur *in vivo*, would have important implications for understanding bacterial colonization of tooth surfaces.

### 3. Mechanism of Action of the PRP as Inhibitors of Secondary Precipitation
### a. Nature of Secondary Precipitation and Its Inhibition

Secondary precipitation, or crystal growth, is considered to proceed by the accretion of ions on crystal surfaces, a process which is relatively well understood in contrast to the understanding of the processes involved in primary precipitation. Typically, crystal growth is considered to occur at specific growth sites such as kinks or dislocations on the surface, rather than by uniform deposition of layers of ions on crystal faces. Adsorption of foreign compounds at these growth sites can strongly inhibit crystal growth, consistent with the finding that, in the case of inhibitors of small molecular size, only a small fraction of the crystal surface need be covered to inhibit crystal growth essentially completely.[30] Consequently, inhibitors of calcium phosphate crystal growth should show exceptional adsorption properties onto surfaces of calcium phosphate salts.

Hay[42] reported that the PRP were among those proteins which were selectively adsorbed from glandular saliva by HA. Thus, in experiments in which the amount of HA added to a series of identical saliva samples was progressively increased, the protein showing the most selective adsorption behavior was statherin,[42] followed by a histidine-rich acidic peptide,[63] and then by the PRP. A small basic protein is adsorbed along with these proteins, possibly in a less selective fashion, and as the amount of HA is increased, the basic parotid glycoprotein[64,65] is also adsorbed.[66] Considering that over 40 proteins have been detected in human glandular salivas,[67,68] the selective adsorption of these 5 proteins indicates that they possess exceptional properties regarding interactions with HA. Of these proteins, only statherin, described earlier, the PRP, and cysteine-rich proteins from submandibular saliva[37] have been identified as inhibitors of precipitation of calcium phosphate salts. The PRP have been extensively studied with respect to their adsorption behavior and ability to inhibit secondary precipitation of calcium phosphate salts.

### b. The PRP as Inhibitors of Calcium Phosphate Crystal Growth; Adsorption Behavior and Structure-Activity Relationships

Inhibition of calcium phosphate crystal growth by the PRP has been shown to be closely related to the adsorption of these molecules onto HA.[8,36,45] Thus, the adsorption coverages of HA seed crystals by the PRP matched very closely the reductions in crystal growth rates of calcium phosphate on the treated seeds, from defined supersaturated solutions.[45] From these experiments it was shown that concentrations of PRP in glandular salivas were in excess of those required to inhibit crystal growth under oral conditions, an observation which supported the proposed role of these proteins. A single molecular segment of the PRP was found to be associated with inhibitory activity. Thus, tryptic digestion of all four major PRP, followed by separation of the tryptic peptides by anion exchange chromatography, showed that inhibition of crystal growth was associated with a single peak. Isolation and

## Table 4
## CONCENTRATION OF PRP IN HUMAN SALIVARY
## SECRETIONS

| No. of subjects | Secretion | PRP concentration (mg%) | | | Ref. |
| --- | --- | --- | --- | --- | --- |
| | | Mean | Range | S.D. | |
| 42 | Parotid | 48.9 | 19—80 | 14.5 | 78 |
| | Whole | 7.7 | 0—18 | 4.6 | |
| 220 | Parotid | 45 | 10—90 | | 76 |
| 92 | Parotid | 43 | 14—103 | | 77 |
| | Submandibular | 43 | | | |

characterization of this material showed it to be the phosphoserine-containing amino-terminal tryptic peptide (Figure 2, residues 1 to 30) of these molecules.[26,34]

Adsorption of this molecular segment onto HA has been studied in detail, and a close relationship was found between adsorption and inhibition of crystal growth.[44] Also, removal of the two phosphate groups caused a major reduction in its inhibitory activity,[44,69] emphasizing the importance of the bound phosphate groups in inhibitory activity. The identification of the amino-terminal segment of the molecule as the segment which bound to HA was also reported by Bennick and co-workers,[70] who also studied adsorption and calcium ion binding behavior of the PRP to HA.[71-75] It can be concluded from these results that it is this molecular segment which mediates adsorption of the intact molecule to HA. Also, adsorption mechanisms and the thermodynamics of the adsorption process of the PRP and other molecules have been studied.[27,28] Evidence was obtained that, for the PRP, the adsorption process is entropically driven and probably involves changes in the configuration of these molecules on adsorption as well as desorption of water molecules from the adsorbent and the protein. Such changes in configuration may be important in other biological activities, noted next

### 4. Biological Aspects
### a. Normal Concentration Range of PRP in Human Saliva

Table 4 gives the results of three studies in which the concentrations of PRP were determined in the glandular secretions. These studies gave essentially similar results, and no significant variations were observed with respect to health status[76] or age.[77] Levels measured in whole saliva, however, were considerably lower and negatively related to plaque accumulation and gingival index scores,[78] presumably associated with microbial degradation of these proteins by the oral microflora.

### b. Consideration of Likely Sites of Action

Consideration of the states of supersaturation of human salivary secretions, with respect to calcium phosphate salts, suggests a virtually absolute requirement for the presence of inhibitor(s) of calcium phosphate crystal growth on tooth surfaces, to prevent otherwise inevitable deposition of calcium phosphate salts. Based on studies on the inhibitory activities of the PRP[8,44] there appears to be a significant excess of PRP in glandular secretions for this function (Table 4). The fact that PRP are detectable using immunological methods on tooth surfaces exposed to the oral environment[78,79] supports the likelihood that this is the site of action of the PRP. The long-term survival of PRP on tooth surfaces, however, is not established. In one study[78] PRP were found in long-term pellicle on extracted teeth. In another study[79] it was found that although the PRP made up over one third of the total protein in short-term pellicle (up to 24 h) formed on enamel blocks placed in the mouth, little PRP could be detected in pellicle material recovered from extracted teeth. It may be significant in this connection that only a monomolecular layer formed from the amino-terminal segment of the PRP, present on the tooth surface, would be sufficient to inhibit secondary precipitation of calcium phosphates. Such films may not be readily detected in older pellicle material, part of which at least undergoes degradation in the oral cavity.[79]

### c. Other Biological Aspects of the PRP

Recently, the PRP were found to inhibit precipitation of calcite, and this was proposed as a further biological activity for the PRP.[80] The state of saturation of human salivary secretions with respect to calcite, however, has not been clearly established. Investigation of this problem[81] showed that a significant proportion of 70 saliva samples examined were supersaturated with respect to calcite, suggesting that inhibition of calcite precipitation would be a necessary biological activity in human saliva. Calcite precipitation, however, is strongly inhibited by inorganic phosphate at concentrations well below those found in human salivary secretions.[82,83] Salivary concentrations of phosphate appear to be high enough to inhibit fully calcite precipitation from saliva for time periods of biological significance, and, although the PRP, statherin, and inorganic phosphate all act as inhibitors of calcite precipitation,[80,81] quantitatively, phosphate is by far the most important inhibitor present, and the contributions made by the macromolecules appear to be minor.

The present state of knowledge regarding the biological function of human PRP is consistent with the proposal that their major function is to act as inhibitors of calcium phosphate crystal growth on tooth surfaces. There are, however, clearly several unanswered questions relating to this proposal. Thus the proposed function could be fulfilled by the phosphoserine-containing amino-terminal segment of these molecules, adsorbed to the tooth surface. Considering this, what is the function of the major part of the molecule? This amounts to four fifths of the residues in PRP-1 and -2, and two thirds of the residues in PRP-3 and -4. Also, what are the implications of the remarkable degree of genetic polymorphism found with these proteins? This is in contrast to statherin, for which no genetic variants have yet been detected, and most of the other proteins in human saliva. Since the PRP form a significant fraction of the early pellicle[78,79] it may be worth considering that the proline-, glycine-, and glutamine-rich carboxy-terminal part of the molecule plays some as yet undefined role in mediating adsorption of a further layer or layers of protein to form the mature pellicle, a process which may involve processing of the initially adsorbed protein.

It is interesting in this connection that salivary proteins, including the PRP, adsorbed onto HA surfaces, appear to play an important role in mediating selective bacterial colonization of such surfaces *in vitro* and, presumably, tooth surfaces *in vivo*.[84,85] Thus, recent studies have shown that PRP, adsorbed to HA, strongly enhance adhesion of certain strains of *Actinomyces viscosus*. Remarkably, this organism does not appear to interact to a significant extent with PRP in solution, suggesting that the conformational change which appears to occur on adsorption of PRP onto HA[28] exposes previously hidden receptors for bacterial attachment.[85] This suggests a further level of biological activity for the PRP and other salivary proteins adsorbed to the tooth surface, which remains a topic for future studies.

### C. Formation of Salivary Gland and Dental Calculi

Although statherin and the PRP are present in salivary secretions at concentrations which appear to be more than adequate to inhibit completely calcium phosphate precipitation in the oral environment, calcium phosphate calculi still form in the salivary glands and on the teeth. Formation of these concretions appears to represent a failure of the inhibitory activities considered here. It is appropriate, therefore, to consider possible mechanisms involved in the formation of these calculi and to attempt to identify the reasons for the apparent ineffectiveness of the inhibitors under circumstances in which salivary gland and dental calculi form.

A highly significant observation regarding dental calculi is that their formation evidently requires the presence of dental plaque.[86,87] Thus the first appearance of crystalline calcium phosphate deposits were reported to occur within established bacterial plaques, and the mineral of dental calculi does not form or exist in direct contact with the mineral phase of the teeth.[86] This clearly precludes a mechanism of formation involving crystal growth of calcium phosphates on tooth surfaces, consistent with the presence of inhibitors of calcium phosphate crystal growth such as the PRP, known to be present on natural tooth surfaces.[78,79]

A further significant observation is that both statherin and the PRP are degraded on prolonged exposure to the oral microflora,[43] presumably by extracellular or surface-bound microbial proteases. This implies that even if these salivary macromolecules are present in the initial stages of dental plaque formation, they will not survive there for long. Also, it seems highly unlikely that the macromolecules will diffuse into bacterial plaques, because of their relatively large molecular size. It seems reasonable to expect, therefore, that compartments will develop in plaque from which statherin, the PRP, and other possible inhibitors are excluded, but to which salivary calcium and phosphate have access. In those compartments, precipitation of calcium phosphate salts is likely to occur, to form dental calculi. In addition, the complex chemistry of plaque may well make its own contribution to calculus formation, a process which appears to involve a relatively high degree of supersaturation with respect to calcium phosphate salts, since DCPD is often found as a constituent of early dental calculi.[87]

These considerations provide a reasonable working hypothesis for the formation of calcium phosphate concretions in the oral environment, in spite of the presence of inhibitory macromolecules. A similar explanation can be proposed tentatively to explain the formation of salivary gland calculi. This situation would require formation of a compartment in the salivary gland to which inorganic ions have access, but from which statherin and the PRP are excluded. No experimental verification for such a model exists at present, but it seems significant that formation of salivary gland concretions appears to be associated with salivary gland injury or infection, conditions which would appear to favor creation of such compartments, and degradation of the inhibitors.

## NOTE ADDED IN PROOF

Sequences of additional proline-rich proteins Db-s, Db-f, Pa (Azen, E. A., et al., *Am. J. Hum. Genet.*, 41, 1035, 1987), PIF-s and PIF-f, and corrected sequences of PRP-1, PRP-2, PRP-3, and PRP-4 (Hay, D. I., et al., *Biochem. J.*, 255, 15, 1988) have recently been reported.

## REFERENCES

1. **Hay, D. I., Schluckebier, S. K., and Moreno, E. C.,** Equilibrium dialysis and ultrafiltration studies of calcium and phosphate binding by human salivary proteins. Implications for salivary supersaturation with respect to calcium phosphate salts, *Calcif. Tissue Int.*, 34, 531, 1982.
2. **Gregory, T. M., Moreno, E. C., and Brown, W. E.,** Solubility of $CaHPO_4 \cdot 2H_2O$ in the system $Ca(OH)_2$-$H_3PO_4$-$H_2O$ at 5, 15, 25 and 37.5°C, *J. Res. Natl. Bur. Stand.*, 74A, 461, 1970.
3. **Moreno, E. C., Gregory, T. M., and Brown, W. E.,** Preparation and solubility of hydroxyapatite, *J. Res. Natl. Bur. Stand.*, 72A, 773, 1974.
4. **Lagerlof, F.,** Determination of ionized calcium in parotid saliva, *Clin. Chim. Acta*, 102, 127, 1980.
5. **Lagerlof, F.,** Effect of flow rate and pH on calcium phosphate saturation in human parotid saliva, *Caries Res.*, 17, 403, 1983.
6. **Gron, P.,** Saturation of human saliva with calcium phosphates, *Arch. Oral Biol.*, 18, 1385, 1973.

7. **Hay, D. I., Smith, D. J., Schluckebier, S. K., and Moreno, E. C.,** Relationship between concentration of human salivary statherin and inhibition of calcium phosphate precipitation in stimulated human parotid saliva, *J. Dent. Res.,* 63, 857, 1984.

8. **Moreno, E. C., Kresak, M., and Hay, D. I.,** Adsorption of two human parotid salivary macromolecules on hydroxy-, fluorhydroxy- and fluorapatites, *Arch. Oral Biol.,* 23, 525, 1978.

9. **Backer-Dirks, O.,** Post-eruptive changes in enamel, *J. Dent. Res.,* 45, 503, 1966.

10. **von der Fehr, F. R., Loe, H., and Theilade, E.,** Experimental caries in man, *Caries Res.,* 4, 131, 1970.

11. **Koulourides, T., Feagin, F., and Pigman, W.,** Effect of pH, ionic strength, and cupric ions on the rehardening rate of buffer-softened human enamel, *Arch. Oral Biol.,* 13, 335, 1968.

12. **Margolis, H., Varughese, K., and Moreno, E. C.,** Effect of fluoride on crystal growth of calcium apatites in the presence of a salivary inhibitor, *Calcif. Tissue Int.,* 34, S33, 1982.

13. **Blomfield, J., van Lennep, E. W., Shorey, C. D., Malin, A. S., Dascalu, J., and Brown, J. M.,** Ultrastructure of the *in vitro* formation of hydroxy-apatite in submandibular saliva of children with cystic fibrosis, *Arch. Oral Biol.,* 19, 1153, 1974.

14. **Tomazic, B., Tomson, M., and Nancollas, G. H.,** The growth of calcium phosphates on natural enamel, *Calcif. Tissue Res.,* 12, 193, 1976.

15. **Feagin, F. F., Walker, A. A., and Pigman, W.,** Evaluation of the calcifying characteristics of biological fluids and inhibitors of calcification, *Calif. Tissue Res.,* 4, 231, 1969.

16. **Fleisch, H. and Bisaz, S.,** Mechanism of calcification: inhibitory role of pyrophosphate, *Nature (London),* 195, 911, 1962.

17. **Nakagawa, Y., Margolis, H. C., Yokoyama, S., Kezdy, F. J., Kaiser, E. T., and Coe, F. L.,** Purification and characterization of a calcium oxalate monohydrate crystal growth inhibitor from human kidney tissue culture medium, *J. Biol. Chem.,* 256, 3936, 1981.

18. **Edmondson, H. A., Bullock, W. K., and Mehl, J. W.,** Chronic pancreatitis and lithiasis. II. Pathology and pathogenesis of pancreatic lithiasis, *Am. J. Pathol.,* 26, 37, 1950.

19. **Multigner, L., De Caro, A., Lombardo, D., Campese, D., and Sarles, H.,** Pancreatic stone protein, a phosphoprotein which inhibits calcium carbonate precipitation from human pancreatic juice, *Biochem. Biophys. Res. Commun.,* 110, 69, 1983.

20. **Gron, P. and Hay, D. I.,** Inhibition of calcium phosphate precipitation by human salivary secretions, *Arch. Oral Biol.,* 21, 201, 1976.

21. **Hay, D. I. and Schlesinger, D. H.,** Human salivary statherin; a peptide inhibitor of calcium phosphate precipitation, in *Calcium-Binding Proteins and Calcium Function,* Proc. Int. Symp. on Calcium-Binding Proteins and Calcium Functions, Wasserman et al., Eds., North-Holland, New York, 1977, 401.

22. **Hay, D. I.,** The isolation from human parotid saliva of a tyrosine-rich acid peptide which exhibits high affinity for hydroxyapatite surfaces, *Arch. Oral Biol.,* 18, 1531, 1973.

23. **Schlesinger, D. H. and Hay, D. I.,** Complete covalent structure of statherin, a tyrosine-rich acidic peptide which inhibits calcium phosphate precipitation from human parotid saliva, *J. Biol. Chem.,* 252, 1689, 1977.

24. **Williams, G. and Sallis, J. D.,** Structure-activity relationship of inhibitors of hydroxyapatite formation, *Biochem. J.,* 184, 181, 1979.

25. **Williams, G. and Sallis, J. D.,** Structural factors influencing the ability of compounds to inhibit hydroxyapatite formation, *Calcif. Tissue Int.,* 34, 169, 1982.

26. **Hay, D. I., Moreno, E. C., and Schlesinger, D. H.,** Phosphoprotein-inhibitors of calcium phosphate precipitation from salivary secretions, *Inorg. Perspect. Biol. Med.,* 2, 271, 1979.

27. **Moreno, E. C., Kresak, M., and Hay, D. I.,** Adsorption thermodynamics of acidic proline-rich human salivary proteins onto calcium apatites, *J. Biol. Chem.,* 257, 2981, 1982.

28. **Moreno, E. C., Kresak, M., and Hay, D. I.,** Adsorption of molecules of biological interest onto hydroxyapatite, *Calcif. Tissue Int.,* 36, 48, 1984.

29. **Meyer, J. L.,** Can biological calcification occur in the presence of pyrophosphate? *Arch. Biochem. Biophys.,* 231, 1, 1984.

30. **Meyer, J. L. and Nancollas, G. H.,** The influence of multidentate organic phosphonates on the crystal growth of hydroxyapatite, *Calif. Tissue Res.,* 13, 295, 1973.

31. **Thomas, W. C.,** Trace metal-citric acid complexes as inhibitors of calcification and crystal formation, *Proc. Soc. Exp. Biol. Med.,* 170, 321, 1982.

32. **Tew, W. P., Mahle, C., Benavides, J., Howard, J. E., and Lehninger, A. L.,** Synthesis and characterization of phosphocitric acid, a potent inhibitor of hydroxylapatite crystal growth, *Biochemistry,* 19, 1983, 1980.

33. **Meyer, J. L., McCall, J. T., and Smith, L. H.,** Inhibition of calcium phosphate crystallization by nucleoside phosphates, *Calcif. Tissue Res.,* 15, 287, 1974.

34. **Schlesinger, D. H. and Hay, D. I.,** Primary structure of the active tryptic fragments of human and monkey salivary anionic proline-rich proteins, *Int. J. Pept. Protein Res.,* 17, 34, 1981.

35. **Schluckebier, S. K. and Hay, D. I.,** Structural studies and chemical modifications of human salivary statherin, *J. Dent. Res.,* 60, 574, Abstr. 1058, 1981.

Volume I **149**

36. **Hay, D. I. and Moreno, E. C.,** Differential adsorption and chemical affinities of proteins for apatitic surfaces, *J. Dent. Res.,* 58(B), 930, 1979.

37. **Shomers, J. P., Tabak, L. A., Levine, M. J., Mandel, I. D., and Hay, D. I.,** Properties of cysteine-containing phosphoproteins from human submandibular-sublingual saliva, *J. Dent. Res.,* 61, 397, 1982.

38. **Varughese, K. and Moreno, E. C.,** Crystal growth of calcium apatites in dilute solutions containing fluoride, *Calcif. Tissue Int.,* 33, 431, 1981.

39. **Hay, D. I.,** Some observations on human saliva proteins and their role in the formation of the acquired enamel pellicle, *J. Dent. Res.,* 48, 806, 1969.

40. **Oppenheim, F. G.,** Preliminary observations on the presence and origin of serum albumin in human saliva, *Helv. Odontol. Acta,* 14, 10, 1970.

41. **Hay, D. I.,** The adsorption of salivary proteins by hydroxyapatite and enamel, *Arch. Oral Biol.,* 12, 937, 1967.

42. **Hay, D. I.,** The interaction of human parotid salivary proteins with hydroxyapatite, *Arch. Oral Biol.,* 20, 1517, 1973.

43. **Hay, D. I. and Gron, P.,** Inhibitors of calcium phosphate precipitation in human whole saliva, in Proceedings, *Microbiological Aspects of Dental Caries,* Vol. 1, Stiles, H. M., Loesche, W. J., and O'Brien, T. C., Eds., Sp., Microbiology Abstracts, Information Retrieval, Washington, D. C. and London, 1976.

44. **Aoba, T., Moreno, E. C., and Hay, D. I.,** Inhibition of apatite crystal growth by the amino-terminal segment of human salivary acidic proline-rich proteins, *Calcif. Tissue Int.,* 36, 651, 1984.

45. **Moreno, E. C., Varughese, K., and Hay, D. I.,** Effect of human salivary proteins on the precipitation kinetics of calcium phosphate, *Calcif. Tissue Int.,* 28, 7, 1979.

46. **Oppenheim, F. G., Hay, D. I., and Franzblau, C.,** Proline-rich proteins from human parotid saliva. Isolation and partial characterization, *Biochemistry,* 10, 4233, 1971.

47. **Bennick, A. and Connell, G. E.,** Purification and partial characterization of four proteins from human parotid saliva, *Biochem. J.,* 123, 455, 1971.

48. **Hay, D. I. and Oppenheim, F. G.,** The isolation from human parotid saliva of a further group of proline-rich proteins, *Arch. Oral Biol.,* 19, 627, 1974.

49. **Bennick, A.,** Chemical and physical characteristics of a phosphoprotein from human parotid saliva, *Biochem. J.,* 145, 557, 1975.

50. **Bennick, A.,** The binding of calcium to a salivary phosphoprotein, protein A, common to human parotid and submandibular secretions, *Biochem. J.,* 155, 163, 1976.

51. **Bennick, A.,** The binding of calcium to a salivary phosphoprotein, protein C, and comparison with calcium binding to protein A, a related salivary phosphoprotein, *Biochem. J.,* 163, 241, 1977.

52. **Bennick, A.,** Chemical and physical characterization of a phosphoprotein, protein C, from human saliva and comparison with a related protein A, *Biochem. J.,* 163, 229, 1977.

53. **Schlesinger, D. H., Jacobs, R., and Hay, D. I.,** Primary structure of protein inhibitors of calcium phosphate precipitation from human salivary secretions, in *Peptides,* Proc. 5th Am. Peptide Symposium, Goodman and Meienhofer, Eds., Halsted Press, John Wiley & Sons, New York, 1977, 56.

54. **Bennick, A., Wong, R., and Cannon, M.,** Structure and biological activities of salivary acidic proline-rich proteins, in *Calcium-Binding Proteins and Calcium Function,* Proc. Int. Symp. on Calcium-Binding Proteins and Calcium Function, Wasserman et al., Eds., North-Holland, New York, 1977, 391.

55. **Wong, R. S., Hofmann, T., and Bennick, A.,** The complete primary structure of a proline-rich phosphoprotein from human saliva, *J. Biol. Chem.,* 254, 4800, 1979.

56. **Schlesinger, D. H. and Hay, D. I.,** Complete primary structure of a proline-rich phosphoprotein (PRP-4), a potent inhibitor of calcium phosphate precipitation in human parotid saliva, in *Peptides, Structure and Biological Function,* Proc. 6th Am. Peptide Symp., Gross, G. and Meienhofer, J., Eds., Pierce Chemical, Rockford, IL, 1979, 133.

57. **Wong, R. S. and Bennick, A.,** The primary structure of a salivary calcium-binding proline-rich phosphoprotein (protein C), a possible precursor of a related salivary protein A, *J. Biol. Chem.,* 255, 5943, 1980.

58. **Schlesinger, D. H. and Hay, D. I.,** Complete covalent structure of a proline-rich phosphoprotein, PRP-2, an inhibitor of calcium phosphate crystal growth from human parotid saliva, *Int. J. Pept. Protein Res.,* 27, 373, 1986.

59. **Isemura, S., Saitoh, E., and Sanada, K.,** The amino-acid sequence of a salivary proline-rich peptide, P-C, and its relation to a salivary proline-rich phosphoprotein, protein C, *J. Biochem. (Tokyo),* 87, 1071, 1980.

60. **Maeda, N., Kim, H. S., Azen, E. A., and Smithies, O.,** Differential RNA splicing and post-translational cleavages in the human salivary proline-rich protein gene system, *J. Biol. Chem.,* 260, 11123, 1985.

61. **Wong, R. S. C., Madapallimattam, G., and Bennick, A.,** The role of glandular kallikrein in the formation of a salivary proline-rich protein A by cleavage of a single bond in salivary protein C, *Biochem. J.,* 211, 35, 1983.

62. **Azen, E. A. and Denniston, C.,** Genetic polymorphism of PIF (parotid isoelectric focusing variant) proteins with linkage to the PPP (parotid proline-rich protein) gene complex, *Biochem. Genet.,* 19, 475, 1981.

63. **Hay, D. I.,** Fractionation of human parotid salivary proteins and the isolation of an histidine-rich acidic peptide which shows high affinity for hydroxyapatite surfaces, *Arch. Oral Biol.,* 20, 553, 1975.

64. **Levine, M. J., Weill, J. C., and Ellison, S. A.,** The isolation and analysis of a glycoprotein from parotid saliva, *Biochim. Biophys. Acta,* 188, 165, 1969.

65. **Levine, M. J., Ellison, S. A., and Bahl, O. P.,** The isolation from human parotid saliva and partial characterization of the protein core of a major parotid glycoprotein, *Arch. Oral Biol.,* 18, 827, 1973.

66. **Hay, D. I., Schluckebier, S. K., and Moreno, E. C.,** Adsorption of proteins by hydroxyapatite from human parotid, submandibular and whole salivas, *J. Dent. Res.,* 64, 379, Abstr. 1838, 1985.

67. **Meyer, T. S. and Lamberts, B. L.,** The use of wool fast blue BL for the electrophoresis of human parotid salivary proteins in acrylamide gel, *Arch. Oral Biol.,* 13, 839, 1968.

68. **Steiner, J. C. and Keller, P. J.,** An electrophoretic analysis of the protein components of human parotid saliva, *Arch. Oral Biol.,* 13, 1213, 1968.

69. **Carlson, E. R. and Hay, D. I.,** Structure-activity studies of the acidic proline-rich proteins, *J. Dent. Res.,* 62, 242, Abstr. 659, 1983.

70. **Bennick, A., Cannon, M., and Madapallimattam, G.,** The nature of the hydroxyapatite-binding site in salivary acidic proline-rich proteins, *Biochem. J.,* 183, 115, 1979.

71. **Bennick, A. and Cannon, M.,** Quantitative study of the interaction of salivary acidic proline-rich proteins with hydroxyapatite, *Caries Res.,* 12, 159, 1978.

72. **Bennick, A., McLaughlin, A. C., Grey, A. A., and Madapallimattam, G.,** The location and nature of calcium-binding sites in salivary acidic proline-rich phosphoproteins, *J. Biol. Chem.,* 265, 4741, 1981.

73. **Bennick, A., Cannon, M., and Madapallimattam, G.,** Factors affecting the adsorption of salivary acidic proline-rich proteins to hydroxyapatite, *Caries Res.,* 15, 9, 1981.

74. **Bennick, A.,** Salivary proline-rich proteins, *Mol. Cell. Biochem.,* 45, 83, 1982.

75. **Bennick, A., Kells, D., and Madapallimattam, G.,** Interaction of calcium ions and salivary acidic proline-rich proteins with hydroxyapatite. A possible aspect of inhibition of hydroxyapatite formation, *Biochem. J.,* 213, 11, 1983.

76. **Mandel, I. D. and Bennick, A.,** Quantitation of human salivary acidic proline-rich proteins in oral diseases, *J. Dent. Res.,* 62, 943, 1983.

77. **Baum, B. J., Kousvelari, E. E., and Oppenheim, F. G.,** Exocrine protein secretion from human parotid glands during aging: stable release of the acidic proline-rich proteins, *J. Gerontol.,* 17, 392, 1982.

78. **Kousvelari, E. E., Baratz, R. S., Burke, B., and Oppenheim, F. G.,** Immunochemical identification and determination of proline-rich proteins in salivary secretions, enamel pellicle and glandular tissue specimens, *J. Dent. Res.,* 59, 1430, 1980.

79. **Bennick, A., Chau, G., Goodlin, R., Abrams, S., Tustian, D., and Madapallimattam, G.,** The role of human salivary acidic proline-rich proteins in the formation of acquired dental pellicle *in vivo* and their fate after adsorption to the human enamel surface, *Arch. Oral Biol.,* 28, 19, 1983.

80. **Saitoh, E., Isemura, S., and Sanada, K.,** Inhibition of calcium carbonate precipitation by human salivary proline-rich phosphoproteins, *Arch. Oral Biol.,* 30, 641, 1985.

81. **Schluckebier, S. K., Hay, D. I., and Moreno, E. C.,** Supersaturation of human saliva with respect to calcite, and inhibition of its precipitation by salivary constituents, *J. Dent. Res.,* 65, 808, Abstr. 741, 1986.

82. **Reddy, M. M.,** Crystallization of calcium carbonate in the presence of trace amounts of phosphorus-containing anions, *J. Cryst. Growth,* 41, 287, 1977.

83. **Reitemeier, R. F. and Buehrer, T. F.,** The inhibiting action of minute amounts of sodium hexametaphosphate on the precipitation of calcium carbonate from ammoniacal solutions. I. Quantitative studies of the inhibition process, *J. Phys. Chem.,* 44, 535, 1940.

84. **Gibbons, R. J., Hay, D. I., and Schluckebier, S. K.,** Proline-rich proteins are pellicle receptors for type 1 fimbriae of *A. viscosus, J. Dent. Res.,* 65, 179, Abstr. 84, 1986.

85. **Hay, D. I., Gibbons, R. J., and Schluckebier, S. K.,** Evidence that type 1 fimbriae of *A. viscosus* bind to determinants exposed due to a conformational change in adsorbed proline-rich proteins, *J. Dent. Res.,* 65, 179, Abstr. 85, 1986.

86. **Schroeder, H. E.,** Crystal morphology and gross structures of mineralizing plaque and calculus, *Helv.Odontol. Acta,* 9, 73, 1965.

87. **Schroeder, H. E. and Bambauer, H. U.,** Stages of calcium phosphate crystallization during calculus formation, *Arch. Oral Biol.,* 11, 1, 1966.

Chapter 6

## SALIVARY HISTIDINE-RICH PROTEINS

**Frank G. Oppenheim**

## TABLE OF CONTENTS

## I. IDENTIFICATION, ISOLATION, AND CHARACTERIZATION

The history of the human salivary histidine-rich proteins (HRPs) is complex, since the proteins or peptides composing this group have been identified by several investigators which led to the assignment of different names for the same component(s). Adding to the complexity is the fact that the approaches used for the electrophoretic identification and chromatographic separation of HRPs differ extensively between laboratories. In the absence of complete characterization data it is difficult at best to establish the identity or the degree of relatedness of similar components. As will be seen later, the confusion regarding the number and relationship of HRPs is becoming untangled as progress is made in isolating and characterizing each member peptide.

When protein from human parotid secretion is subjected to electrophoresis under acidic conditions at relatively high densities of the support medium, several small molecular weight components can be noted to move faster toward the cathode than the very basic protein lysozyme.[1,2] In addition these proteins exhibit a high affinity for a stain used to visualize arginine-rich proteins such as histones.[3] Chromatographic separation of these proteins into three fractions indicated that these proteins show a higher affinity for cation exchangers than lysozyme and are enriched with the amino acids histidine, arginine, and lysine.[4] From these observations it was concluded that the components comprised in these fractions represent the most basic proteins of human parotid secretion and that they belong to the well-characterized class of histone proteins.

Cationic electrophoretic systems specifically suited to separate HRPs were developed by Azen[2] and Baum et al.[5] The work conducted in both laboratories indicated that human parotid secretion displays upon cationic electrophoresis at least seven components which were shown to contain histidine as their predominant amino acid.[6-8] Figure 1 shows schematically that six of these components migrate cathodically as three pairs of three double bands, with the seventh, being the fastest component, migrating close to the buffer front. With increasing order of cathodic mobility the seven HRPs were named HRP-1 to HRP-7 by Baum,[5] whereas Azen[6,7,9] used the labels PPb (HRP-1, HRP-2), Pbe (HRP-3), Pbd (HRP-4), Pbb (HRP-5), Pba (HRP-6), and Pl (HRP-7).

The first purification and partial characterization of a salivary histidine-rich protein, labeled Component II, was reported by Hay.[10] Leading to this isolation was previous work indicating that some salivary proteins show a high degree of selectivity with regard to their affinity for hydroxyapatite surfaces.[11] The principal components showing such selectivity are the anionic proline-rich proteins,[12] a tyrosine-rich peptide,[13] later called statherin,[14] and Component II.[10] This Component II behaved more like an acidic protein or peptide, since it was well retained on anion exchangers at pH 8.0 and migrated at pH 8.3 to the midsection of anionic polyacrylamide gels.[15] Using a salt gradient to elute salivary proteins from an anion exchange resin (DEAE Sephadex A25) at pH 8, Component II was retained longer than the anionic proline-rich proteins (pI 4.09 to 4.71[12]) and released just before statherin (pI 4.2[13]). Contrary to expectations, however, Component II was found not to be anionic peptide since its pI was determined to be 7.04.[10] The composition revealed a high content of basic amino acids (histidine 19%, arginine 11%, and lysine 8%) concomitant with a high level of dicarboxylic acids (aspartic acid 14% and glutamic acid 9%) and significant amounts of aromatic amino acids (tyrosine 9% and phenylalanine 8%) (cf. Table 1). Because of the affinity for hydroxyapatite surfaces, its electrophoretic and chromatographic behavior, and a pI close to neutrality, Component II was considered to be significantly different from the basic HRPs described by Azen and Baum. Amino acid analysis of HRP preparations purified by gel filtration and cation exchangers[6-8] led to compositional data, however, which are very similar to those of Component II (Table 1). From a careful comparison of electrophoretic and amino acid composition data it can be concluded that Component II, HRP-1 and PPb

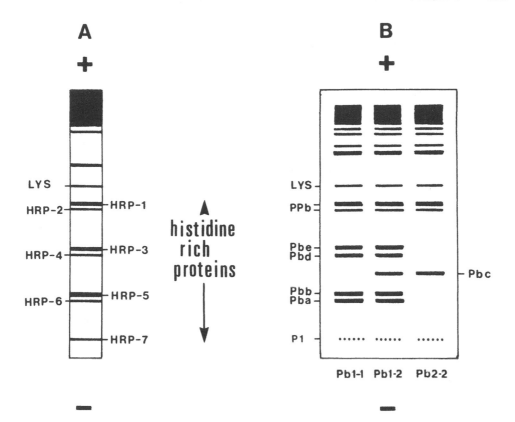

FIGURE 1. Schematic electrophoretic patterns of salivary HRP. (A): Separation of human parotid saliva protein on cationic polyacrylamide gel, 15%, pH 2.74, according to Baum et al.[5] and MacKay et al.;[22] histidine-rich proteins are labeled HRP-1 to HRP-7; (B): Separation of parotid saliva protein from 3 individuals with the phenotypes Pb1-1, Pb-1-2, and Pb2-2 on acid-urea starch gel, pH 2.4, according to Azen[2,9] and Peters et al.;[7] HRPs are labeled PPb, Pbe, Pbd, Pbc, Pbb, and Pba; P1 is observed after autoincubation of sample; + anode; − cathode; LYS, lysozyme.

constitute the same histidine-rich protein. This is the neutral histidine-rich polypeptide which has recently been isolated to homogeneity and fully characterized by Oppenheim et al.[16,17] The composition of HRP-2 is almost identical with that of HRP-1.[8] The proteins composing the second pair (HRP-3/HRP-4), the third pair (HRP-5/HRP-6), and HRP-7 have not yet been isolated to homogeneity. The composition of the mixture of HRP-3 and HRP-4 (Pbe and Pbd) shows that this pair is very similar to HRP-1 or HRP-2 but differs by the presence of alanine, an increase in basic residues, lower levels of glutamic acid and phenylalanine, and the absence of proline. The composition of the fastest-moving pair (HRP-5/HRP-6, or Pbb/Pba) exhibits again strong similarities with that of HRP-1 but contains even higher levels of basic residues at the expense of aspartic acid and aromatic residues. Again the absence of proline and the presence of alanine can be noted. For the fastest-moving HRP-7 no compositional data are as yet available. Current evidence indicates that all seven HRPs lack carbohydrates and are present in both human parotid and submandibular secretions but cannot be found in other body fluids.[9] The similarity in their composition and their immunological cross-reactivity[7,18] suggests that they are closely related.

The neutral histidine-rich polypeptide (HRP-1) contains 38 amino acid residues and is the first HRP for which the primary structure has been determined[17] (Figure 2). The molecular weight of HRP-1, calculated from its amino acid sequence, is 4929. This value is considerably lower than many of the values which had been based on minimum molecular weight estimates (Table 1). As can be seen from its amino acid sequence, HRP-1 contains many polar side

**Table 1**
**AMINO ACID COMPOSITIONS OF HRP PREPARATIONS (RESIDUES PER 100 RESIDUES)**

| Amino acid | HRP-1[a] | HRP-2[a] | PPb[b] | Pbe + Pbd[c] | Pbb + Pba[c] | Component II[d] | Neutral | HRP[e] |
|---|---|---|---|---|---|---|---|---|
| Aspartic acid | 12.9 | 11.0 | 13.1 | 11.5 | 4.9 | 14.4 | 14.1 | (5)* |
| Threonine | — | — | 0 | 0.2 | 0.2 | 0 | 0 | (0) |
| Serine | 8.3 | 9.5 | 4.6 | 6.6 | 5.7 | 7.3 | 7.7 | (3)** |
| Glutamic acid | 8.7 | 10.0 | 9.1 | 4.3 | 5.6 | 8.9 | 8.2 | (3) |
| Proline | 2.4 | 2.4 | 2.6 | 0.2 | 0.2 | 2.6 | 3.2 | (1) |
| Glycine | 8.9 | 9.0 | 9.3 | 7.6 | 8.9 | 8.6 | 7.4 | (3) |
| Alanine | 0.5 | 1.3 | — | 3.5 | 4.2 | 0 | 0 | (0) |
| Valine | — | — | 0 | 0.2 | 0.3 | 0 | 0 | (0) |
| Cysteine | 0 | 0 | 0 | 0.4 | 0.3 | 0 | 0 | (0) |
| Methionine | — | — | 0 | 0 | 0 | 0 | 0 | (0) |
| Isoleucine | — | — | 0 | 0.1 | 0.1 | 0 | 0 | (0) |
| Leucine | 2.6 | 2.1 | 3.0 | 3.1 | 0.6 | 3.1 | 2.9 | (1) |
| Phenylalanine | 7.6 | 7.3 | 7.8 | 3.1 | 4.1 | 8.3 | 7.4 | (3) |
| Tyrosine | 12.0 | 9.1 | 12.6 | 11.2 | 7.9 | 8.5 | 12.2 | (5) |
| Lysine | 8.0 | 9.2 | 7.6 | 12.0 | 15.5 | 8.1 | 8.2 | (3) |
| Histidine | 17.2 | 17.3 | 18.6 | 20.7 | 25.9 | 19.0 | 18.0 | (7) |
| Arginine | 10.0 | 9.8 | 10.4 | 12.4 | 13.1 | 11.1 | 10.5 | (4) |
| Min mol wt | 5733 | 5879 | 8275 | 7708 | 6426 | 4520 | 4675 | (4929)*** |

[a]    Baum et al.[8]
[b]    Peters et al.[7]
[c]    Peters and Azen.[6]
[d]    Hay.[10]
[e]    Oppenheim et al.,[17] values in parentheses are based on amino acid sequence of neutral HRP (total 38 residues);
       *2 asparagine + 3 aspartic acid; **1 phosphoserine + 2 serine; ***$M_r$ computed from amino acid sequence.

```
1           5                    10                   15                   20
Asp-Pse-His-Glu-Lys-Arg-His-His-Gly-Tyr-Arg-Arg-Lys-Phe-His-Glu-Lys-His-His-Ser-
—→     —→  —→  —→  —→  —→  —→  —→  —→  —→  —→  —→  —→  —→  —→  —→  —→  —→
←——————————T-1——————————→  ←————— T-2 —————→  ←——— T-3 ———→  ←— T-4 —
←——SA-1——→                                                 ←—— SA-2 —

21          25                   30                   35        38
His-Arg-Glu-Phe-Pro-Phe-Tyr-Gly-Asp-Tyr-Gly-Ser-Asn-Tyr-Leu-Tyr-Asp-Asn
—→  —→  —→  —→  —→                                   ←—  ←—  ←—  ←—
—T-4—→  ←———————————————— T-5 ———————→
—SA-2—→       ←——————— SA-3 ——————→  ←————— SA-4 —————→
```

FIGURE 2.    Amino acid sequence of neutral HRP (HRP-1). Designations are: T, tryptic peptides; SA, *S. aureus* V8 protease peptides; —→, automated Edman degradation of intact HRP; ←—, sequence obtained by carboxypeptidase A digestion; Pse, phosphoserine (From Oppenheim, F. G., Yang, Y. C., Diamond, R. D., Hyslop, D., Offner, G. D., and Troxler, R. F., *J. Biol. Chem.*, 261, 1177, 1986. With permission.)

chains, with 7 histidine, 4 arginine, 3 lysine, 3 aspartic acid, 3 glutamic acid, and 1 phosphoserine residue. Its content in aromatic residues (5 tyrosine, 3 phenylalanine) is 21%. Disregarding the minimal charge contributions made by histidine at pH 7, the neutral characteristics of this peptide are not surprising, since acidic and basic residues are well balanced. Furthermore, HRP-1 lacks threonine, alanine, valine, isoleucine, cysteine, and methionine. In the case of the anionic proline-rich proteins and statherin, the negatively charged residues are localized in the amino-terminal portion, whereas proline, glycine, and glutamine are almost exclusively found in the carboxyl-terminal segment of the polypeptide. HRP-1 is different from statherin or proline-rich proteins, since it lacks such structural polarity by virtue of a more uniform distribution of hydrophobic and hydrophilic residues. This is further supported by the results obtained from the hydropathy analysis by the method of Kyte and Doolittle,[19] which indicates that the overall nature of the polypeptide is hydrophilic. The secondary structure of HRP-1 has not been determined, but a predictive analysis based on its primary structure[20,21] suggests the presence of two segments of α-helix (residues 2-7 and 12-19), two short segments of β-pleated sheet (residues 26-29 and 35-38), and three reverse turns (residues 8-11, 20-23, and 31-34). There is a strong probability that HRP-1 contains significant amounts of higher-ordered structure. Furthermore, no sequence homology could be found using the data bank of the National Biomedical Research Foundation between the sequence of HRP-1 and the sequence of any other protein. This is not too surprising considering that histidine is among the least common amino acids found in proteins.[19]

## II. GENETIC POLYMORPHISM AND BIOSYNTHESIS

A certain variability in the electrophoretic pattern of HRPs obtained from different individuals or of aliquots of the same sample stored for different time periods was noted by several investigators. Furthermore, MacKay et al.[22] observed electrophoretically seven additional components belonging to the HRP group which are on electrophoretograms interspersed among the major HRPs. The variability associated with HRPs is in part due to a genetic polymorphism and in part due to proteolytic fragmentation of larger HRPs giving rise to smaller histidine-rich peptides. Azen[2,9,23] described a genetic polymorphism for histidine-rich proteins which is almost exclusively found among blacks. This polymorphism comprises the peptides Pbe, Pbd, Pbc, Pbb, and Pba (Figure 1) and is dictated by two autosomal codominant alleles, Pb1 and Pb2. The common homozygote, Pb1-1, displays phenotypically the peptides Pbe, Pbd, Pbb, and Pba, whereas the less common homozygote, Pb2-2, expresses only one component, the peptide Pbc. The electrophoretic mobility of Pbc is intermediate to those of Pbd and Pbb (Figure 1). The gene frequencies calculated from 90 American blacks were 0.84 and 0.16 for Pb1 and Pb2, respectively. Among 101 Caucasians, 100 were found to be common homozygotes, and only 1 heterozygous pattern could be identified, indicating a very low gene frequency of 0.005 for the allele Pb2. It should be noted that this genetic polymorphism is restricted to the faster-moving Pb peptides (HRP-3 to HRP-6) and does not control the expression of the slower PPb proteins (HRP-1 and HRP-2).[7]

Electrophoretic changes due to proteolysis were observed by both Baum et al.[8] and Azen.[9] Baum conducted incubation studies with mixtures of parotid and whole saliva at a ratio of 4:1 and observed a gradual conversion of HRP-1 to products which exhibited electrophoretic mobilities identical with those of HRP-3 and HRP-4 and subsequently also of HRP-5 and HRP-6. Boiling of whole saliva or the use of proteolytic inhibitors slowed this breakdown process but could not totally prevent it. The degree of conversion was proportional to the time and temperature of incubation. HRPs could also be isolated from whole saliva, but the preparation obtained from whole saliva resembled electrophoretically and compositionally the most cationic or smaller forms of HRPs.[8] The breakdown products studied by Baum showed not only the characteristic electrophoretic mobilities of the faster-moving HRPs but also compositions consistent with the hypothesis that they originate from the larger and less basic HRP-1 or HRP-2. From the increase in histidine and lysine and the reduction in aspartic acid, phenylalanine, and tyrosine, he concluded that HRP-1 is the progenitor protein giving rise to the smaller and more basic HRP species. Azen[9] also observed variations in band intensities and mobilities of HRPs, but these observations were restricted to the Pb peptides (HRP-3 to HRP-7). He showed that autoincubation of parotid saliva samples led to the conversion of the peptides Pbe, Pbd, Pbb, Pba to a fast-moving component labeled P1.

Several proteolytic inhibitors prevented this conversion while incubation of parotid saliva with various proteolytic enzymes mimicked the results seen after autoincubation. Based on the amino acid composition and partial sequence data of purified Pb proteins, a hypothesis was formulated which took into account both genetic control and posttranslational modifications, such as proteolysis and deamidation, to explain the variabilities observed.[6,23] This hypothesis, however, differs significantly from the conclusions drawn by Baum in that the largest HRPs (HRP-1, HRP-2, or PPb proteins) are not considered to bear any direct precursor relationship with the smaller and more cationic HRPs. Azen's hypothesis is based on the observation that the PPb proteins (HRP-1, HRP-2) show no genetic polymorphism and display despite their overall similarities some significant differences in composition and structure (partial sequence data) when compared with those of the Pb proteins (HRP-3 to HRP-6). It was postulated that PPb and Pb proteins are not directly related, since they appear to be controlled by different loci. The structural kinship of the PPb to the Pb proteins, however, could be explained by a gene duplication event. In this case the PPb proteins would have evolved from the Pb proteins during evolution.[7,23]

The precise mechanism giving rise to the various species of HRPs has not been elucidated, but the similarities in their composition, their immunological cross-reactivity,[7,18] and their progressive decrease in aspartic acid, proline, and aromatic residues and relative increase in basic residues the further an HRP component moves toward the cathode is strong support for the posttranslational proteolysis model. The only inconsistency in this model is the reported presence of alanine in the smaller HRPs, which is not present in HRP-1 or HRP-2. From the amino acid sequence of HRP-1 (Figure 2) it can readily be seen, for example, that a loss of the carboxyl-terminal tryptic peptide T-5 would result in a compositional change consistent with a relative increase of basic residues, while significant losses of dicarboxylic acids, proline, leucine, and aromatic residues would become evident. Progressive proteolysis from the carboxyl-terminal end could possibly account for the various HRP species observed. From this it is also tempting to speculate that the more cathodically migrating HRPs do so because of a reduction in size and to a lesser degree because of an increase in their cationic nature. Discounting the possibility of negative-charge contributions from ester-linked phosphate groups, an overestimation of their apparent molecular weights and an overestimation of the positive charge contributions made by histidine residues seem to be responsible for an exaggeration of their cationic nature. Structural analysis of each HRP component will be necessary to clarify these unanswered questions.

Several histidine-rich peptides with electrophoretic mobilities and amino acid compositions similar to those of man have been identified in parotid saliva of subhuman primates.[7,9,24] Antiserum to human HRPs cross-reacted with macaque HRPs providing further support for the notion that they are the phylogenetic equivalent of the human HRPs. Primate models have been useful in proving that HRPs are not histones[25] and that HRPs are synthesized *in vitro* and *in vivo* by the parotid gland. The latter studies represent convincing evidence that HRPs are true secretory products.[26] Circular dichroic spectra of purified macaque HRPs indicated the presence of higher-ordered structure under conditions prevailing in the oral cavity.[24] Of phylogenetic interest is the finding that the PPb-like proteins have so far not been found in monkeys. What has been found are proteins with electrophoretic behavior and amino acid compositions very similar to those of the human Pb proteins. These proteins were detected in several species of old-world monkeys but not in new-world monkeys. It is therefore possible that the alleles of the PPb proteins have arisen from gene duplication relatively recently, whereas the alleles for the Pb proteins appeared after the divergence of new-world monkeys from the evolutionary path about 50 million years ago.[7,9,23]

## III. FUNCTION

As pointed out earlier, interest in the neutral histidine-rich protein originated from its high affinity for hydroxyapatite surfaces.[10,11] HRP-1 is therefore implicated in the formation of the acquired enamel pellicle. Similar to the well-characterized pellicle precursor proteins, the anionic proline-rich proteins, and statherin, HRP-1 is a phosphoprotein and an active inhibitor of crystal growth in calcium phosphate solutions supersaturated with respect to hydroxyapatite.[17] In contrast to the proline-rich proteins and statherin, HRP-1 exhibits only one phosphate group, has a considerably higher pI of 7.04, and does not show the characteristic structural polarity consisting of strongly negatively charged amino-terminal portion and a larger neutral carboxyl-terminal segment. The inhibition of crystal growth by proline-rich proteins and statherin has been shown to be related directly to adsorption of protein to the hydroxyapatite mineral.[27] There is good evidence for the functional importance of the negatively charged amino-terminal segments containing both phosphoserine residues.[28] Recent evidence, however, emhasizes the additional role of secondary structure contributions in the adsorption process.[29] Thermodynamic studies of the adsorption of proline-rich proteins indicate that the mineral protein interactions are an entropically driven process involving both changes in the structure of the macromolecule as well as the displacement of water. The established primary structure and the predicted secondary structure of HRP-1 are consistent with the possibility of both electrostatic interactions and conformational changes upon adsorption to hydroxyapatite.

An unusual but important feature of the HRPs is their antimicrobial activity.[16,17,30,31] Partly purified preparations of HRPs were shown to inhibit both the growth and the cell viability of several strains of *Streptococcus mutans in vitro*.[30] Preincubation of bacteria with HRPs at pH 5.2 was most effective in inhibiting both growth and viability. Bacterial lethality was maintained for 48 h at an HRP concentration of 250 μg/ml, whereas 76 to 81% killing was noted over a 24-h period at 50 μg/ml. The time period of preincubation, pH of the buffer, and the concentration of HRPs appear to be related directly to the degree of inhibition observed. Furthermore, nongrowing cells were more sensitive than growing cells, showing 100% lethality at an HRP concentration of 50 μg/ml. Hen egg white lysozyme displayed similar antibacterial effects but was less effective than HRPs. Subtle differences were noted, particularly with respect to growth inhibition of specific strains, suggesting a different mechanism for the action of lysozyme. Interestingly, after preincubation with HRPs, the exposure to enriched media favors the recovery of some HRP-treated cells. It would appear that under marginal nutritive states and low growth conditions, HRPs could constitute a highly effective antibacterial agent *in vivo*. The molecular mechanism underlying these antibacterial activities is not clear, but it is possible that HRPs can activate intrinsic autolysins.

Contrasting these findings is an earlier study of Holbrook and Molan,[32] who reported on a histidine-, lysine-, and arginine-rich protein preparation obtained from parotid saliva which enhanced the glycolytic activity of selected oral bacteria. There are, however, differences in the amino acid composition between this partially purified salivary fraction and HRPs. The effect observed, therefore, cannot be directly related to a specific HRP.

The second and possibly more important antimicrobial property of HRPs is their antifungal effect.[16,17,31] Using partly purified preparations containing mixtures of several HRPs, Pollock et al.[31] noted complete growth inhibition of *Candida albicans* when both preincubation buffer and growth medium contained 250 μg of HRP per milliliter. HRPs were also more effective than hen egg white lysozyme. The inhibitory effects of HRPs added directly to the medium of growing cells was proportional to the HRP concentration but inversely proportional to the cell density. At an HRP concentration of 25 μg/ml in the medium more than 99% killing of growing yeast cells could be observed after 24 h. For nongrowing cells viability losses of more than 93% resulted from preincubation with HRPs at a concentration of 100 μg/ml for 30 min. Similar to what is known for imidazole antibiotics,[33,34] loss of viability was concomitant with loss of potassium from exposed yeast cells, suggesting that HRPs can cause membrane damage. Synthetic homopolymers of poly-L-histidine and poly-L-lysine exhibited similar growth inhibitory effects, but in contrast to the HRPs their maximum inhibitory effect was more dependent on their presence in the growth medium.

Pure preparations of HRP-1, though, were shown to be highly effective in inhibiting germination of *C. albicans*.[16,17] Fungicidal activity was not present or could only be observed at unphysiologically high concentrations. At concentrations of 2 and 8 μg/ml, HRP-1 inhibited the germination of *C. albicans* by 50% and 80%, respectively. These values are well within the estimated physiological concentration range of HRPs in glandular secretions. Lysozyme inhibited germination to a minimal degree (20%) even at a high concentration of 2 mg/ml. In addition, salivary protein fractions not retained on anion exchange resins which should contain most other cationic proteins of saliva were found to lack inhibitory activity. The inhibition of mycelial transformation is significant, since germ tube formation has been shown to optimize fungal adherence to oral mucous membranes,[35,36] and there is considerable evidence indicating a direct relationship between germination and infection.[37] Homopolymers of histidine have recently been shown to reduce both the number and the size of germ tubes formed in culture.[38]

The elucidation of the primary structure of HRP-1 allows meaningful comparisons with other nonsalivary proteins displaying antimicrobial activities. It is well known that macrophages and polymorphonuclear leukocytes contain cationic proteins or peptides with microbicidal activity.[39-45] The primary structures of the 2 cationic peptides MCP-1 and MCP-2 from rabbit lung macrophages and of the 6 cationic peptides NP-1, NP-2, NP-3a, NP-3b, NP-4, and NP-5 from rabbit peritoneal neutrophils have been determined.[46,47] These peptides are enriched with arginine and cysteine and are closely related in size and structure. Their polypeptide chains contain 32 to 34 amino acid residues. The amino acid sequences of the macrophage-derived peptides MCP-1 and MCP-2 are identical with those of the neutrophil-derived peptides NP-1 and NP-2, respectively. In addition, comparison of the individual peptide structures indicates a high degree of sequence homology. While there is no similarity between the composition and structure of HRP-1 and the peptides derived from these phagocytic cells, both display short polypeptide chains and exhibit anti-*Candida* activity.

There is considerable evidence for an increase in the incidence of candidosis in recent years which appears to be related to the widespread use of antibiotics, immunosuppressive agents, aggressive cancer chemotherapy, parenteral nutrition, and surgical prosthetic devices.[48] The steps responsible for the pathway from a harmless commensal existence of *C. albicans* in the oral cavity to pathogenicity are not clearly understood. While cellular and humoral immunity are important in the host defense, other factors have gained increased attention. Among these are factors controlling the transition from the yeast to the mycelial state. Such a transition favors adhesion of certain fungi to host tissues over elimination from epithelial surfaces. Playing a role in this process the salivary histidine-rich proteins may represent an important part of the nonimmune host defense system.

## ACKNOWLEDGMENTS

This work was supported by grants DEO5672-04 and DEO7652-01 from the National Institutes of Health.

# REFERENCES

1. **Bonilla, C. A. and Stringham, R. M.,** Electrophoresis of human salivary secretions at acid pH, *J. Chromatog.,* 50, 345, 1970.
2. **Azen, E. A.,** Genetic polymorphism of basic proteins from parotid saliva, *Science,* 176, 673, 1972.
3. **Sung, M. and Smithies, O.,** Differential elution of histones from gel-trapped nuclei, *Biopolymers,* 7, 39, 1969.
4. **Balekjian, A. Y. and Longton, R. W.,** Histones isolated from human parotid fluid, *Biochem. Biophys. Res. Commun.,* 50, 676, 1973.
5. **Baum, B. J., Bird, J. L., and Longton, R. W.,** Polyacrylamide gel electrophoresis of human salivary histidine-rich polypeptides, *J. Dent. Res.,* 56, 1115, 1977.
6. **Peters, E. H. and Azen, E. A.,** Isolation and partial characterization of human parotid basic proteins, *Biochem. Genet.,* 15, 925, 1977.
7. **Peters, E. H., Goodfriend, T., and Azen, E. A.,** Human Pb, human post-Pb, and nonhuman primate Pb proteins: immunological and biochemical relationships, *Biochem. Genet.,* 15, 947, 1977.
8. **Baum, B. J., Bird, J. L., Millar, D. B., and Longton, R. W.,** Studies on histidine-rich polypeptides from human parotid saliva, *Arch. Biochem. Biophys.,* 177, 427, 1976.
9. **Azen, E. A.,** Properties of salivary basic proteins showing polymorphism, *Biochem. Genet.,* 9, 69, 1973.
10. **Hay, D. I.,** Fractionation of human parotid salivary proteins and the isolation of an histidine-rich acidic peptide which shows high affinity for hydroxyapatite surfaces, *Arch. Oral Biol.,* 20, 553, 1975.
11. **Hay, D. I.,** The interaction of human salivary proteins with hydroxyapatite, *Arch. Oral Biol.,* 18, 1517, 1973.
12. **Oppenheim, F. G., Hay, D. I., and Franzblau, C.,** Proline-rich proteins from human parotid saliva. I. Isolation and characterization, *Biochemistry,* 10, 4233, 1971.
13. **Hay, D. L.,** The isolation from human parotid saliva of a tyrosine rich acidic peptide which exhibits high affinity for hydroxyapapatite surfaces, *Arch. Oral Biol.,* 18, 1531, 1973.
14. **Schlesinger, D. H. and Hay, D. I.,** Complete covalent structure of statherin, a tyrosine-rich acidic peptide which inhibits calcium phosphate precipitation from human parotid saliva, *J. Biol. Chem.,* 252, 1689, 1977.
15. **Davis, B. J.,** Disc electrophoresis. II. Method and application to human serum proteins, *Ann. N.Y. Acad. Sci.,* 121, 404, 1964.
16. **Oppenheim, F. G., Yang, Y. C., and Troxler, R. F.,** Structural and functional characterization of human parotid histidine-rich protein, *J. Dent. Res.,* 64, 239 (Sp. Issue), Abstr. 571, 1985.
17. **Oppenheim, F. G., Yang, Y. C., Diamond, R. D., Hyslop, D., Offner, G. D., and Troxler, R. F.,** The primary structure and functional characterization of the neutral histidine-rich polypeptide from human parotid secretion, *J. Biol. Chem.,* 261, 1177, 1986.
18. **Baum, B. J., Ellison, S. A., and Levine, M. J.,** Differential antigenicity of human salivary histidine-rich polypeptides in goats and rabbits, *Arch. Oral Biol.,* 22, 457, 1977.
19. **Kyte, J. and Doolittle, R. F.,** A simple method for displaying the hydropathic character of a protein, *J. Mol. Biol.,* 157, 105, 1982.
20. **Chou, P. Y. and Fasman, G. E.,** Prediction of the secondary structure of proteins from their amino acid sequence, *Adv. Enzymol. Relat. Areas Mol. Biol.,* 47, 45, 1978.
21. **Chou, P. Y. and Fasman, G. E.,** Prediction of -turns, *Biophys. J.,* 26, 367, 1979.
22. **MacKay, B. J., Pollock, J. J., Iacono, V. J., and Baum, B. J.,** Isolation of milligram quantities of a group of histidine-rich polypeptides from human parotid saliva, *Infect. Immun.,* 44, 688, 1984.
23. **Azen, E. A.,** Genetic protein polymorphisms in human saliva: an interpretive review, *Biochem. Genet.,* 16, 79, 1978.
24. **Baum, B. J., Bird, J. L., Millar, D. B., and Longton, R. W.,** Isolation and partial characterization of an histidine-rich polypeptide from parotid saliva of the monkey, *Macaca nemestrina, Comp. Biochem. Physiol.,* 56A, 115, 1977.
25. **Baum, B. J., Bird, J. L., and Longton, R. W.,** Histidine-rich polypeptides in macaque parotid saliva are not nuclear histones, *Arch. Oral Biol.,* 22, 455, 1977.
26. **Baum, B. J., Bird, J. L., Berzinskas, V. J., and Longton, R. W.,** Synthesis of histidine-rich polypeptides by monkey parotid glands, *Proc. Saliva and Dental Caries,* Kleinberg, I., Ellison, S. A., and Mandel, I. D., Eds., Information Retrieval, New York, Microbiol. Abstr. 89, 1979.
27. **Moreno, E. C., Varughese, K., and Hay, D. I.,** Effect of human salivary proteins on the precipitation kinetics of calcium phosphate, *Calcif. Tissue Int.,* 28, 7, 1979.
28. **Aoba, T., Moreno, E. C., and Hay, D. I.,** Inhibition of apatite crystal growth by the amino-terminal segment of human salivary acidic proline-rich proteins, *Calcif. Tissue Int.,* 36, 651, 1984.
29. **Moreno, E. C., Kresak, M., and Hay, D. I.,** Adsorption of molecules of biological interest onto hydroxyapatite, *Calcif. Tissue Int.,* 36, 48, 1984.

30. **MacKay, B. J., Denepitiya, L., Iacono, V. J., Krost, S. B., and Pollock, J. J.,** Growth-inhibitory and bactericidal effects of human parotid salivary histidine-rich polypeptides on *Streptococcus mutans, Infect. Immun.,* 44, 695, 1984.

31. **Pollock, J. J., Denepitiya, L., MacKay, B. J., and Iacono, V. J.,** Fungistatic and fungicidal activity of human parotid salivary histidine-rich polypeptides on *Candida albicans, Infect. Immun.,* 44, 702, 1984.

32. **Holbrook, I. B. and Molan, P. C.,** The identification of a peptide in human parotid saliva particularly active in enhancing the glycolytic activity of the salivary microorganisms, *Biochem. J.,* 149, 489, 1975.

33. **Iwata, K., Yamaguchi, H., and Hiratani, T.,** Mode of action of clotrimazole, *Sabouraudia,* 11, 158, 1973.

34. **Sud, I. J. and Feingold, D. S.,** Action of antifungal imidazoles on *Staphylococcus aureus, Antimicrob. Agents Chemother.,* 22, 470, 1982.

35. **Kimura, L. H. and Pearsall, N. N.,** Adherence of *Candida albicans* to human buccal epithelial cells, *Infect. Immun.,* 28, 464, 1980.

36. **Sobel, J. D., Meyers, P. G., Kaye, D., and Lesion, M. E.,** Adherence of *Candida albicans* to human vaginal and buccal epithelial cells, *J. Infect. Dis.,* 143, 76, 1981.

37. **Odds, F. C.,** *Candida and Candidosis,* Odds, F. C., Ed., Leicester University Press, Leicester, 1979.

38. **Brant, E. C. and Pollock, J. J.,** Inhibition of *Candida albicans* germ tube formation by histidine peptides, *J. Dent. Res.,* (Sp. Issue), 65, 268 (Abstr. 888), 1986.

39. **Hocking, W. G. and Golde, D. W.,** The pulmonary-alveolar macrophage, *N. Engl. J. Med.,* 301, 580, 639, 1979.

40. **Carrol, S. F. and Martinez, R. J.,** Purification and properties of rabbit alveolar macrophage lysozyme, *Infect. Immun.,* 24, 460, 1979.

41. **Weiss, J., Elsbach, P., Olsson, I., and Odeberg, H.,** Purification and characterization of a potent bacteridical and membrane-active protein from the granules of human polymorphonuclear leukocytes, *J. Biol. Chem.,* 253, 2664, 1978.

42. **Drazin, R. E. and Lehrer, R. I.,** Fungicidal properties of a chymotrypsin-like cationic protein from human neutrophils: adsorption to *Candida parapsilosis, Infect. Immun.,* 17, 382, 1977.

43. **Odeberg, H. and Olsson, I.,** Antibacterial activity of cationic proteins from human granulocytes, *J. Clin. Invest.,* 56, 1118, 1975.

44. **Patterson-Delafield, J., Sklarek, D., Martinez, R. J., and Lehrer, R. I.,** Microbicidal cationic proteins of rabbit alveolar macrophages: amino acid composition and functional attributes, *Infect. Immun.,* 31, 723, 1981.

45. **Selsted, M. E., Szklarek, D., and Lehrer, R. I.,** Purification and antibacterial activity of antimicrobial peptides of rabbit granulocytes, *Infect. Immun.,* 45, 150, 1984.

46. **Selsted, M. E., Brown, D. M., DeLange, R. J., and Lehrer, R. I.,** Primary structures of MCP-1 and MCP-2, natural peptide antibiotics of rabbit lung macrophages, *J. Biol. Chem.,* 258, 14485, 1983.

47. **Selsted, M. E., Brown, D. M., DeLange, R. J., Harwig, S. S. L., and Lehrer, R. I.,** Primary structures of six antimicrobial peptides of rabbit peritoneal neutrophils, *J. Biol. Chem.,* 260, 4579, 1985.

48. **Shepherd, M. G., Poulter, R. T. M., and Sullivan, P. A.,** *Candida albicans:* biology, genetics, and pathogenicity, *Ann. Rev. Microbiol.,* 39, 579, 1985.

Chapter 7

# GENETIC PROTEIN POLYMORPHISMS OF HUMAN SALIVA

**Edwin A. Azen**

## TABLE OF CONTENTS

# I. INTRODUCTION

Human saliva is an easily obtained source of material for genetic and biochemical analysis.[1] In particular, there are several advantages of the parotid saliva component (collected with the Curby cup) over whole saliva for analyzing many proteins. These advantages are a more uniform composition, less tendency for enzymatic degradation of proteins, and less extraneous contamination with food and bacteria. There are about 25 to 35 proteins in stimulated parotid saliva (150 to 264 mg/100 ml total protein[2]) that can be stained in acid polyacrylamide or SDS gels with Coomassie Brilliant Blue R-250. Most of these components are proline-rich proteins (PRPs) and amylase. The PRPs, representing about two thirds of the parotid salivary proteins, show numerous genetically determined polymorphisms.[3] In addition, there are numerous enzymes and other proteins (such as the $B_{12}$ binding R proteins) that can also be identified by sensitive techniques.

In this chapter I will report recent advances in the understanding of human salivary protein polymorphisms since the subject was last reviewed.[4-6] First, the more recently described studies of salivary protein polymorphisms (mainly among PRPs) will be briefly discussed. Second, advances in genetic understanding of the exceedingly complex PRP gene family will be examined. Finally, electrophoretic characterization of many different PRPs will be described in several gel systems.

# II. RECENT STUDIES OF SALIVARY PROTEIN POLYMORPHISMS

Representative population data of newly described as well as previously studied polymorphisms are given in Table 1, and some striking racial differences in gene frequencies of polymorphic variants are shown. For example, PIF$^+$ is much less frequent in blacks than in whites; however, Db$^+$ is much more frequent in blacks than in whites, while Pb$^2$ and Pr$^{1\prime}$ and some Amy variants are virtually confined to blacks. The Rs$^2$ variant, commonly seen in whites, is not seen in Chinese; however, Pm$^+$ is much more frequent in Orientals than in whites, and Gl$^5$ and Gl$^6$ are seen at low frequencies in Japanese, but not in whites.

## A. Salivary Amylase (Amy)

Merritt and Karn[7] summarized genetic variants that were detected by alkaline polyacrylamide slab gel electrophoresis. The combined frequency of these autosomal variants is low in whites (less than 1%) and only reaches polymorphic proportions (7%) in blacks. In contrast, Pronk[8] and Pronk and Frants[9] found, by isoelectric focusing in slab gels, evidence for two new alleles (Amy$_1$ R$^1$ and Amy$_1$R$^2$) in the Dutch population, with frequencies of 0.06 and 0.03, respectively. These Amy variants are probably of the fast electrophoretic type, Amy$_1$R$^1$, as described by Merritt and Karn.[7] They recognized rare Amy$_1$R$^1$ homozygotes but were unable to resolve the more common heterozygote phenotypes. It is also likely[99] that previously described amylase variants[91,92] are of the same general type as those more recently described by Pronk.[8] De Soyza[10] independently made similar observations in a white population by isoelectric focusing in slab gel and described six Amy phenotypes representing four alleles. Kühnl and Tischberger[11] studied salivary amylase in a white population by isoelectric focusing in slab gels and found that the gene frequencies of the three common alleles were very similar to those recorded by Pronk and Frants.[9] Using isoelectric focusing in slab gels, Eckersall and Beeley[12] described, in a white population, several amylase variants with a combined frequency of 11.7%. They used a starch-iodine procedure which is more sensitive than protein staining for detecting amylase variants. Pronk et al.[93] found evidence for duplication of the human salivary amylase gene. The evidence was based on analysis of a puzzling electrophoretic pattern interpreted to represent three different amylase gene products in each of four individuals.

## Table 1
## GENE FREQUENCIES OF SALIVARY PROTEIN POLYMORPHISMS IN DIFFERENT POPULATIONS

| System | Population | $S^a$ | n | $Amy^A$ | Others | Ref. |
|---|---|---|---|---|---|---|
| $Amy_1$ (amylase[b]) (in alkaline PAGE) | Whites (America) | WS | 961 | 0.995 | 0.005 | 7 |
| | Blacks (America) | WS | 208 | 0.961 | 0.039 | |
| | Japanese (Japan) | WS | 529 | 0.988 | 0.012 | 41 |
| | Whites (Japan) | PS | 96 | 1.000 | | 25 |

| System | Population | $S^a$ | n | $Amy_1^1$ | $Amy_1^2$ | $Amy_1^3$ | Others | Ref. |
|---|---|---|---|---|---|---|---|---|
| $Amy_1$ (in isoelectric focusing gels)[c] | Whites (England) | WS | 160 | 0.891 | 0.069 | 0.038 | 0.00 | 10 |
| | Whites (Netherlands) | PS | 330 | 0.907 | 0.067 | 0.027 | | 13 |
| | Blacks (West Africa, Bozo) | | 71 | 0.875 | 0.015 | | 0.101 | |
| | Blacks (Kenya) | | 200 | 0.959 | 0.008 | | 0.051 | 11 |
| | Whites (Germany) | WS | 170 | 0.909 | 0.070 | | | |
| | Whites (Scotland) | WS | 368 | 0.933 | 0.044 | 0.021 | 0.067 | 12 |

| System | Population | $S^a$ | n | $Con\ 1^+$ | $Con\ 1^-$ | Ref. |
|---|---|---|---|---|---|---|
| Con 1 (Concanavalin A) | Whites (America) | PS | 134 | 0.396 | 0.604 | 29 |
| | Chinese (America) | | 79 | 0.580 | 0.420 | |
| | Blacks (America) | | 74 | 0.581 | 0.419 | |

| System | Population | $S^a$ | n | $Con\ 2^+$ | $Con\ 2^-$ | Ref. |
|---|---|---|---|---|---|---|
| Con 2 (Concanavalin A) | Whites (America) | PS | 134 | 0.034 | 0.966 | 29 |
| | Chinese (America) | | 79 | 0 | 1.000 | |
| | Blacks (America) | | 74 | 0.007 | 0.993 | |

## Table 1 (continued)
## GENE FREQUENCIES OF SALIVARY PROTEIN POLYMORPHISMS IN DIFFERENT POPULATIONS

| System | Population | S$^a$ | n | Db$^+$ | Db$^-$ | Others | Ref. |
|---|---|---|---|---|---|---|---|
| Db (double band) | Whites (America) | PS | 100 | 0.12 | 0.88 | | 42 |
| | Blacks (America) | | 100 | 0.56 | 0.44 | | |
| | Chinese (America) | | 54 | 0.07 | 0.93 | | |
| | Japanese (Japan) | PS | 350 | 0.033 | 0.967 | | 41 |
| | Whites (Japan) | PS | 94 | 0.143 | 0.857 | | 25 |
| | Whites (Netherlands) | PS | 100 | 0.19 | 0.81 | | 13 |
| | Blacks (Kenya) | | 200 | 0.55 | 0.45 | | |
| | Whites (America) | PS | 685 | 0.179 | 0.821 | | 43 |

| System | Population | S$^a$ | n | Gl$^1$ | Gl$^2$ | Gl$^3$ | Gl$^4$ | Gl$^0$ | Others | Ref. |
|---|---|---|---|---|---|---|---|---|---|---|
| Gl (major salivary glycoprotein) | Whites (America) | PS | 143 | 0.742 | 0.040 | 0.155 | 0.017 | 0.046 | | 21 |
| | Blacks (America) | | 82 | 0.459 | 0.050 | 0.337 | 0.044 | 0.110 | | |
| | Japanese (Japan) | PS | 104 | 0.555 | 0.033 | 0.245 | 0.033 | 0.105 | 0.029 | 23 |

| System | Population | S$^a$ | n | Pa$^1$(+) | Pa$^0$(−) | Pa$^2$(+) | Ref. |
|---|---|---|---|---|---|---|---|
| Pa (acidic protein) | Whites (America) | PS | 330 | 0.21 | 0.79 | | 44 |
| | Blacks (America) | | 122 | 0.14 | 0.86 | | |
| | Orientals (America) | | 6 | 0.42 | 0.58 | | |
| | Whites (America) | PS | 101 | 0.208 | 0.787 | 0.005 | 45 |
| | Whites (America) | PS | 685 | 0.211 | 0.789 | | 43 |
| | Japanese (Japan) | PS | 554 | 0.221 | 0.779 | | 41 |
| | Whites (Japan) | PS | 96 | 0.158 | 0.842 | | 25 |
| | Whites (Netherlands) | PS | 100 | 0.12 | 0.88 | | 13 |
| | Blacks (Kenya) | PS | 200 | 0.18 | 0.82 | | |

| Pb (parotid basic protein) | S* | n | Pb¹ | Pb² | Ref. |
|---|---|---|---|---|---|
| Whites (America) | PS | 101 | 0.995 | 0.005 | 46 |
| Blacks (America) | PS | 90 | 0.840 | 0.160 | 41 |
| Japanese (Japan) | PS | 435 | 1.000 | | 13 |
| Whites (Netherlands) | PS | 110 | 1.000 | | |
| Blacks (West Africa, Bozo) | | 71 | 0.800 | 0.200 | |
| Blacks (Kenya) | PS | 200 | 0.880 | 0.120 | 25 |
| Whites (Japan) | PS | 91 | 1.000 | | |

| Pc (protein) | S* | n | Pc¹ | Pc² | Ref. |
|---|---|---|---|---|---|
| Whites (America) | PS | 178 | 0.461 | 0.539 | 37 |
| Blacks (America) | PS | 47 | 0.670 | 0.330 | |

| Pe (protein) | S* | n | Pe⁺ | Pe⁻ | Ref. |
|---|---|---|---|---|---|
| Whites (America) | PS | 317 | 0.76 | 0.24 | 30 |
| Blacks (America) | PS | 51 | 0.76 | 0.24 | |

| Ph (parotid heavy band) | S* | n | Ph⁺ | Ph⁻ | Ref. |
|---|---|---|---|---|---|
| Japanese (Japan) | PS | 440 | 0.029 | 0.971 | 41 |
| Whites (Japan) | PS | 96 | 0 | 1.000 | 25 |
| Malays (Malaysia) | WS | 147 | 0.082 | 0.918 | 47 |
| Chinese (Malaysia) | | 189 | 0.109 | 0.891 | |
| Indians (Malaysia) | | 175 | 0.062 | 0.938 | |

| PIF (parotid isoelectric focusing variant) | S* | n | PIF⁺ | PIF⁻ | Ref. |
|---|---|---|---|---|---|
| Whites (America) | PS | 148 | 0.66 | 0.34 | 38 |
| Blacks (America) | | 90 | 0.35 | 0.65 | |
| Chinese (America) | | 78 | 0.56 | 0.44 | |
| Japanese (Japan) | PS | 257 | 0.721 | 0.279 | 41 |

## Table 1 (continued)
## GENE FREQUENCIES OF SALIVARY PROTEIN POLYMORPHISMS IN DIFFERENT POPULATIONS

| System | Population | S* | n | Pm+ | Pm− | Others | Ref. |
|---|---|---|---|---|---|---|---|
| Pm (parotid middle band — also called PmF[26] | Japanese (Japan) | PS | 426 | 0.399 | 0.601 | | 41 |
| | Whites (America) | PS | 140 | 0.15 | 0.85 | | 26 |
| | Noraini et al | WS | | | | | 47 |
| | Malays (Malaysia) | | 172 | 0.385 | 0.615 | | |
| | Chinese (Malaysia) | | 186 | 0.282 | 0.718 | | |
| | Indians (Malaysia) | | 180 | 0.289 | 0.711 | | |
| | Whites (Japan) | PS | 86 | 0.14 | 0.86 | | 25 |

| System | Population | S* | n | PmS+ | PmS− | | Ref. |
|---|---|---|---|---|---|---|---|
| PmS (parotid middle band, slow) | Whites (America) | PS | 140 | 0.12 | 0.88 | | 26 |
| | Blacks (America) | | 101 | 0.24 | 0.76 | | d |
| | Japanese (Japan) | PS | 254 | 0.354 | 0.646 | | |

| System | Population | S* | n | Po+ | Po− | | Ref. |
|---|---|---|---|---|---|---|---|
| Po (protein) | Whites (America) | PS | 408 | 0.75 | 0.25 | | 30 |
| | Blacks (America) | | 59 | 0.77 | 0.23 | | |

| System | Population | S* | n | Pr1 | Pr2 | Pr1' | Ref. |
|---|---|---|---|---|---|---|---|
| Pr (proline-rich proteins) | Whites (America)e | PS | 100 | 0.640 | 0.355 | 0.005 | 42 |
| | Blacks (America)e | | 100 | 0.700 | 0.250 | 0.050 | |
| | Oriental (America)e | | 54 | 0.770 | 0.230 | | |
| | Japanese (Japan) | PS | 453 | 0.741 | 0.259 | | 41 |
| | Whites (Netherlands) | PS | 100 | 0.81 | 0.19 | | 13 |

| | $S^{[a]}$ | n | $Ps^1$ | $Ps^2$ | $Ps^0$ | Others | Ref. |
|---|---|---|---|---|---|---|---|
| Blacks (Kenya) | PS | 200 | 0.66 | 0.34 | | | 25 |
| Whites (Japan) | PS | 95 | 0.721 | 0.279 | | | 43 |
| Whites (America) | PS | 685 | 0.718 | 0.282 | | | |

| $Ps$ (parotid size variant) | $S^{[a]}$ | n | $Ps^1$ | $Ps^2$ | $Ps^0$ | Others | Ref. |
|---|---|---|---|---|---|---|---|
| Whites (America) | PS | 150 | 0.598 | 0.101 | 0.301 | | 26 |
| Blacks (America) | PS | 101 | 0.185 | 0.126 | 0.689 | | |
| Japanese (Japan) | PS | 317 | 0.298 | | 0.652 | 0.047 | d |

| $Rs$ ($B_{12}$ binding R proteins) | $S^{[a]}$ | n | $Rs^1$ | $Rs^2$ | Ref. |
|---|---|---|---|---|---|
| Whites (America) | PS | 143 | 0.88 | 0.12 | 15 |
| Blacks (America) | WS | 104 | 0.94 | 0.06 | 16 |
| Chinese (America) | | 75 | 1.00 | | |
| Whites (America) | | 452 | 0.88 | 0.12 | |
| Blacks (America) | | 48 | 0.99 | 0.01 | |
| Chinese (America) | | 136 | 1.00 | | |

| $Sal_I$ (proteins)[f] | $S^{[a]}$ | n | $Sal_I^F$ | $Sal_I^r$ | Ref. |
|---|---|---|---|---|---|
| Whites (Hawaii) | WS | 154 | 0.403 | 0.597 | 48 |
| Japanese (Hawaii) | | 42 | 0.364 | 0.636 | |

| $Sal_{II}$ (proteins)[f] | $S^{[a]}$ | n | $Sal_{II}^S$ | $Sal_{II}^s$ | Ref. |
|---|---|---|---|---|---|
| Whites (Hawaii) | WS | 154 | 0.573 | 0.427 | 48 |
| Japanese (Hawaii) | | 42 | 0.591 | 0.409 | |

| $Sap_A$ (acid phsophatase) | $S^{[a]}$ | n | $Sap_A^A$ | $Sap_A^{A'}$ | $Sap_A^O$ | Ref. |
|---|---|---|---|---|---|---|
| Whites (Hawaii) | WS | 213 | 0.698 | 0.009 | 0.293 | 20 |
| Japanese (Hawaii) | | 72 | 0.731 | 0.014 | 0.255 | |

## Table 1 (continued)
## GENE FREQUENCIES OF SALIVARY PROTEIN POLYMORPHISMS IN DIFFERENT POPULATIONS

| System | Population | Sᵃ | n | s-AcPᴬ | s-AcPᴮ | | Others | Ref. |
|---|---|---|---|---|---|---|---|---|
| s-AcP (acid phosphatase) | Japanese (Japan) | PS | 183 | 0.227 | 0.773 | | | 19 |

| System | Population | Sᵃ | n | SAPX¹ | SAPX² | SAPX³ | Others | Ref. |
|---|---|---|---|---|---|---|---|---|
| SAPX (salivary peroxidase) | Whites (America) | PS | 101 | 0.787 | 0.208 | 0.005 | | 45 |
| | Malays (Malaysia) | WS | 143 | 0.762 | 0.238 | | | 47 |
| | Chinese (Malaysia) | | 151 | 0.755 | 0.245 | | | |
| | Indians (Malaysia) | | 180 | 0.723 | 0.277 | | | |

| System | Population | Sᵃ | n | Sgd¹ | Sgd² | Others | Ref. |
|---|---|---|---|---|---|---|---|
| Sgd (glucose-6-phosphate dehydrogenase) | Whites (Hawaii) | WS | 190 | 0.755 | 0.245 | | 49 |
| | Japanese (Hawaii) | | 104 | 0.659 | 0.341 | | |

| System | Population | Sᵃ | n | Set_iᶠ | Set_iˢ | Others | Ref. |
|---|---|---|---|---|---|---|---|
| Set_i (carboxylesterase) | Whites (Hawaii) | WS | 96 | 0.609 | 0.391 | | 50 |
| | Japanese (Hawaii) | | 53 | 0.500 | 0.500 | | |

a Saliva source: WS is whole saliva; PS is parotid saliva.

b An extensive compilation of allelic frequencies of Amy tested by alkaline PAGE is presented by Merritt and Karn.[7]

c The nomenclature of Kühnl and Tischberger[11] is used.

d Minaguchi, K. and Suzuki, K., personal communication.

e These data were recalculated by assuming that the phenotypes of all Pr 2' individuals are both Pr 2 and Pa⁺.

f These polymorphisms studied in whole saliva are probably among acidic Pr proteins.[4]

It is difficult to compare the new amylase variants found by the different investigators, since isoelectric points were not always given. The biochemical basis of the variant phenotypes has not been determined, but their polymorphic frequencies extend the usefulness of salivary amylase for further genetic studies.

## B. B₁₂ Binding Protein (Rs)

Human $B_{12}$ binding proteins can be divided into three classes: gastric intrinsic factor, which facilitates $B_{12}$ absorption from the small intenstine; plasma transcobalamin II (TC II), which facilitates cellular uptake of $B_{12}$ by tissues; and R proteins, which are found in several body fluids and tissues. It is hypothesized that the R proteins may subserve antibacterial, transport, or protective binding functions. Based on current evidence, summarized by Allen,[14] all R proteins share a common protein backbone and differ from each other only in the amount and proportion of attached carbohydrates. From current biochemical and genetic evidence, these three classes of $B_{12}$ binding proteins are probably products of three genes.

Azen and Denniston[15] found in parotid saliva a polymorphism of $B_{12}$ binding R proteins in blacks and whites, and the polymorphism (Rs) is determined by autosomal inheritance of two codominant alleles. After neuraminidase treatment and radiolabeling ($^{57}CoB_{12}$) of the Rs proteins in parotid saliva, the Rs polymorphism is determined by isoelectric focusing in slab gels (ph 4 to 6.5). The Rs polymorphism is shared by $B_{12}$ binding R proteins of milk, tears, and leukocytes. In a later study, using similar methods, Yang et al.[16] found the same polymorphism in whole saliva and granulocytes.

Genetic polymorphism of the plasma $B_{12}$ binder, TC II, has also been described by Daiger et al.[17] and Fráter-Schröeder et al.[18] We found no evidence for close linkage between Rs and TC II or between Rs and several PRP genetic determinants.[15]

## C. Salivary Acid Phosphatase (s-AcP)

Ikemoto et al.[19] described in a Japanese population genetic polymorphism of human parotid salivary acid phosphatase (s-AcP) in isoelectric focusing slab gels (pH 4.0 to 6.5) stained enzymatically for acid phosphatase. Three variant protein patterns are determined by two codominant alleles at an autosomal locus. The relationship of this polymorphism to that described in whole saliva by Tan and Ashton[20] is unclear.

## D. PRP Polymorphisms

Four PRP polymorphisms — namely, Pr,[42,55] Db,[42] Pa,[44] and Pm(PmF)[31] — were found before the period of this review. Nine new PRP polymorphisms were discovered subsequently and will be described individually next. The general features of the PRP polymorphisms and gene family will be discussed later. Studies of PRP polymorphisms have led to the concept of a closely linked multigene family that is located on a single autosome and that determines all of the salivary PRPs.

### 1. Major Parotid Salivary Glycoprotein (Gl)

Earlier studies (summarized in Reference 21) had identified a heterogeneous group of salivary basic PRPs, and some of these were glycosylated. The major parotid salivary glycoprotein contains about 40% carbohydrate, is especially rich in proline, glycine, and glutamic acid, has an isoelectric point of greater than pH 8.2, and has a molecular weight of around 36,000. Levine et al.[22] state that this glycoprotein accounts for 21 to 25% of stimulated parotid salivary proteins and 75% of the total carbohydrate.

Azen et al.[21] stained parotid salivary proteins in acid polyacrylamide slab gels (Figure 5) with the periodic acid-Schiff stain for glycoproteins and described genetic polymorphism of Gl. Gl is the same as the IA glycoprotein of Kauffman and Keller[32] (Table 2). The polymorphism is determined by autosomal inheritance of at least four expressed alleles and one

**Table 2**
**ELECTROPHORETIC IDENTITIES OF PURIFIED PRPs WITH PRP GENETIC POLYMORPHISMS**

| Basic PRPs[32a] | Genetic PRP polymorphisms | | Basic PRPs[a] (other workers) | | Acidic PRPs[3,57] |
| --- | --- | --- | --- | --- | --- |
| | System | Ref. | System | Ref. | |
| IB-1 | | | | | |
| IB-4 | | | P-H | 89 | |
| IB-5 | Po | 30 | P-D | 36 | |
| IB-6 | PmS | 26 | P-I | 89 | |
| IB-7 | | | P-G | 89 | |
| IB-8a | Pc | 37 | | | |
| IB-8b | | | P-F | 35 | |
| IB-9 | PMF | 31 | P-E | 33 | |
| IIB-1 | | | | | |
| IIB-2 | Pe | 30 | | | |
| IA | Gl[b] | 21 | | | |
| | Ps | 26 | | | |
| | Con 1 | 29 | | | |
| | Con 2 | 29 | | | |
| | | | P-B | 73 | |
| | | | P-C | 62 | |
| | Pr | 55 | | | PrI, PrII, PrIII, Pr IV |
| | Pa | 44 | | | |
| | Db | 42 | | | |
| | PIF | 38 | | c | |

[a]   Although electrophoretically identical, there are biochemically unresolved amino acid differences between PRPs IB-4 and P-H, between PRPs IB-5 and P-D, between PRPs IB-6 and P-I, and between PRPs IB-8b and P-F.[101]
[b]   Ph[24] may be an allele of Gl (see text).
[c]   PIF polymorphic proteins were probably copurified with PRPs C and A.[39,102]

unexpressed allele in blacks and whites. Minaguchi et al.[23] recently studied a Japanese population of Gl variants. They found two new very slow migrating variants in acid polyacrylamide slab gels, and this will be discussed later with relationship to the Ph protein polymorphism. From family studies, there was strong evidence for close linkage of Gl to genetic determinants for other PRPs.[21] This was the first evidence that the closely linked multigene PRP family includes genetic determinants for basic as well as acidic PRPs, and it strongly suggested that genes determining other salivary PRPs would also be linked to the same gene family. Amino acid compositions of Gl 1 and Gl 4 variant proteins strongly resembled the compositions of the major basic glycoprotein and acidic PRPs described by others. The Gl protein polymorphism is determined by apparent differences in molecular weights of the variant proteins. This is an unusual finding, since most previously described protein polymorphisms are due to charge differences. The molecular basis for the apparent molecular weight differences of Gl variant proteins is not known, although data from DNA analysis of PRP genes (to be discussed later) suggest unequal crossing over as a possible mechanism.

### 2. Salivary Parotid Heavy Protein (Ph)

Ikemoto et al.[24] described, in a Japanese population, genetic polymorphism of a large glycoprotein in SDS urea gels. The polymorphism is characterized by autosomal dominant (Ph$^+$) and recessive (Ph$^-$) forms. Since the Ph and Gl proteins are of similar molecular size in SDS gels and both are well stained for carbohydrate with the periodic acid-Schiff stain, it is possible that the Ph protein is an allelic form of the Gl protein. Additionally, as Minaguchi et al.[23] point out in a later paper, two very slow migrating Gl variant proteins observed in the acid polyacrylamide gel system are seen in Japanese but not in whites. It is thus likely that one or both of these Gl variants might represent the Ph protein(s), since the Ph$^+$ variant (like the slow Gl variants) was also not seen in whites.[25]

### 3. Parotid Size Variant (Ps)

Azen and Denniston[26] described in blacks and whites genetic polymorphism of the basic Ps protein in acid polyacrylamide slab gels stained with Coomassie Brilliant Blue R-250. The electrophoretic polymorphism (as with Gl) is manifested by apparent differences in molecular weights in acid polyacrylamide and SDS gels (Figure 3, 4, 6, and 7A). Goodman and Karn[27] have confirmed these molecular weight differences by subjecting purified Ps proteins to limited proteolysis with several enzymes. Digestion patterns indicate considerable homology between Ps isoproteins.

The Ps polymorphism is determined by autosomal inheritance of expressed and unex- pressed alleles. In the initial report, only two expressed alleles were found, but Minaguchi and Suzuki[100] later found, in a Japanese population, evidence for other Ps variants. There is strong evidence for close linkage between Ps and other genetic determinants for PRPs.[26,28] Amino acid analysis of the Ps proteins indicates that they have the typical amino acid composition of the PRP family.[28] Furthermore, Ps proteins cross-react immunologically with other PRPs when tested with antisera to several specific PRPs[26,29,30] (Figure 7B). The Ps proteins have not been identified with any of the basic PRPs purified from saliva by other workers (Table 2).

### 4. Slow Parotid Middle Band (PmS)

Azen and Denniston[26] described in blacks and whites genetic polymorphism of the basic protein PmS in acid polyacrylamide slab gels stained with Coomassie Brilliant Blue R-250 (Figures 3 and 4). The polymorphism is manifested by autosomal inheritance of one expressed (PmS$^+$) and one unexpressed (PmS$^-$) allele. Phenotypically, it is closely associated with the smaller Pm(PmF) protein described by Ikemoto et al.[31] Thus, the PmS$^+$ type is always associated with PmF$^+$, and the PmS$^-$ type is almost always associated with PmF$^-$ (Table 3). The nature of this strong association of PmS and PmF proteins is unclear. The Pm genetic determinants are closely linked to those for other PRPs,[26,28] and the Pm proteins are im- munologically related to other PRPs[26,29,30] (Figure 7B). Minaguchi et al.[34] showed that the amino acid composition of the Pm protein is typical for a PRP. The PmF and PmS proteins are electrophoretically the same as the PRPs IB-9 and IB-6, respectively, of Kauffman and Keller[32] and PRPs P-E[33] and P-I[89] (Table 2). However, biochemically there are unresolved amino acid differences between PRPs IB-6 and P-I.[101]

### 5. Concanavalin A Binding Salivary Proteins (Con 1 and Con 2)

In parotid saliva of blacks and whites, Azen and Yu[29] found two basic protein poly- morphisms (Con 1 and Con 2), each of which is determined by autosomal inheritance of one expressed ($+$) and one unexpressed ($-$) allele. The Con proteins are typed after electrophoretic transfer of salivary proteins from SDS gels to nitrocellulose and identification with peroxidase labeled concanavalin A (Figure 8B). The genetic determinants for these proteins are tightly linked to those for other PRPs.[29] The Con proteins cross-react immu- nologically with other PRPs when tested with antisera to several specific PRPs.[29] They have not been identified, however, with basic PRPs of other workers (Table 2).

### 6. Pe Protein

This polymorphism, described in parotid saliva of blacks and whites by Azen and Yu,[30]

### Table 3
### SOME SIGNIFICANTLY POSITIVE ASSOCIATION (OBS./EXP.) IN RANDOMLY COLLECTED PAROTID SALIVA SAMPLES FROM WHITES

|  | Pa+ | Pa− |  |
|---|---|---|---|
| Pr 2 types | 37/13.9 | 0/23.1 | 37 |
| Other Pr types | 1/24.1 | 63/39.9 | 64 |
|  | 38 | 63 | 101 |

$X^2 = 92.7, p < 0.0001$

|  | Con 2+ | Con 2− |  |
|---|---|---|---|
| PmF+ | 9/2.3 | 25/31.7 | 34 |
| PmF− | 0/6.7 | 100/93.3 | 100 |
|  | 9 | 125 | 134 |

$X^2 = 24.31, p < 0.0001$

|  | PmS+ | PmS− |  |
|---|---|---|---|
| PmF+ | 25/6.5 | 9/27.5 | 34 |
| PmF− | 0/18.5 | 96/77.5 | 96 |
|  | 25 | 105 | 130 |

$X^2 = 82.7, p < 0.0001$

*Note:* Association data for Pa/Pr are from Azen;[45] for Con 2/Pm F and PmS/Pm F, from Azen and Yu.[29]

is determined by autosomal inheritance of one expressed (Pe$^+$) and one unexpressed (Pe$^-$) allele. The Pe protein polymorphism is typed in alkaline polyacrylamide slab gels stained with Coomassie Brilliant Blue R-250 (Figure 1). The genetic determinant for Pe is probably closely linked to those of other PRPs, and the Pe protein cross-reacts immunologically with other PRPs.[30] The Pe protein is electrophoretically the same as the IIB-2 PRP of Kauffman and Keller[32] (Table 2), and it has an isoelectric point of approximately pH 6.1 to 6.3. This isoelectric point is unusual for a PRP which is usually much more basic or acidic.

### 7. Po Protein

This basic protein polymorphism,[30] found in parotid saliva of blacks and whites, is determined by autosomal inheritance of one expressed (Po$^+$) and one unexpressed (Po$^-$) allele. After electrophoretic transfer of salivary proteins from SDS gels to nitrocellulose (Figure 7), the polymorphism is typed by immunologic reactivity to anti-PRP serum or by protein staining. The Po protein is electrophoretically the same as the PRPs IB-5[32] and P-D[36] (Table 2). Biochemically, however, there are unresolved amino acid differences between PRPs IB-5 and P-D.[101]

### 8. Pc Protein

Karn et al.[37] described this polymorphism in parotid saliva of blacks and whites, and it is determined by autosomal inheritance of two expressed alleles. The polymorphism is typed after electrophoresis and protein staining in acid polyacrylamide slab gels (Figure 9). The Pc protein immunologically cross-reacts with the Pr 1 and Ps 1 proteins by Ouchterlony analysis when tested against an antiserum to whole parotid salivary proteins. The amino acid compositions of the Pc proteins are very similar to those of other basic PRPs,[37] and by electrophoretic analysis (Table 2) the Pc protein is the same as the IB-8a PRP of Kauffman and Keller.[32] There is suggestive but not conclusive evidence of linkage of the Pc genetic determinant to those of other PRPs.

### 9. Parotid Isoelectric Focusing Variant (PIF)

Azen and Denniston[38] found this genetic polymorphism in parotid salivary proteins of blacks, whites, and Chinese. The polymorphism is detected after separation in urea isoelectric focusing slab gels (pH 3.5 to 5.2) and staining with Coomassie Brilliant Blue R-250 (Figure 2), or more conveniently by simply precipitating the proteins in the slab gel with trichloracetic acid. The phenotypes (which are determined by autosomal inheritance) consist of a pair of bands (PIF S and PIF F) that are either present (PIF$^+$) or absent (PIF$^-$) from all salivas. The genetic determinant for the PIF proteins is closely linked to that for Gl, a known PRP.[38] In addition, PIF proteins show unusual staining reactions that are typical for acidic PRPs (to be discussed later). The cDNA for the PIF protein has probably been isolated from a cDNA library prepared from the human parotid gland, and its structure is clearly that of an acidic PRP.[39] As will be discussed later, the PIF F protein may be derived from the PIF S protein by posttranslational proteolytic cleavage. The PIF S and PIF F proteins have isoelectric points that are very close to those for the acidic PRPs, Pr 1 and Pr 3, respectively. Therefore, the PIF and Pr proteins would have been difficult to separate during previous attempts at purification of Pr proteins.[40] Indeed, the PIF proteins were probably inadvertently copurified with acidic PRPs C and A.[39,102]

## III. THE PRP GENE FAMILY

### A. Studies of Genetic Polymorphisms Among Proline-Rich Proteins (PRPs)

The PRPs constitute about 70% of the proteins of human saliva, and proline alone accounts for 25 to 42% of amino acids of PRPs.[3] Proline, glycine, and glutamine (glutamic acid) together constitute 70 to 88% of amino acids of PRPs. Although there is some overlap between glycosylated and basic PRPs, the PRPs can be roughly subdivided into three groups: glycosylated, basic, and acidic accounting for approximately 17%, 23%, and 30%, respectively, of the total protein in parotid saliva. PRPs have also been found in acinic cell carcinomas of the parotid salivary glands.[94] Some probable tooth-related functions[3] have been assigned to acidic PRPs in saliva: these include binding to calcium and maintaining it in the supersaturated state (thus avoiding calcium precipitation in saliva ducts or in the oral cavity); forming a part of the dental pellicle; and binding to hydroxyapatite. Since PRPs are found in serous cells of the submucosal glands of the respiratory tract, they may subserve other functions such as effects of viscosity.[51,52] In the rat and mouse, the production of PRPs is stimulated by feeding sorghums containing the high levels of tannins.[53,54] Apparently tannins are toxic, carcinogenic, and bind strongly to salivary PRPs. Therefore, it was proposed that salivary PRPs may tightly bind tannins and thus protect dietary proteins, digestive enzymes, and the gastrointestinal tract from these detrimental effects.

The many PRPs show complex electrophoretic patterns that vary markedly between individuals. Some of these variations are due to numerous genetic polymorphisms, and others to posttranslational processes such as proteolysis. Polymorphisms for acidic PRPs include Pr (proline rich),[42,55] Pa (acidic protein),[4,44,45] Db (double band),[42] and PIF (parotid isoelectric-focusing variant).[38] Polymorphisms for basic PRPs are Pm (parotid middle band),[31] PmS (parotid middle slow band),[26] Ps (parotid size variant),[26] Gl (major glycoprotein),[21] Con 1 and Con 2 (Concanavalin A binding),[29] and Pc.[37] Polymorphism for the almost neutral Pe protein has also been described.[30]

Some workers have isolated PRPs from saliva for biochemical studies, and others have characterized them genetically. Therefore, several different terminologies were applied to the PRPs by these different workers. Previously, Anderson et al.[56] found that the PmS polymorphic protein is the same as the basic PRP IB-6, and the PmF polymorphic protein is the same as the basic PRP IB-9. In addition, Azen and Oppenheim[55] established the identity of the polymorphic acidic Pr proteins 1, 2, 3, and 4 with purified PRPs I, II, III, and IV.[57] Among other acidic PRPs, the PIF polymorphic proteins were probably inadvertently copurified with acidic PRPs C and A,[39,102] and Db and Pa polymorphic proteins may be among other acidic PRPs described by Hay and Oppenheim.[58] To further match polymorphic PRPs with other biochemically purified PRPs, E. Saitoh, D. Kauffman, and P. Keller kindly provided a number of purified basic PRPs for electrophoretic comparisons (in more than one gel system) with polymorphic PRPs, and the results are shown in Table 2. Thus, all of the available PRPs (including those not yet correlated with genetic polymorphisms) are shown in Table 2. Among the PRP polymorphisms only Ps, Con 1, and Con 2 proteins could not be electrophoretically identified with the available purified PRPs. However, although electrophoretically identical, there are biochemically unresolved amino acid differences between PRPs IB-4 and P-H, between PRPs IB-5 and P-D, between PRPs IB-6 and P-I, and between PRPs IB-8b and P-F.[101]

The PRP polymorphisms show several unusual phenotypic features which will now be described. These features include double-banded patterns among the acidic PRPs, molecular size variants among two of the basic PRPs, and frequent null (unexpressed) forms among a number of the PRP polymorphisms. The first described PRP genetic polymorphism was that called Pr.[42,55] Each Pr allele determines a double-banded phenotype (Figures 1 and 2). Three alleles (Pr 1, Pr 1', and Pr 2) at an autosomal locus could account for the variant double-banded phenotypes.[42] The allele Pr 2'[42] was later found to be the Pr 2 allele associated with the Pa+ allele.[45] Therefore, the designation Pr 2' is no longer appropriate. It was proposed that the double-banded pattern of the Pr proteins is due to proteolytic cleavage. Thus, Karn et al.[88] found that the more rapidly migrating Pr 3 and Pr 4 proteins are derived from the Pr 1 and Pr 2 proteins, respectively, by posttranslational cleavages by a salivary protease. Wong et al.[59] and Wong and Bennick[60] determined that amino acid sequences of protein A (Pr 3) and protein C (Pr 1). The sequence of protein A is identical to the N-terminal 106 residues of protein C, which is 150 residues in length. Wong et al.[61] found that the salivary protease kallakrein could cleave protein C (Pr 1) on the carboxyl side of Arg-106 *in vitro*. Isemura et al.[62] found a peptide, P-C, in saliva, and this peptide is identical to the C-terminal 44 residues of protein C (Pr 1). Although kallikrein is present in the saliva, Wong et al.[61] found no evidence that the proteolytic cleavage occurs primarily in the saliva or salivary ducts, implying that this process occurs mainly in the acinar cell of the gland.

The acidic PRPs, PIF,[38] and Db[42] also show double-banded patterns (Figures 1 and 2), and it is postulated that the smaller protein is generated from the larger one by proteolytic cleavage at Arg-106. There is strong evidence for this idea, at least for the PIF protein, since Maeda et al.[39] have isolated and sequenced the cDNAs for both the Pr 1 and PIF proteins. The derived amino acid sequences are identical except for two differences, and both proteins possess the Arg-106 residue.

The acidic Pa protein polymorphism[44] (unlike the Pr, Db, and PIF polymorphisms) shows only a single-banded rather than a double-banded pattern (Figures 1 and 2), and thus the Pa protein is probably not cleaved by proteolysis. Unlike all other known PRPs, the Pa protein is probably a dimer and contains cysteine residues[28] with a disulfide linkage between monomeric subunits.[4,45] The Pa protein monomer may also bind to salivary peroxidase through disulfide bond formation.[45,77,90] As will be discussed later, Maeda[67] proposed that $Pa^+$, $Db^+$, and $PIF^+$ phenotypes may be determined by expressed alleles at one locus. To account for the single-banded $Pa^+$ type as opposed to the double-banded $Db^+$ and $PIF^+$ types, she further proposed that the Pa protein monomer may contain an allelic amino acid substitution (cysteine) at the Arg-106 residue which may interfere with proteolytic cleavage at this site.

Two of the basic PRP polymorphisms (Gl and Ps) are unusual, since their allelic variants (Figures 5 and 7A) are characterized by molecular size rather than the usual charge differences.[21,26] Although there are other possibilities, the findings (to be discussed later) of similar and frequent tandem repeats in the PRPs suggest that unequal crossing over at the gene level might lead to deletions and duplications of DNA in coding regions, with consequent protein size differences. With the exception of Pr and Pc, all of the PRP polymorphisms show null phenotypes — that is, apparent lack of protein expression in saliva. The molecular basis for the null phenotypes among PRPs is unknown. As will be discussed later in more detail, Maeda[67] proposed for the acidic PRPs that $Pa^-$, $Db^-$, and $PIF^-$ null alleles may actually not exist if $Pa^+$, $Db^+$, and $PIF^+$ represent expressed alleles at a single locus without null alleles.

It was suggested that each of the recognized 13 PRP polymorphisms is determined by a different gene, 4 for the acidic PRPs and 9 for the others. Data from numerous family linkage studies (summarized by Goodman et al.[28]) indicate that the PRP polymorphisms are determined by a closely linked multigene family (on a single autosome) which may span 15 map units. The overall physical size of the PRP gene complex, however, remains undetermined pending completion of the DNA analysis to be described. Additionally, many studies (summarized by Goodman et al.[28]) show nonrandom associations between phenotypes determined by different loci. The exact nature of these associations is unknown, although in some cases linkage disequilibrium (related to closely linked genes) may be occurring. Several of the more striking associations are shown in Table 3 between PmS and PmF, Con 2 and PmF, and $Pa^+$ and Pr. Thus, samples are usually of the $PmF^+S^+$ or $PmF^-S^-$ types; samples of the $Con\ 2^+$ type are always also of the $PmF^+$ type; and samples of the $Pa^+$ type are usually also of the Pr 2 type.

The evolutionary implications of many protein studies suggest that the PRP multigene family probably evolved by a process of gene duplication. This conclusion seems likely, since there is good biochemical and immunologic evidence that the various PRPs are closely related. To summarize these data, many studies indicate that the various PRPs are strikingly similar in amino acid compositons.[3,28] The PRPs also show marked similarities in amino acid sequences. Thus, Kauffman et al.[63] showed that, with one exception, the first 54 residues in the amino acid sequence of IB-9 (PmF) and IB-6 (PmS) are identical. Furthermore, there is a high degree of homology between the amino acid sequences of IB-9 and IB-6 with the C-terminal portion of the acidic PRP, protein C. Additionally, amino acid sequence data[35,60,63] show an exceptional degree of internal repetition in different PRPs and indicate that these tandem repeats are very similar. Thus, it is not surprising that Azen and Denniston[26] and Azen and Yu,[29,30] using polyclonal rabbit antisera prepared to different basic and acidic PRPs, showed extensive immunologic cross-reactivity between many acidic and basic PRPs, underscoring the close biochemical relationships of the PRPs. Therefore, the hypothesized process of gene duplication within the PRP gene family may have occurred in part through unequal crossing over facilitated by the similar tandem repeats.

## B. DNA Studies of the PRP Gene Family

In order to determine the molecular organization of the PRP gene family and to further understand the complex expressions of PRPs in saliva, DNA cloning and nucleotide sequencing were initiated.[64] This was facilitated by using a PRP cDNA, PRP 33, synthesized and cloned from PRP mRNAs from parotid glands of isoproterenol-treated rats.[65] Isoproterenol dramatically increases the synthesis of PRPs. Rat PRP mRNAs and their protein products are homologous to human PRPs, since amino acid sequences deduced from the rat PRP cDNA clone show considerable homology to human PRP amino acid sequences.[65]

A library of human genomic DNA fragments in bacteriophage lambda Charon 4A was screened with the rat PRP cDNA probe.[64] Two phages (PRP 1 and PRP 2) were isolated and shown to contain related but not identical DNAs that hybridized to the probe. Preliminary nucleotide seqeunce data indicate that both of the DNAs include regions composed of nearly identical tandemly repeated sequences, each able to code for 21 amino acids. These repeat regions were cut frequently by BstNI endonuclease digestion. The decoded consensus repeat sequence is homologous to the repeating amino acid units found by others in human PRPs.[60,63,66] Thus, it is likely that the PRP 1 and PRP 2 genomic clones contain members of the PRP gene family. Polymorphic differences between DNAs of different individuals were observed after probing digests of human genomic DNA with a fragment from the repetitive region of the PRP 1 clone. These DNA polymorphisms reflect size differences, possibly caused by unequal crossing over between the repetitive units in the PRP genes. There was no evidence, however, for missing or half-intensity bands to explain the null alleles observed with the protein polymorphisms.

The nucleotide sequences of cDNAs for human PRPs were then determined.[39] A human cDNA library (prepared from mRNA from a normal human parotid gland) was screened with a DNA probe made from the region that contains tandem repeats in the human PRP gene clone, PRP 1. Two classes of cDNA were found, and they differ reproducibly in the structure of the repeat region they contain. Members of one class (BstNI type) have BstNI sites spaced approximately every 63 bp. The cDNAs with these BstNI-type repeats code for basic PRPs. Members of the other class (HaeIII type) have HaeIII sites which occur repeatedly and thus are named HaeIII-type repeats. HaeIII-type cDNAs code for acidic PRPs. The BstNI and HaeIII repeats show only slight differences in sequence. Seven different types of cDNA clones were isolated, two of the HaeIII type and five of the BstNI type. Three of the BstNI clones are the same except that one of them is missing 399 bp, and a second one 459 bp from the repetitive region of the third one. The sequences at the deletion end points are homologous to consensus sequences of RNA splicing donor and acceptor splice sites, strongly suggesting that the three cDNAs are derived from a transcript of a single gene by differential RNA splicing. The BstNI-type cDNAs code for PRPs that are larger than those found in the saliva, and from the decoded amino acid sequences each presumed precursor could generate multiple PRPs by posttranslational proteolytic cleavages on the carboxylic side of specific arginine residues. From these data, it is likely that differential RNA splicing and posttranslational cleavages could generate a large number of basic PRPs (such as those found in saliva) from a much smaller number of genes.

Further evidence for a limited number of PRP genes to account for many salivary PRPs came from further studies of the PRP genes. Previously, Azen et al.[64] found six hybridizing fragments after Southern blotting and hybridization of EcoRI digests of total human DNA with a DNA probe made from the repetitive region of the PRP 1 genomic clone. Maeda[67] determined that each of the six hybridizing fragments contains only one gene sequence (hybridizing region), and thus the PRPs are probably determined by six loci, rather than at least 13 loci as previously suggested from studies of the protein polymorphisms.

Furthermore, Maeda[67] could divide the six genes into two subfamilies by hybridizing Southern blots of EcoRI digests of human DNA with DNA probes containing either BstNI or HaeIII-type repeats and then washing the blots under stringent conditions. Two of the loci (HaeIII type) code for the four acidic PRPs (Pr, Db, Pa, PIF) and are called PRH1 and PRH2. The other four loci (BstNI type) code for the numerous basic PRPs and are called PRB1, PRB2, PRB3, and PRB4. Maeda[67] hypothesized that the acidic PRPs Pa, Db, and PIF are coded by three expressed alleles (without nulls) at one HaeIII-type locus (PRH1) and that the acidic Pr proteins are determined by the other HaeIII-type locus (PRH2). This hypothesis is supported by study of the phenotypes of 300 random samples from whites and 92 random samples from blacks. As predicted, none lacks all of the three proteins (Pa, Db, PIF), and none has all of the three. Furthermore, as predicted, the sum of gene frequencies for Pa$^+$, Db$^+$, and PIF$^+$ is approximately 1 in black and white populations. Studies of 72 family pedigrees are also explicable with the single-locus model for Pa, Db, and PIF alleles. Thus, the discrepancy in the number of loci (when comparing the protein and DNA data) is partly resolved at least for the acidic PRPs. As mentioned before, the likelihood of differential RNA processing and posttranslational cleavages by proteolysis[39] may further resolve the discrepancy between the nine basic PRP polymorphisms and the four BstNI-type genes.

The two HaeIII-type genes, PRH1 and PRH2, have been isolated and completely sequenced, and they code for acidic PRPs.[68] They both have four exons spanning about 3.5 kbp of DNA. Exon 1 encodes mainly the secretory signal; exon 2 composes part of the N-terminal sequence; exon 3 encodes the proline-rich part composed of five 63-bp tandem repeats; and exon 4 encodes the 3' untranslated region including the poly-A addition signal sequence. The entire 4-kbp region of sequenced DNA from PRH1 and PRH2 differs by 8.7% on the average, but a portion of the coding region containing exon 3 differs by only 0.2% between the two genes. This result suggests the occurrence of a recent gene conversion event.

The seven cDNAs that were sequenced by Maeda et al.[39] have been tentatively assigned to five of the six PRP loci: one each to PRH1 and PRH2; three of them to PRB1 (two transcripts are derived from the third by differential RNA processing); one to PRB4 and one to PRB2. The cDNA for PRB3 was not isolated from the cDNA library. It is likely that the PRP1 and PRP2 genomic clones previously isolated[64] contain the PRB1 and PRB2 genes, respectively.

Currently (because of incomplete DNA and protein sequence data), only a few specific PRPs can be assigned to the six genes. The PRH1 gene probably codes for the PIF, Db, and Pa proteins, and the PRH2 gene codes for the Pr proteins. The PRB3 gene probably codes for the major glycosylated protein, Gl, because there is a perfect correlation between different DNA-length polymorphisms of the PRB3 gene and Gl-protein-size variants in the salivas of a number of individuals.[103]

The human PRP gene family has been localized on chromosome 12. To determine chromosomal location, a DNA probe from the repetitive region of the PRP1 genomic clone was used to analyze segregation of human PRP genes in human × mouse somatic cell hybrids by hybridizing the probe to endonuclease-digested and Southern-transferred DNAs from the hybrids.[71] Mamula et al.[72] used the same probe and localized the PRP gene complex to a single band on chromosome 12 (12p13.2) by *in situ* hybridization. The localization of PRP genes to a single band on chromosome 12 is consistent with the extensive data from previous studies of PRP polymorphisms, indicating close linkage of this multigene family on a single autosome. Since the PRP gene probe detects frequent DNA-length polymorphisms in the four BstNI-type genes,[64,67] the probe may prove especially useful for genetic linkage studies with other chromosomal 12 markers.

Proline-rich proteins, cDNAs, and genes have also been studied in rodents, and there is evidence for multiple PRP genes in the rat and mouse[69] which are inducible with tannins and isoproterenol.[53,54] As in the human, all of the PRP genes have been localized to a single autosome by probing Southern blots of endonuclease-digested DNAs of mouse × hamster somatic cell hybrids with the rat PRP33 cDNA probe.[70] A cDNA clone, PRP33, from rat contains 6 repeats of 19 amino acids.[65] A mouse PRP gene, MP 2, contains 13 repeats of 14 amino acids.[69] Consensus nucleotide sequences of the rat and mouse repeats show a strong relationship to that of the HaeIII- and BstNI-type human repeats.[68] The HaeIII- and BstNI-type repeats of the human, however, are more related to each other than either is to the rat or mouse repeats. It is thus likely that partial gene duplications, gene conversions, and unequal crossing over occurred frequently among the repeated regions of exon 3 of human PRP genes.

In summary, only a skeletal outline of the human PRP gene family can be given at this time. The overall physical size of the PRP gene complex, its organization, detailed structure, evolutionary relationships, and assignment of all of the PRPs to specific loci remain to be established.

## IV. ELECTROPHORETIC STUDIES OF PRP POLYMORPHISMS

In this section I will describe characterization of PRP polymorphisms in various electrophoretic systems and emphasize some practical aspects in their identification and analysis. Table 2 give the nomenclature for protein polymorphisms and purified PRPs, and Table 4 gives some details of the electrophoretic systems to be discussed. The PRPs shown in the electrophoretograms (Figures 1 to 9) are identified in two ways: for polymorphic PRPs, the terminology for polymorphisms is used; and for the other PRPs, the terminology for the purified proteins is employed. We generally use parotid saliva (often concentrated by lyophilization and reconstitution in a smaller volume) for reasons previously discussed.

The acidic Pr, Db, Pa, and PIF proteins show some unusual staining properties. In alkaline gels they stain intensely blue with "Stains All"[4] and negatively against a dark-brown background with 3-3' dimethoxybenzidine.[42,55] The acidic PRPs can also be stained for phosphate after alkaline hydrolysis.[87] All of the PRPs show an unusual pink-violet color when stained with Coomassie Brilliant Blue R-250 in a solution of methanol-water-acetic acid.[30,74] For routine purposes, though, most PRPs can be readily identified by staining with Coomassie Brilliant Blue R-250 in the presence of trichloracetic acid.

### A. Electrophoresis of Acidic PRPs

When interpreting Pr, Db, and PIF phenotypes, it should be noted that each allele determines a pair of proteins. For example, $Pr^1$ determines Pr 1 and Pr 3 proteins, $Pr^2$ determines Pr 2 and Pr 4 proteins, and $Pr^{1'}$ determines Pr 1' and Pr 3 proteins. Db and PIF each determine a different pair of proteins. In contrast, Pe and Pa determine only single proteins.

**Table 4**
**ELECTROPHORETIC SYSTEMS FOR ANALYSES OF PRPs**

| System | Gel | Reservoir buffer | Sample solution |
|---|---|---|---|
| Alkaline PAGE[30] (0.1 × 15 × 20 cm); for acidic PRPs (Pr, Db, Pa) and Pe | Stacking: 4% acrylamide/0.2% bis; 0.062 $M$ Tris/HCl (pH 6.7); 0.05% TEMED; 0.1% AP Separating: 6.8% acrylamide/0.37% bis; 0.38 $M$ Tris/HCl, pH 8.9; 0.05% TEMED; 0.1% AP | 0.038 $M$ glycine/Tris, pH 8.4 | Dried saliva concentrated 5 × in 0.020 ml of 1% glycine with bromphenol blue marker |

| | Running conditions | Stain | Destain |
|---|---|---|---|
| | 100 V for 1 h; then increase to 300 V for ca. 6 h total at 4°C | 0.05% CBB in 20% TCA overnight | 2% HA |

| System | Gel | Electrode buffers | Sample solution |
|---|---|---|---|
| Isoelectric focusing[38] (0.1 × 10 × 11.5 cm); for acidic PRPs (Pr, Db, Pa, PIF) | Dissolve in 15 ml D/W, 2.33 g acrylamide/0.066 g bis; 10 g urea; bring to 30 ml with D/W; suction filter (20 $\mu M$); to 20 ml of this solution add 0.5 ml ampholines (pH 3.5—5.0) and 0.5 ml ampholines (pH 4—6); add 2.2 ml 0.004% riboflavin-5'-phosphate and 0.5% AP; photopolymerize | Anode wick: 1 $M$ phosphoric acid Cathode wick: 2% ampholines, pH 6—8 | Saliva dialyzed at least 1 × (0.01 $M$ ammonium bicarbonate); dried; reconstituted to 0.1 vol in 1% glycine; 0.020 ml applied 2—3 cm from cathode on filter paper strip |

| | Running conditions | Visualize bands | Destain |
|---|---|---|---|
| | Starting V = 200; gradually increase to 1200 V over 50 min; total time, 6 h at 0°C | Rinse and fix: 20% TCA, 24 h; stain: 0.1% CB in 20% TCA; *or* Soak: 20% TCA, 30 min; bands visible by indirect lighting | 20% TCA |

| System | Gel | Reservoir buffer | Sample solution |
|---|---|---|---|
| Acid-lactate PAGE[21] (0.6 × 18 × 12 cm) in E-C apparatus (St. Petersburg, FL); for major glycoprotein [Gl] | 300-ml gel solution containing 6.84% acrylamide/0.36% bis, 0.03 $M$ Tris/lactate (pH 2.4), ascorbic acid, 0.08%, ferrous sulfate, 0.0025%; filter; polymerize cold mixture with 0.090 ml 30% hydrogen peroxide; add quickly to mold | 0.03 $M$ Tris/lactate (pH 2.4) | 0.6 ml dried saliva in 0.6 ml 0.1 $M$ sodium actate/acetic acid (pH 5.0); add 0.010 ml neuraminidase (2.7 U/ml) and 0.020 ml aprotinin (10,000 U/ml); incubate 37° for 18 h; dialyze 2 × (0.01 $M$ ammonium bicarbonate); dry; reconstitute in 0.060 ml sucrose/Tris lactate buffer (15 mg/0.1 ml sucrose in 0.03 $M$ Tris/lactate, pH 2.4) with fuchsin marker; 0.060 ml sample loaded per slot |

**Table 4 (continued)**
**ELECTROPHORETIC SYSTEMS FOR ANALYSES OF PRPs**

| Running conditions | Stain |
|---|---|
| 160 V for 6.5 h at 10°C | Slice gel to produce slab no more than 3.0 mm thick; stain lower slice with periodic acid-Schiff |

| System | Gel | Reservoir buffer | Sample solution |
|---|---|---|---|
| Acid-lactate PAGE (0.3 × 18 × 12 cm) in E-C apparatus;[26] for basic PRPs (Ps, PmS, PmF) | 200-ml gel solution containing 8.55% acrylamide/0.45% bis; composition otherwise as earlier for Gl assay | 0.03 $M$ Tris/lactate (pH 2.4) | 0.075 ml dried saliva in 0.030-ml sample buffer (see Gl assay, earlier); 0.030 ml loaded per slot |

| Running conditons | Stain | Destain |
|---|---|---|
| 100 V for 18 h at 10°C | 0.1% CBB in 20% TCA overnight | 2% HAC |

| System | Gel | Reservoir buffer | Sample solution |
|---|---|---|---|
| SDS PAGE[29] (0.1 × 13 × 17 cm) modified from Laemmli;[76] for western blotting: protein, immunodetection, Con A reactions (Ps, PmS, Con 1, Con 2, Po) | Stacking: 10 × diluted from 30%/0.8% (acrylamide/bis) stock; 0.125 $M$ Tris/HCl (pH 6.8); 0.1% SDS; 0.03% AP; 0.1 TEMED | 0.025 $M$ Tris/0.192 $M$ glycine (pH 8.3); 0.1% SDS | Dried saliva dissolved and boiled 5 min in original vol of sample buffer: 0.0625 $M$ Tris/HCl (pH 6.8), 2% SDS, 10% glycerol, 5% 2-mercapto-ethanol, 0.001% bromphenol blue |
| | Separting: 2 × diluted from same stock; 0.375 $M$ Tris/HCl (pH 8.8); 0.1% SDS; 0.03% AP; 0.025% TEMED | | |

| Running conditions | Stain |
|---|---|
| 100 V for 1 h; increase to 250—300 V for total of 4—5 h at 4°C; stop when bromphenol blue migrates off end of gel | Transfer electrophoretically to nitrocellulose: stain for protein with amido black; immunoenzymatic staining using anti-PRP sera; Con A binding and staining |

| System | Gel | Reservoir buffer | Sample solution |
|---|---|---|---|
| Acid Tris/citrate (pH 2.9)[a] (0.1 × 16 × 32 cm); for basic PRPs (especially Pc) | 2 × diluted from 30%/0.8% (acrylamide/bis) stock; 0.015 $M$ Tris/citrate (pH 2.9), 0.0025% ferrous sulfate, 0.028% ascorbic acid, 0.04% hydrogen peroxide | 0.28 $M$ glycine/citric acid (pH 4.0) | Dried saliva concentrated 7 × in 50% sucrose with fuchsin marker; 0.01-ml sample per slot |

**Table 4 (continued)**
# ELECTROPHORETIC SYSTEMS OF ANALYSES OF PRPs

| Running conditions | Stain | Destain |
|---|---|---|
| 400 V; gradually increased to 600 V; run overnight; then increased to 1000 V at 4°C | 0.05% CBB in 20% TCA for 2 d | 2% HA |

*Note:* AP (amminoum persulfate); CBB (Coomassie Brilliant Blue R-250); TCA (trichloracetic acid); HA (acetic acid); D/W (distilled water).

[a]  Modified from Karn et al.[37]

Two useful slab gel systems are employed, alkaline polyacrylamide[30] and isoelectric focusing.[38] The alkalaine polyacrylamide slab gel system is slightly modified from that of Posner[75] (Figure 1). In order to enhance resolution of the proteins, a higher than standard voltage gradient is used, and electrophoresis is done at 4°C to reduce heating effects. The Pe protein (with a somewhat higher isoelectric point of approximately pH 6.2 as compared with those of the other acidic PRPs) migrates very close to the orgin. To study this polymorphism, therefore, it may be necessary to extend the time of electrophoresis over that usually required to separate other acidic PRPs.

The Pr proteins 1, 2, 3, and 4 are easily separated in the alkaline polyacrylamide gel, but the Pa protein may overlap the uncommon Pr 1′ protein characteristic of the Pr 1′ types seen mostly in blacks.[4,42,45] The Pr 1′ portein can be separated from the Pa protein by varying the polyacrylamide concentration or more easily by separating the proteins in the isoelectric focusing slab gel system (Figure 2). Since the Pa protein (alone among PRPs) contains a disulfide bond, it will show altered mobility when the sample is treated with a reducing agent,[4,42,45] and this is another way to distinguish it from other PRPs. The PIF S and PIF F proteins overlap the Pr 1 and Pr 3 proteins, respectively, in the alkaline polyacrylamide slab gel (Figure 1) but are easily resolved in the isoelectric focusing slab gel (Figure 2). In the isoelectric focusing gel, the Db S protein is easily typed, whereas the Db F protein is not well separated from the statherin protein, which migrates slightly cathodal to it. I prefer the isoelectric focusing gel system for identification of acidic PRPs other than Pe, since they are more easily typed in this system. The PRPs can be stained in isoelectric focusing gels with Coomassie Brilliant Blue R-250,[38] but they are more conveniently and rapidly identified by precipitating the proteins with trichloracetic acid and visualizing them with indirect light.[29]

## B. Electrophoresis of Basic PRPs in Acid-Lactate Gels

The acid-lactate gel stained with Coomassie Brilliant Blue R-250 is useful for typing Ps, PmF, and PmS polymorphisms[26] (Figures 3 and 4). The PmF and PmS types are scored + or − and the Ps types as either Ps 1, Ps 2, Ps 1-2, or Ps 0. Sometimes it is difficult to type Ps proteins if they overlap adjacent proteins. Therefore, it may be necessary to adjust the polyacrylamide concentration so that the Ps 1 and Ps 2 proteins (which usually stain more sharply than adjacent proteins) can be readily distinguished. To separate the Ps, PmF, and PmS polymorphisms adequately, it may be necessary to electrophorese the fast-migrating PmF protein almost to the end of a 13-cm gel (Figure 3). If the electrophoresis time is extended, with migration of the PmF protein off the end of a 13-cm gel, this will give a somewhat better separation of the slower-migrating PmS and Ps proteins (Figure 4). Other basic PRPs (indicated by arrowheads in Figure 3) are not as well separated in this system and, as will be shown later, are better resolved in the slightly modified acidic tris-citrate system of Karn et al.[37]

## C. Electrophoresis of the Major Glycosylated PRP (Gl) in Acid-Lactate Gels

The Gl proteins, alone among parotid salivary proteins, are easily stained with periodic acid-Schiff (PAS) and are among the slowest-migrating proteins in this gel system[21] (Figure 5). Since the faster allelic forms of Gl proteins overlap other salivary proteins that stain with Coomassie Brilliant Blue R-250, to distinguish the Gl proteins, it is necessary to stain them selectively for carbohydrate with the PAS stain. The resolution of Gl proteins can be improved by treating the salivary proteins with neuramidinase before electrophoresis, thereby reducing the charge heterogeneity due to sialic acid. The heterozygote phenotypes include various combinations of the expressed and unexpressed (null) alleles. We have seen only one homozygote (Gl 0-0) for the null allele. Most of the expressed heterozygote types (with double-band patterns) show the faster-migrating protein to be stained more faintly than the slower-migrating protein (Figure 5).

## D. Electrophoresis of PRP Polymorphisms in SDS Gels

We have found considerable advantages in the SDS gel system[76] for analysis of some PRP polymorphisms including Ps, PmS, Con 1, Con 2, and Po.[29,30] We electrophorese the proteins at higher than standard voltage at 4°C to enhance resolution. The electrophoretic mobilities of the many PRPs are shown in detail in Figure 6, and in less detail in Figures 7A and 8A. We have found the SDS gel system more reproducible than either the acid-lactate[26] or acid tris-citrate[37] gel systems. Furthermore, we obtain excellent electrophoretic transfers to nitrocellulose from SDS gels, and, as will be described later, these transfers are extremely useful for studying the polymorphisms by protein staining, lectin binding, or immunoblotting techniques.

The Ps and PmS polymorphisms can be reliably typed on stained gels or, as we prefer (because of enhanced speed and sensitivity of staining), on nitrocellulose transfers (Figures 6, 7A, and 8A). Unfortunately, the very rapidly migrating PmF protein is not readily separated from several other small PRPs (Figure 6). In our initial studies of the Po protein polymorphism,[30] we typed samples by using an immunoblotting technique (Figure 7B and C). We used polyclonal antisera to both acidic and basic PRPs. These antisera cross-react with many PRPs on the immunoblots as is illustrated in Figures 7B and C. With this technique the Po protein is readily distinguished from another closely adjacent protein (now known to be IB-4) that migrates slightly cathodal to it and does not react on immunoblots. The samples are typed as either Po[+] or Po[−]. After further studies,[104] however, we can now adequately identify the Po protein on nitrocellulose transfers stained for protein and distinguish it from IB-4 (identified by a white spot in Figure 7A, sample 2).

The Con 1 and Con 2 polymorphisms are not easily typed by protein staining because of insensitivity of staining and inability to distinguish these proteins from other closely adjacent PRPs. Concanavalin A, however, binds selectively to the Con 1 and Con 2 proteins on nitrocellulose transfer,[29] and thus the two polymorphisms can be typed as being present (+) or absent (−) from the saliva (Figure 8B).

## E. Electrophoresis of PRP Polymorphisms in Acid Tris-Citrate Gels

As discussed previously, we could not adequately resolve many smaller rapidly migrating PRPs in the acid-lactate or SDS gel systems. Therefore, we modified the acid tris-citrate slab gel system[37] to enhance resolution of these proteins. These modifications[104] include elimination of the stacking gel, doubling the gel length, and electrophoresis (4°C) at higher than standard voltage gradients. A gel stained for protein with Coomassie Brilliant Blue R-250 is shown in Figure 9. The Pc, PmS, and PmF polymorphisms can be seen. As noted by Karn et al.,[37] the Pc 1 protein may be difficult to separate from an adjacent protein that migrates slightly anodally. The Pc protein phenotypes are determined by Pc[1] and Pc[2] alleles without recognized nulls. A high-resolution technique, such as this, will be necessary to study genetic variations of Pc and other PRPs of small molecular weight. As seen in Figure 9, there are electrophoretic variations among PRPs other than those previously identified, as in the region of IB-8B. These variations, however, are difficult to characterize because of overlapping bands and weak staining.

## V. IMPLICATIONS AND CONCLUSIONS

The salivary protein polymorphisms have been and will continue to be valuable genetic tools in studying DNA and protein variations at the molecular and population levels. The possible relationship of some of these genetic variations to altered protein functions has not been established. For example, is there any biologic significance to the probable complexing of the Pa protein monomer to salivary peroxidase,[45,77,90] which is part of a potent antibacterial system? Some investigators[78] have shown that in children the Pa$^+$ phenotype (always associated with the complex form of peroxidase) is correlated with an increase in DMFS (decayed-missing-filled tooth surface) score as compared with the Pa$^-$ phenotype (always associated with the unmodified peroxidase). Other studies, however, show no correlation of PRP phenotypes or levels of acidic PRPs to dental disease.[79-81]

Apart from the possible functional significance of genetic variations of salivary proteins, the normal functions of important salivary proteins such as the many PRPs and histidine-rich basic proteins are still poorly defined. For example, the large number, variety, and overall predominance of PRPs in saliva defy a simple explanation of function. This difficulty is further compounded by the recent finding of PRPs in the respiratory tract.[51,52] Thus, which PRPs are expressed in the respiratory tract and what are their functions? In another context, Shatzman and Henkin[82] previously found that PRP(s) may be complexed to the parotid salivary protein called gustin (which may subserve a taste function). They suggested that this complex may be the functionally active form for tast bud growth and nutrition. Also, genes for PRPs were found to be closely linked to or the same as genes for bitter taste in the mouse.[98] This would suggest a possible role of PRPs in taste function. Does the tight binding of PRPs to tannins[53,54] protect the gastrointestinal tract and digestive enzymes from these toxic phenolic compounds which are found in many plants? Since high tannin diets in some human populations may be etiologic in causing esophageal cancer, Warner and Azen[83] hypothesized that salivary PRPs may possibly protect the esophagus from developing cancer by binding with the tannins.

As another example, the function of the biochemically and genetically related histidine-rich basic proteins (Pb and PPB) that are found in trace amounts in saliva has been likewise unclear.[46,95,96,97] Previous evolutionary studies in primates[84] indicate that there is a good relationship between the electrophoretically determined forms of Pb proteins in salivas of anthropoid primates and the type of diet they consume as well as with certain aspects of their dental structure. Recently, MacKay et al.[85] found growth-inhibitory and bactericidal effects of the histidine-rich polypeptides on *Streptococcus mutans*. In a related study, Pollock et al.[86] found fungistatic and fungicidal activity of these proteins on *Candida albicans*. We suggest there may be interesting surprises in the future when the functional significance of salivary PRPs, histidine-rich basic proteins, and other unique salivary proteins are better understood.

## ACKNOWLEDGMENTS

This work was supported by grant DEO-3658-20 from the National Institutes of Health. I thank Drs. D. Kauffman, P. Keller, and E. Saitoh for providing purified PRPs for electrophoretic comparisons. I appreciate the efforts of G. Larson, who provided technical assistance and aided in the preparation of Table 4. This is paper No. 2975 from the Laboratory of Genetics.

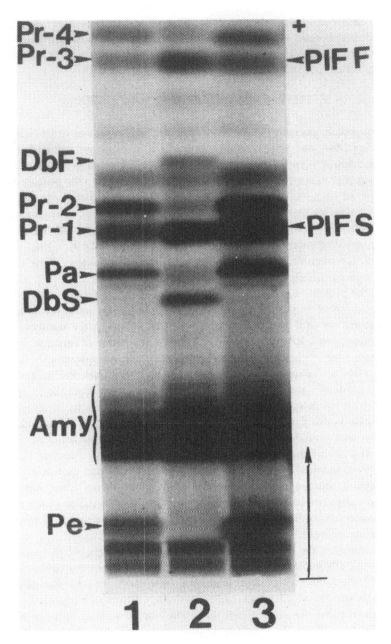

FIGURE 1. Alkaline polyacrylamide slab gel for acidic PRP polymorphisms stained for protein with Coomassie Brilliant Blue R-250. Each parotid saliva sample is from a different individual. Sample 1 is Pr 1-2, Db$^-$, Pa$^+$, Pe$^+$; sample 2 is Pr 1-1, Db$^+$, Pa$^-$, Pe$^-$; sample 3 is Pr 1-2, Db$^-$, Pa$^+$, Pe$^+$. PIF F and PIF S proteins overlap Pr 1 and Pr 3 proteins in this system and cannot be reliably typed. (From Azen, E. A. and Yu, P. L., *Biochem. Genet.*, 22, 1065, 1984. With permission.)

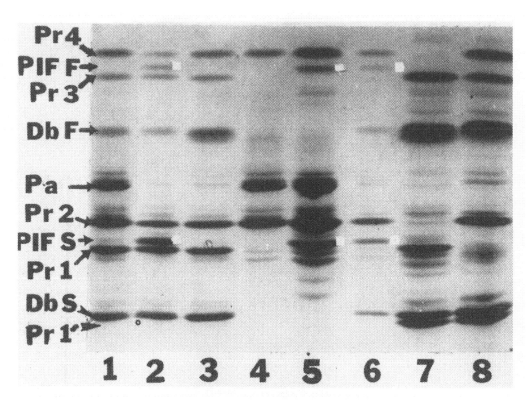

FIGURE 2.   Isoelectric focusing slab gel (pH 3.5 to 5.2) for acidic PRP polymorphisms stained with Coomassie Brilliant Blue R-250. Each parotid saliva sample is from a different individual. PIF F and PIF S proteins are labeled with white spots. Sample 1 is Pr 1-2, Db$^+$, Pa$^+$, PIF$^-$; sample 2 is Pr 1-2, Db$^+$, Pa$^-$, PIF$^+$; sample 3 is Pr 1-2, Db$^+$, Pa$^-$, PIF$^-$; sample 4 is Pr 2-2, Db$^-$, Pa$^+$, PIF$^-$; sample 5 is Pr 2-2, Db$^-$, Pa$^+$, PIF$^+$; sample 6 is Pr 2-2, Db$^+$, Pa$^-$, PIF$^+$; sample 7 is Pr 1-1', Db$^+$, Pa$^-$, PIF$^-$; sample 8 is Pr 1'-2, Db$^+$, Pa$^-$, PIF$^-$. (From Azen, E. A. and Denniston, C., *Biochem. Genet.*, 19, 475, 1981. With permission.)

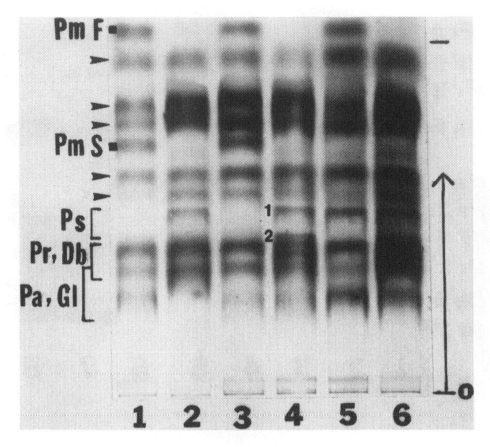

FIGURE 3.    Acid-lactate polyacrylamide slab gel for basic PRP polymorphisms stained with Coomassie Brilliant Blue R-250. This gel is run for a shorter time than the acid-lactate gel in Figure 4, in order to type the fast-migrating PmF as well as slower-migrating PmS and Ps polymorphisms. Other rapidly migrating PRPs (labeled with arrows) are not well resolved in this system. In order of migration from anode to cathode, these PRPs include IB-1, Pe, IB-4 and Pc overlapping, Po, IB-7 and IB-8b overlapping. Each parotid saliva sample is from a different individual. Sample 1 is PmF$^+$, PmS$^+$, Ps O; sample 2 is PmF$^-$, PmS$^-$, Ps 1; sample 3 is PmF$^+$, PmS$^+$, Ps O; sample 4 is PmF$^-$, PmS$^-$, Ps 1-2; sample 5 is PmF$^+$, PmS$^-$, Ps 1; sample 6 is PmF$^-$, PmS$^-$, Ps 1-2. (From Azen, E. A. and Denniston, C., *Biochem. Genet.*, 18, 483, 1980. With permission.)

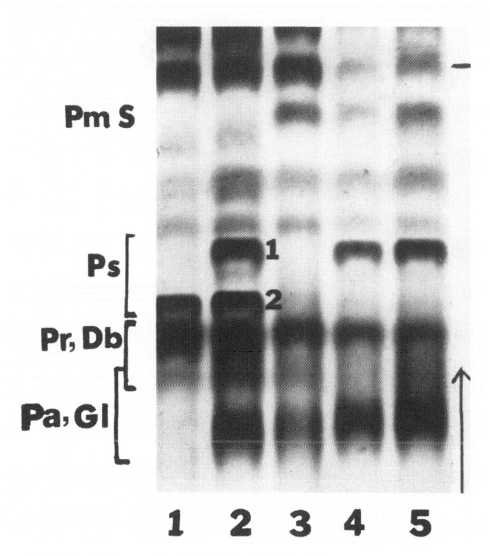

FIGURE 4. Acid-lactate polyacrylamide slab gel for basic PRP polymorphisms, stained with Coomassie Brilliant Blue R-250. PmS and Ps polymorphisms can be typed, but PmF has migrated off the cathodal end. Each parotid saliva sample is from a different individual. Sample 1 is Ps 2, PmS⁻; sample 2 is Ps 1-2, PmS⁻; sample 3 is Ps O, PmS⁺; samples 4 and 5 are Ps 1, PmS⁺. (From Azen, E. A. and Denniston, C., *Biochem. Genet.*, 18, 483, 1980. With permission.)

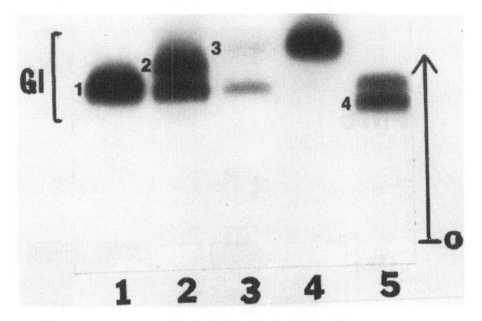

FIGURE 5.    Acid-lactate polyacrylamide slab gel for the Gl protein polymorphism, stained with periodic acid-Schiff. Each parotid saliva sample is from a different individual. Sample 1 is Gl 1; sample 2 is Gl 1-2; sample 3 is Gl 1-3; sample 4 is Gl 3; sample 5 is Gl 1-4. (From Azen, E. A., Hurley, C. K., and Denniston, C., *Biochem. Genet.*, 17, 257, 1979. With permission.)

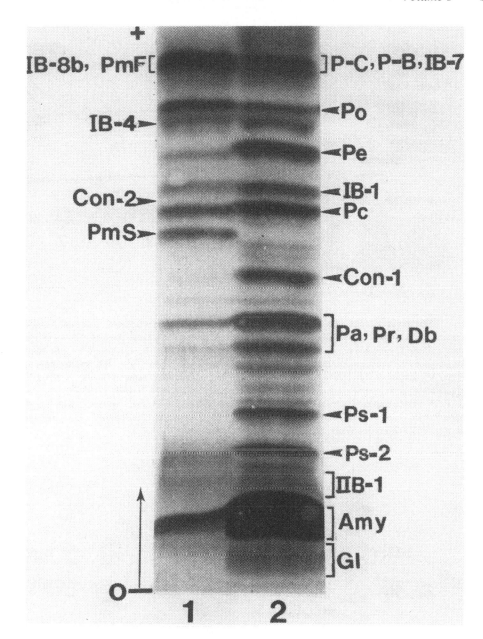

FIGURE 6. SDS polyacrylamide slab gel showing electrophoretic identification of many PRPs, including the PRP polymorphisms Po, Ps, and PmS, which can be easily typed. Proteins are transferred electrophoretically to nitrocellulose and stained with Amido Black. The parotid saliva samples are from two different individuals. The molecular weights of PRPs cannot be reliably determined in SDS gels, but for reference the approximate molecular weights for the Ps 1, PmS, Pe, and Po proteins are 32,500, 16,500, 11,500, and 7,900, respectively. Sample 1 is Ps 0, PmS$^+$, Po$^+$; sample 2 is Ps 1-2, PmS$^-$, Po$^+$.

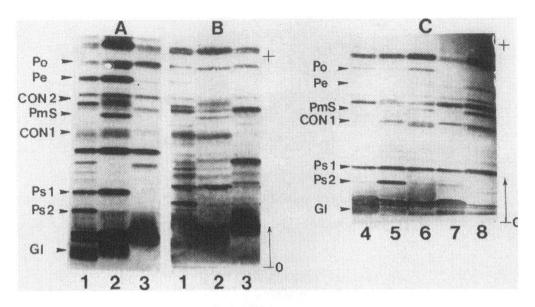

FIGURE 7. SDS polyacrylamide slab gels for typing Ps, PmS, and Po polymorphisms by protein staining and immunoenzymatic reactions on nitrocellulose transfers. The parotid saliva samples are the same in A and B (portions of the same gel), and five other samples are the same in C (from a different gel). A is a protein stain, and B and C are immunoblots with polyclonal anti-Ps serum which cross-reacts with many PRPs. The spotted protein (PRP IB-4) in blot A, channel 2, is closely adjacent to the Po protein and may cause difficulty in typing the Po polymorphism after protein staining unless there is adequate separation. Sample 1 is Ps 1-2, PmS⁻, Po⁺; sample 2 is Ps 1, PmS⁺, Po⁺; sample 3 is Ps 0, PmS⁻, Po⁺; sample 4 is Ps 1, PmS⁻, Po⁺; sample 5 is Ps 1-2, PmS⁻, Po⁺; sample 6 is Ps 1, PmS⁺, Po⁺; sample 7 is Ps 1, PmS⁻, Po⁻; sample 8 is Ps 1, PmS⁺, Po⁻. (From Azen, E. A. and Yu, P. L., *Biochem. Genet.*, 22, 1065, 1984. With permission.)

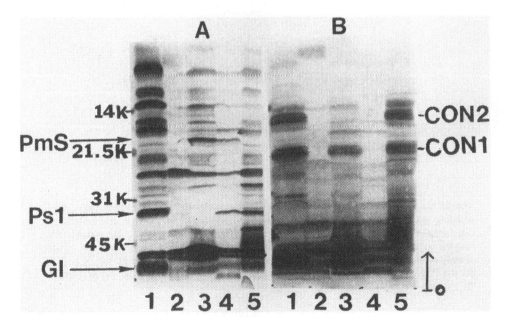

FIGURE 8. SDS polyacrylamide slab gel for typing Con 1 and Con 2 polymorphisms by Concanavalin A staining on nitrocellulose transfers. Blot A is stained for protein (for PmS and Ps polymorphisms), and blot B is stained for Con A binding (for the Con polymorphisms). The parotid salivary proteins are from five different individuals. Sample 1 is Con 1⁺, Con 2⁺, Ps 1, PMS⁻; sample 2 is Con 1⁻, Con 2⁻, Ps 0, PmS⁻; sample 3 is Con 1⁺, Con 2⁻, Ps 0, PmS⁺; sample 4 is Con 1⁻, Con 2⁻, Ps 1, PmS⁺; sample 5 is Con 1⁺, Con 2⁺, Ps 1-2, PmS⁻. (From Azen, E. A. and Yu, P. L., *Biochem. Genet.*, 22, 1, 1984. With permission.)

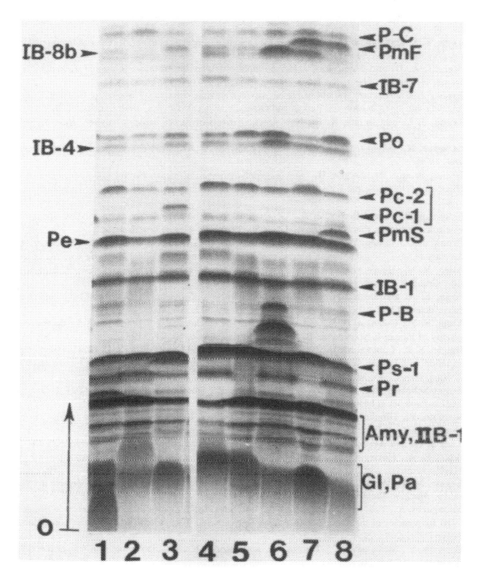

FIGURE 9. Acid tris-citrate polyacrylamide slab gel showing electrophoretic identification of many PRPs. This gel system is used especially to type the Pc polymorphism, although other polymorphisms can be seen in the parotid saliva samples from eight different individuals. Sample 3 is Pc 1-2, and all the other samples are Pc 2-2. Sample 8 is PmS$^+$, and all the other samples are PmS$^-$. Samples 7 and 8 are PmF$^+$, and all the other samples are PmF$^-$. The Ps polymorphism is not well resolved.

## REFERENCES

1. **Boackle, J. and Suddick, R. P.,** Salivary proteins and oral health, in *The Biologic Basis of Dental Caries,* Menaker, L., Ed., Harper & Row, New York, 1980, 113.
2. **Daniels, T. E. and Newburn, E.,** Measurement of protein and free and bound carbohydrate in human parotid saliva, *Arch. Oral Biol.,* 11, 1171, 1966.
3. **Bennick, A.,** Salivary proline-rich proteins, *Mol. Cell. Biochem.,* 45, 83, 1982.
4. **Azen, E. A.,** Genetic protein polymorphisms in human saliva: an interpretive review, *Biochem. Genet.,* 16, 79, 1978.

5. **Tan, S. G. and Teng, Y. S.,** Human saliva as a source of genetic markers. I. Techniques, *Hum. Hered.,* 29, 69, 1979.

6. **Teng, Y. S. and Tan, S. G.,** Human saliva as a source of genetic markers. II. Genetic interpretations and possible utilizations, *Hum. Hered.,* 29, 129, 1979.

7. **Merritt, A. D. and Karn, R. C.,** Human alpha-amylases, in *Advances in Human Genetics.,* Vol. 8, Harris, H. and Hirschhorn, K., Eds., Plenum Press, New York, 1977, 135.

8. **Pronk, J. C.,** A genetic variant of human salivary amylase detected by isoelectric focusing, in *Electrofocusing and Isotachophoresis,* Radola and Graesslin, Eds., de Gruyter, Berlin, 1977, p359.

9. **Pronk, J. C. and Frants, R. R.,** New genetic variants of parotid salivary amylase, *Hum. Hered.,* 29, 181, 1979.

10. **de Soyza, K.,** Polymorphism of human salivary amylase, a preliminary communication, *Hum. Genet.,* 45, 189, 1978.

11. **Kühnl, P. and Tischberger, H.,** Amylase, polymorphism of human parotid saliva: detection of a new allele Amy$^5$ by isoelectric focusing and Amy$_1$ population data from Germany, *Electrophoresis,* 1, 186, 1980.

12. **Eckersall, P. D. and Beeley, J. A.,** Genetic analysis of human salivary alpha-amylase isoenzymes by isoelectric focusing, *Biochem. Genet.,* 19, 1055, 1981.

13. **Pronk, J. C., Jansen, W. W., Pronk, A., Christian, F. A. M., Frants, R. R., and Erickson, A. W.,** Salivary protein polymorphism in Kenya: evidence for a new Amy 1 allele, *Hum. Hered.,* 34, 212, 1984.

14. **Allen, R. H.,** Human vitamin B$_{12}$ transport proteins, in *Progress in Hematology,* Vol. 9, Brown, E. B., Ed., Grune & Stratton, New York, 1975, 57.

15. **Azen, E. A. and Denniston, C.,** Genetic polymorphism of vitamin B$_{12}$ binding (R) proteins of human saliva detected by isoelectric focusing, *Biochem. Genet.,* 17, 909, 1979.

16. **Yang, S. Y., Coleman, P. S., and Dupont, B.,** The biochemical and genetic basis for the microheterogeneity of human R-type vitamin B$_{12}$ binding proteins, *Blood,* 59, 747, 1982.

17. **Daiger, S. P., Labowe, M. L., Parsons, M., Wang, L., and Cavalli-Sforza, L. L.,** Detection of genetic variation with radioactive ligands. III. Genetic polymorphism of transcobalamin II in human plasma, *Am. J. Hum. Genet.,* 30, 202, 1978.

18. **Fráter-Schröder, M., Hitzig, W. H., and Bütler, R.,** Studies of transcobalamin (TC). I. Detection of TCII isoproteins in human serum, *Blood,* 53, 193, 1979.

19. **Ikemoto, S., Hinohara, H., Tsuchida, S., and Tomita, K.,** Phenotype and gene frequencies of acid phosphatase (s-AcP) in the human parotid saliva, *Hum. Genet.,* 71, 30, 1985.

20. **Tan, S. G. and Ashton, G. C.,** Saliva acid phosphatases: genetic studies, *Hum. Hered.,* 26, 81, 1976.

21. **Azen, E. A., Hurley, C. K., and Denniston, C.,** Genetic polymorphism of the major parotid salivary glycoprotein (Gl) with linkage to the genes for Pr, Db and Pa, *Biochem. Genet.,* 17, 257, 1979.

22. **Levine, M. J., Weill, J. C., and Ellison, S. A.,** The isolation and analysis of a glycoprotein from parotid saliva, *Biochim. Biophys. Acta,* 188, 165, 1969.

23. **Minaguchi, K., Takaesu, Y., Tsutsumi, T., and Suzuki, K.,** Studies of genetic markers in human saliva (VII) frequencies of the major parotid salivary glycoprotein (Gl) system in a Japanese population, *Bull. Tokyo Dent. Coll.,* 22, 1, 1981.

24. **Ikemoto, S., Minaguchi, K., Tomita, T., and Suzuki, K.,** A variant protein in human parotid saliva detected by SDS polyacrylamide gel electrophoresis and its inheritance, *Ann. Hum. Genet. (London),* 43, 11, 1979.

25. **Minaguchi, K. and Suzuki, K.,** Frequencies of salivary genetic marker systems in Caucasians with an emphasis on Pm and Ph systems, *Forensic Sci. Int.,* 17, 5, 1981.

26. **Azen, E. A. and Denniston, C.,** Polymorphism of Ps (parotid size variant) and detection of a protein (PmS) related to the Pm (parotid middle band) system with genetic linkage of Ps and Pm to Gl, Db and Pr genetic determinants, *Biochem. Genet.,* 18, 483, 1980.

27. **Goodman, P. A. and Karn, R. C.,** Human parotid size polymorphism (Ps): characterization of the two allelic products, Ps 1 and Ps 2 by limited proteolysis, *Biochem. Genet.,* 21, 405, 1983.

28. **Goodman, P. A., Yu, P. L., Azen, E. A., and Karn, R. C.,** The human salivary protein complex (SPC): a large block of related genes, *Am. J. Hum. Genet.,* 37, 785, 1985.

29. **Azen, E. A. and Yu, P. L.,** Genetic polymorphism of Con 1 and Con 2 salivary proteins detected by immunologic and concanavalin A reactions on nitrocellulose with linkage of Con 1 and Con 2 genes to the SPC (salivary protein gene complex), *Biochem. Genet.,* 22, 1, 1984.

30. **Azen, E. A. and Yu, P. L.,** Genetic polymorphisms of Pe and Po salivary proteins with probable linkage of their genes to the salivary protein gene complex (SPC), *Biochem. Genet.,* 22, 1065, 1984.

31. **Ikemoto, S., Minaguchi, K., Suzuki, K., and Tomita, K.,** New genetic marker in human parotid saliva, *Science,* 197, 278, 1977.

32. **Kauffman, D. L. and Keller, P. J.,** The basic proline-rich proteins in human parotid saliva from a single subject, *Arch. Oral Biol.,* 24, 249, 1979.

33. **Isemura, S., Saitoh, E., and Sanada, K.,** Fractionation and characterization of basic proline-rich peptides of human parotid saliva and the amino acid sequence of proline-rich peptide P-E, *J. Biochem. (Tokyo),* 91, 2067, 1982.

34. **Minaguchi, K., Ikemoto, S., and Suzuki, K.,** Isolation and partial characterization of a polymorphic protein (Pm) in human parotid saliva, *Biochem. Genet.,* 19, 617, 1981.

35. **Saitoh, E., Isemura, S., and Sanada, K.,** Complete amino acid sequence of a basic proline-rich peptide P-F, from human parotid saliva, *J. Biochem. (Tokyo),* 93, 883, 1983.

36. **Saitoh, E., Isemura, S., and Sanada, K.,** Complete amino acid sequence of a basic proline-rich peptide, P-D, from human parotid saliva, *J. Biochem. (Tokyo),* 93, 495, 1983.

37. **Karn, R. C., Goodman, P. A., and Yu, P. L.,** Description of a genetic polymorphism of a human proline-rich salivary protein, Pc, and its relationship to other proteins in the salivary protein complex (SPC), *Biochem. Genet.,* 23, 37, 1985.

38. **Azen, E. A. and Denniston, C.,** Genetic polymorphism of PIF (parotid isoelectric focusing variant) proteins with linkage to the PPP (parotid proline-rich protein) gene complex, *Biochem. Genet.,* 19, 475, 1981.

39. **Maeda, N., Kim, H.-S., Azen, E. A., and Smithies, O.,** Differential RNA splicing and post translational cleavages in the proline-rich protein gene system, *J. Biol. Chem.,* 260, 11123, 1985.

40. **Bennick, A.,** Chemical and physical characterization of a phosphoprotein, protein C, from human saliva and comparison with a related protein A, *Biochem. J.,* 163, 229, 1977.

41. **Ikemoto, S., Tsuchida, S., Hinohara, H., Nishiumi, A., and Tomita, K.,** Genetic polymorphisms of the human parotid salivary proteins and isozymes among Japanese population, *Forensic Sci. Int.,* 35, 119, 1987.

42. **Azen, E. A. and Denniston, C. L.,** Genetic polymorphism of human salivary proline-rich proteins: further genetic analysis, *Biochem. Genet.,* 12, 109, 1974.

43. **Yu, P.-L., Karn, R. C., Merritt, A. D., Azen, E. A., and Conneally, P. M.,** Linkage relationships and multipoint mapping of the human parotid salivary proteins (Pr, Pa, Db), *Am. J. Hum. Genet.,* 32, 555, 1980.

44. **Friedman, R. D., Merritt, A. D., and Rivas, M. L.,** Genetic studies of human acidic salivary protein (Pa), *Am. J. Hum. Genet.,* 27, 292, 1975.

45. **Azen, E. A.,** Salivary peroxidase (SAPX): genetic modification and relationship to the proline-rich (Pr) and acidic (Pa) proteins, *Biochem. Genet.,* 15, 9, 1977.

46. **Azen, E. A.,** Genetic polymorphism of basic proteins from parotid saliva, *Science,* 176, 673, 1972.

47. **Noraini, I., Tan, S. G., Gan, Y. Y., and Teng, Y. S.,** Salivary peroxidase, Pm and Ph protein polymorphisms in Malaysians, *Hum. Genet.,* 56, 205, 1980.

48. **Balakrishnan, C. R. and Ashton, G. C.,** Polymorphism of human salivary proteins, *Am. J. Hum. Genet.,* 26, 145, 1974.

49. **Tan, S. G. and Ashton, G. C.,** An autosomal glucose-6-phosphate dehydrogenase (hexose-6-phosphate dehydrogenase) polymorphism in human saliva, *Hum. Hered.,* 26, 113, 1976.

50. **Tan, S. G.,** Human salivary esterases: genetic studies, *Hum. Hered.,* 26, 207, 1976.

51. **Warner, T. F. and Azen, E. A.,** Proline-rich proteins are present in serous cells of the submucosal glands of the respiratory tract, *Am. Rev. Respir. Dis.,* 130, 115, 1984.

52. **Ito, S., Suzuki, T., Momotsu, T., Isemura, S., Saitoh, E., Sanada, K., and Shibata, A.,** Presence of salivary protein C and salivary peptide P-C-like immunoreactivity in the laryngo-tracheo-bronchial glands, *Acta Endocrinol.,* 108, 130, 1985.

53. **Mehansho, H., Hagerman, A., Clements, S., Butler, L., Rogler, J., and Carlson, D. M.,** Modulation of proline-rich protein biosynthesis in rat parotid glands by sorghums with high tannin levels, *Proc. Natl. Acad. Sci. U.S.A.,* 80, 3948, 1983.

54. **Mehansho, H., Clements, S., Sheares, B. T., Smith, S., and Carlson, D. M.,** Induction of proline-rich glycoprotein synthesis in mouse salivary glands by isoproterenol and by tannins, *J. Biol. Chem.,* 260, 4418, 1985.

55. **Azen, E. A. and Oppenheim, F. G.,** Genetic polymorphism of proline-rich human salivary proteins, *Science,* 180, 1067, 1973.

56. **Anderson, L. C., Kauffman, D. L., and Keller, P. J.,** Identification of Pm and PmS human parotid salivary proteins as basic proline-rich proteins, *Biochem. Genet.,* 20, 1131, 1982.

57. **Oppenheim, F. G., Hay, D. I., and Franzblau, C.,** Proline-rich proteins from human parotid saliva. I. Isolation and partial characterization, *Biochemistry,* 10, 4233, 1971.

58. **Hay, D. I. and Oppenheim, F. G.,** The isolation from human parotid saliva of a further group of proline-rich proteins, *Arch. Oral Biol.,* 19, 627, 1974.

59. **Wong, R. S. C., Hoffman, T., and Bennick, A.,** The complete primary structure of a proline-rich phosphoprotein from human saliva, *J. Biol. Chem.,* 254, 4800, 1979.

60. **Wong, R. S. C. and Bennick, A.,** The primary structure of a salivary calcium-binding proline-rich phosphoprotein (protein C), a possible precursor of a related salivary protein A, *J. Biol. Chem.,* 255, 5943, 1980.

61. **Wong, R. S. C., Madapallimattam, G., and Bennick, A.,** The role of glandular kallakrein in the formation of a salivary proline-rich protein by cleavage of a single bond in salivary protein C, *Biochem. J.,* 211, 35, 1983.

62. **Isemura, S., Saitoh, E., and Sanada, K.,** The amino acid sequence of a salivary proline-rich peptide, P-C, and its relation to a salivary proline-rich phsophoprotein, protein C, *J. Biochem. (Tokyo),* 87, 1071, 1980.

63. **Kauffman, D., Wong, R., Bennick, A., and Keller, P.,** Basic proline-rich proteins from human parotid saliva: complete covalent structure of protein IB-9 and partial structure of protein IB-6, members of a polymorphic pair, *Biochemistry,* 21, 6558, 1982.

64. **Azen, E., Lyons, K. M., McGonigal, T., Barrett, N. L., Clements, L. S., Maeda, N., Vanin, E. F., Carlson, D. M., and Smithies, O.,** Clones from the human gene complex coding for salivary proline-rich proteins, *Proc. Natl. Acad. Sci. U.S.A.,* 81, 5561, 1984.

65. **Ziemer, M. A., Swain, W. F., Rutter, W. J., Clements, S., Ann, D. K., and Carlson, D. M.,** Nucleotide sequence analysis of a proline-rich protein cDNA and peptide homologies of rat and human proline-rich proteins, *J. Biol. Chem.,* 259, 10475, 1984.

66. **Shimomura, H., Kanai, Y., and Sanada, K.,** Amino acid sequences of glycoproteins obtained from basic proline-rich glycoprotein of human parotid saliva, *J. Biochem. (Tokyo),* 93, 857, 1983.

67. **Maeda, N.,** Inheritance of human salivary proline-rich proteins: a reinterpretation in terms of six loci forming two subfamilies, *Biochem. Genet.,* 23, 455, 1985.

68. **Kim, H.-S. and Maeda, N.,** Structure of two HaeIII-type genes in the human salivary proline-rich protein multigene family, *J. Biol. Chem.,* 261, 6712, 1986.

69. **Ann, D. K. and Carlson, D. M.,** The structure and organization of a proline-rich protein gene of a mouse multigene family, *J. Biol. Chem.,* 260, 15863, 1985.

70. **Azen, E. A., Carlson, D. M., Clements, S., Lalley, P. A., and Vanin, E.,** Salivary proline-rich protein genes on chromosome 8 of mouse, *Science,* 226, 967, 1984.

71. **Azen, E. A., Goodman, P. A., and Lalley, P. A.,** Human salivary proline-rich protein genes on chromosomal 12, *Am. J. Hum. Genet.,* 37, 418, 1985.

72. **Mamula, P. W., Heerema, N. A., Palmer, C. G., Lyons, K. M., and Karn, R. C.,** Localization of the human salivary proteins complex (SPC) to chromosome band 12p13.2, *Cytogenet. Cell Genet.,* 39, 279, 1985.

73. **Isemura, S., Saitoh, E., and Sanada, K.,** Isolation and amino acid sequences of proline-rich peptides of human whole saliva, *J. Biochem. (Tokyo),* 86, 79, 1979.

74. **Henkin, R. I., Lippoldt, R. E., Belstad, J., Wolf, R. O., Lum, C. K. L., and Edelhoch, H.,** Fractionation of human parotid saliva proteins, *J. Biol. Chem.,* 253, 7556, 1978.

75. **Posner, I.,** A new apparatus for recovery of macromolecules from polyacrylamide gel slabs following preparative vertical electrophoresis, *Anal. Biochem.,* 72, 491, 1976.

76. **Laemmli, U.,** Cleavage of structural proteins during the assembly of the head bacterophage T4, *Nature (London),* 227, 680, 1970.

77. **Azen, E. A.,** Genetic variation of salivary peroxidase, in *The Lactoperoxidase System, Chemistry and Biologic Significance,* Pruitt, K. M. and Tenovuo, J. O., Eds., Marcel Dekker, New York, 1985, 89.

78. **Yu, P.-L., Bixler, D., Goodman, P. A., Azen, E. A., and Karn, R. C.,** Human parotid proline-rich proteins: correlation of genetic polymorphisms to dental caries, *Genet. Epidemiol.,* 3, 147, 1986.

79. **Anderson, L. C., Lamberts, B. L., and Bruton, W. F. J.,** Salivary protein polymorphisms in caries-free and caries-active adults, *J. Dent. Res.,* 61, 393, 1982.

80. **Anderson, L. C. and Mandel, I. D.,** Salivary protein polymorphisms in caries-resistant adults, *J. Dent. Res.,* 61, 1167, 1982.

81. **Mandel, I. D. and Bennick, A.,** Quantitation of human salivary acidic proline-rich proteins in oral disease, *J. Dent. Res.,* 62, 943, 1983.

82. **Shatzman, A. R. and Henkin, R.,** Metal-binding characteristics of the parotid salivary protein gustin, *Biochim. Biophys. Acta,* 623, 107, 1980.

83. **Warner, T. F. and Azen, E. A.,** Tannins, salivary proline-rich proteins and esophageal cancer, *Med. Hypothesis,* 26, 99, 1988.

84. **Azen, E. A., Leutenegger, W., and Peters, E. H.,** Evolutionary and dietary aspects of salivary basic (Pb) and post Pb (PPb) proteins in anthropoid primates, *Nature (London),* 273, 775, 1978.

85. **MacKay, B. J., Denepitiya, L., Iacono, V. J., Krost, S. B., and Pollock, J. J.,** Growth-inhibitory and bactericidal effects of human parotid salivary histidine-rich polypeptides on *Streptococcus mutants, Infect. Immun.,* 44, 695, 1984.

86. **Pollock, J. J., Denepitiya, L., MacKay, B. J., and Iacono, V.,** Fungistatic and fungicidal activity of human parotid salivary histidine-rich polypeptides on *Candida albicans, Infect. Immun.,* 44, 702, 1984.

87. **Azen, E. A.,** Phosphorylation of proline-rich, double band, acidic and post-Pb proteins of human saliva, *Arch. Oral Biol.,* 23, 1173, 1978.

88. **Karn, R. C., Friedman, R. D., and Merritt, A. D.,** Human salivary proline-rich (Pr) proteins: a post translational derivation of the phenotypes, *Biochem. Genet.,* 17, 1061, 1979.
89. **Saitoh, E., Isemura, S., and Sanada, K.,** Further fractionation of basic proline-rich peptides from human parotid saliva and complete amino acid sequence of basic proline-rich peptide P-H, *J. Biochem. (Tokyo),* 94, 1991, 1983.
90. **Azen, E. A.,** Salivary peroxidase activity and thiocyanate concentration in human subjects with genetic variants of salivary peroxidase, *Arch. Oral Biol.,* 23, 801, 1978.
91. **Kamarýt, J. and Laxová, R.,** Amylase heterogeneity variants in man, *Humangenetik,* 3, 41, 1966.
92. **Boettcher, B. and de la Lande, F. A.,** Electrophoresis of human saliva and identification of inherited variants of amylase isoenzymes, *Aust. J. Exp. Biol. Med. Sci.,* 47, 97, 1969.
93. **Pronk, J. C., Frants, R. R., Jansen, W., Eriksson, A. W., and Tonino, G. J. M.,** Evidence for duplication of the human salivary amylase gene, *Hum. Genet.,* 60, 32, 1982.
94. **Warner, F. C. S., Seo, I. S., Azen, E. A., Hafez, G. R., and Zarling, T. A.,** Immunocytochemistry of acinic carcinomas and mixed tumors of salivary glands, *Cancer,* 56, 2221, 1985.
95. **Azen, E. A.,** Properties of salivary basic proteins showing polymorphism, *Biochem. Genet.,* 9, 69, 1973.
96. **Peters, E. H. and Azen, E. A.,** Isolation and partial characterization of human parotid basic proteins, *Biochem. Genet.,* 15, 925, 1977.
97. **Peters, E. H., Goodfriend, T., and Azen, E. A.,** Human Pb, human post-Pb and non human primate Pb proteins: immunological and biochemical relationships, *Biochem. Genet.,* 15, 947, 1977.
98. **Azen, E. A., Lush, I. E., and Taylor, B. J.,** Close linkage of mouse genes for salivary proline-rich proteins (PRPs) and taste, *Trends in Genet.,* 2, 199, 1986.
99. **Pronk, J.,** personal communication.
100. **Minaguchi, K. and Suzuki, K.,** personal communication.
101. **Kauffman, D. L. and Keller, P. J.,** personal communication.
102. **Azen, E. A. and Bennick, A.,** unpublished.
103. **Lyons, K. and Azen, E.,** unpublished.
104. **Azen, E. A. and Larson,** unpublished.

# INDEX

Lightning Source UK Ltd.
Milton Keynes UK
UKOW06n0252300115

245399UK00013B/143/P